The Royal Victoria Hospital
Belfast

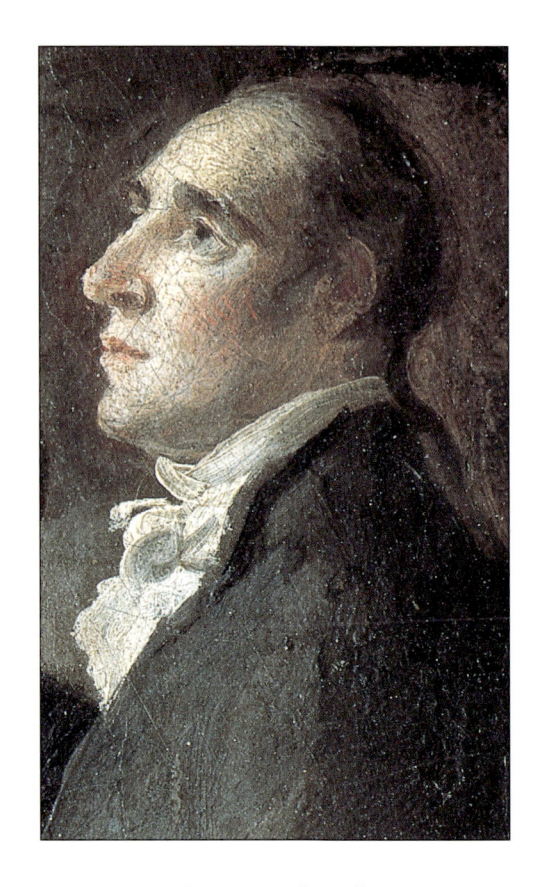

Dr James McDonnell
Attending Physician to the Belfast Fever Hospital, 1797–1837;
detail from *Review of the Belfast Yeomanry by the Lord Lieutenant,
the Earl of Hardwicke, 27 August 1804;* painting by Thomas Robinson
BELFAST HARBOUR COMMISSIONERS

Ulster Bank

The Royal Victoria Hospital Belfast

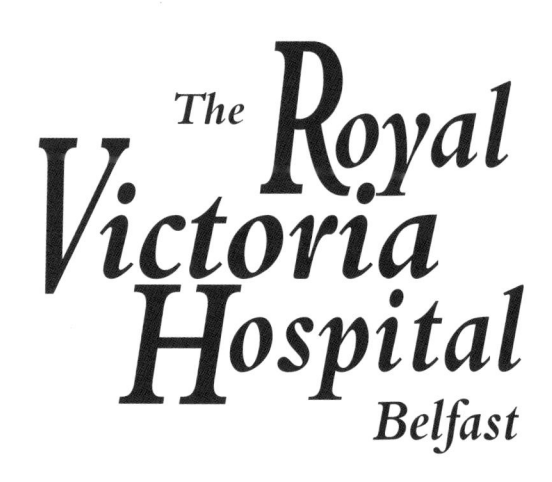

A HISTORY
1797–1997

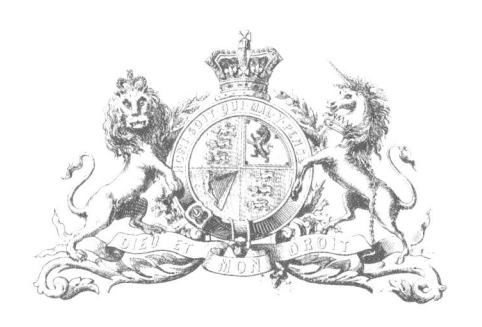

RICHARD
CLARKE

THE
BLACKSTAFF
PRESS

BELFAST

First published in 1997 by
The Blackstaff Press Limited
3 Galway Park, Dundonald, Belfast BT16 0AN, Northern Ireland
for the Royal Victoria Hospital
sponsored by
the Ulster Bank Limited
and supported by
the Esmé Mitchell Trust
and the Royal Victoria Hospital Bicentenary Committee

© Richard Clarke, 1997
All rights reserved

Typeset by Techniset Typesetters, Newton-le-Willows, Merseyside

Printed in Northern Ireland by W. & G. Baird Limited

A CIP catalogue record for this book
is available from the British Library

ISBN 0-85640-601-5

CONTENTS

FOREWORD by J.S. Logan		IX
PREFACE		XI
ABBREVIATIONS		XIII
CHRONOLOGY		XV
1	A General Hospital for Belfast	1
2	The Belfast General Hospital and Belfast Royal Hospital, 1850–1903	27
3	The Royal Victoria Hospital: Building and Administration, 1903–1948	65
4	Medicine and Surgery in the Royal Victoria Hospital, 1903–1948	95
5	The National Health Service: Hospital Changes and the Medical Specialities	137
6	The Surgical Specialities and the Impact of the Troubles	178
7	Other Caring Professions and Fundraising Committees	224
8	Trust Status and Rebuilding	244

APPENDICES

1	Chronological List of the Visiting Physicians and Surgeons (Consultants after 1948) of the Dispensary and Fever Hospital, the Belfast General Hospital, Belfast Royal Hospital and Royal Victoria Hospital	250
2	Chairmen of the Medical Staff Committee	281
3	Honorary Secretaries of the Medical Staff Committee	281
4	Orators of the Annual Winter Oration	282
5	Medical Superintendents and Related Posts	285
6	Matrons and Related Posts	285
7	Presidents of the Hospital (pre-1948)	286
8	Honorary Treasurers of the Hospital (pre-1948)	286
9	Honorary Secretaries of the Hospital (pre-1948) and Senior Administrative Officers after 1948	287

SOURCES & BIBLIOGRAPHY	288
INDEX	295

Diseases desperate grown
By desperate appliance are reliev'd,
Or not at all.

Hamlet, IV, iii, 9

*To all those who have worked
for the sick in this hospital
over the years*

FOREWORD

PROFESSOR RICHARD CLARKE, at the request of the Royal Victoria Hospital and all its staffs, undertook the formidable task of writing the bicentenary history of the hospital. The hospital began in a very small way in 1797, but great oaks grow from little acorns. Professor Clarke brought to his task his very considerable literary and historical abilities, cultivated over many years, along with his great professional skills. He has brought it to a happy conclusion.

When the newly built Belfast Fever Hospital opened in Frederick Street in 1817 it was dedicated by its founders, in stately Latin, to the care of the sick and dying, to the comforting of the brokenhearted, to the improvement of the arts of medicine and surgery, to the study of disease, and to the advancement of public health. The reader must decide how far its successor, the Royal Victoria Hospital, has fulfilled these aims, enjoined by those early citizens of Belfast. Within the walls of the old hospital in Frederick Street, and within those of the newer, well-known and much-loved hospital on the Grosvenor Road, there has been a great and continuing endeavour to live up to them. The nobility of the task has attracted many of the best men and women of Ulster and beyond. But, of course, the Royal Victoria Hospital could not bear the burden alone, and Belfast has cause to be grateful to the old Belfast Union Infirmary (now Belfast City Hospital), for so many years a refuge for the ill and unfortunate. This hospital also commanded the service of devoted staffs. So did the Mater Infirmorum Hospital. And they still do.

As you read the biographical details of so many of the Royal's staff, you may feel that we are encompassed by a cloud of witnesses to the work of generations. You may also feel that the Royal Victoria Hospital is more than just a hospital. It is one manifestation of the spirit of Northern Ireland. Long may it flourish and do good, and may this book convey that inspiration to the generations to come.

J.S. LOGAN
HONORARY CONSULTING PHYSICIAN
TO THE ROYAL VICTORIA HOSPITAL
APRIL 1997

PREFACE

A BICENTENARY HISTORY OF THE Royal Victoria Hospital had been contemplated by the medical staff for many years and it seemed obvious to tie in the writing of such a history with the post of honorary Archivist, which was vacated by Dr J.S. Logan in 1993. I took over at this time but could do little until I retired from the chair of Anaesthetics in 1994, and even then the period of familiarising myself with the contents of the Archive Office delayed any serious writing at first.

My main debt is to former writers of the hospital's history: Dr Andrew Malcolm, Dr Sydney Allison and Dr Robert Marshall, whose work conveniently covers three fifty-year periods. However, the history of the past fifty years, while made easier by my own memories and also by colleagues' memories, is harder to piece together because of the major changes in the National Health Service and in the administration of the hospital. At the same time, medicine as a whole diversified into many fields and the small number of powerful figures in charge of wards in Frederick Street and the Grosvenor Road has been replaced by a host of consultants, in specialities ranging from immunology to accident and emergency medicine. The last and most serious difficulty (noted even in 1953 by Dr Marshall) is that printed annual reports, with staff lists, details of new buildings, medical and surgical advances, and administrative changes, which had existed from 1818 to 1947, ceased after 1948 and have never been replaced.

I am deeply grateful to the large number of friends in the hospital who have read sections of this book, saved me from many errors and pointed out serious omissions. I must in particular thank Dr J.S. Logan who read a late draft of the text and has written the Foreword; also Dr Jennifer Adgey, Professor Desmond Archer, Dr Patrick Bell, Professor John Bridges, Dr Desmond Burrows, Mr Gerry Carson, Mr John Colville, Dr Dennis Coppel, Dr Christine Dearden, Professor Desmond Eccles, Mr Roy Gibson, Mr Derek Gordon, Mr John Gorman, Mr John Gray, Sister Sara Gray, Professor David Hadden, Mr Billy Henry, Professor Gary Love, Dr Alec Lyons, Dr Morrell Lyons, Professor John McGimpsey,

Mr Joe McClelland, Dr Teddy McIlrath, Mr William McKee, Dr Raymond Maw, Dr George Murnaghan, Mr Hugh O'Kane, Professor Jack Pinkerton, Miss Kathleen Robb, Professor Brian Rowlands, Mr Morris Stevenson and Dr Michael Swallow. In Chapter 7 the following have written sections on their own fields which I have used extensively: the Reverend Eric Gallagher (chaplains), René Boyd (social work), Colette McBride (pharmacy), Rita Fox (physiotherapy), Mairead McGowan (occupational therapy), Kathleen Acheson and Anne Wilson (dietetics), Margaret Newman (speech therapy), Julia Shaw (podiatry), Patricia Donnelly (clinical psychology) and Eleanor Menary (Ladies' Committee). All these people have given great assistance but are in no way responsible for any views expressed or any mistakes made.

Finding suitable illustrations for a book covering two hundred years of Belfast and hospital history has not been easy but again I have been considerably helped by the material collected by past honorary Archivists. I have tried to resist the temptation to fill the book with too many images of doctors past and present and instead have attempted to find less formal groups. Many of the above have lent material for reproduction and, in addition, Mr Derek Gordon, Dr Mazhar Khan and Dr Steven McKinstry have lent clinical photographs. Peter Conlon and Therese Gorman have generously allowed me to use many illustrations they had collected, intended for another publication, and I am very grateful to them. The Department of Media Services (photography) has taken many photographs in the period 1995–97 of staff, artefacts and buildings, and I am very grateful for their help. The Trustees of the Ulster Museum, the Belfast Habour Board, the Linen Hall Library, Robert McKelvey, Raymond Piper, Colin Gibson, Carol Graham, Kieran Doyle O'Brien, the Bell Gallery, Queen's University Belfast and the Lord Brock Memorial Trust have permitted the use of copyrighted and other material.

Thanks are also due to our sponsors, the Ulster Bank, who have helped to meet the high cost of producing this book, which has also been supported by the Esmé Mitchell Trust and the Royal Victoria Hospital Bicentenary Committee.

Michelle Dwyer typed the manuscript and other staff in the King Edward Building have also made their contributions, and I must thank them all.

Finally, I would like to thank all those at Blackstaff Press who have played such a large part in finalising the text and the appearance of this history and who gently kept up the pressure to have it ready for our rather rushed deadline.

RICHARD CLARKE
APRIL 1997

ABBREVIATIONS

Aber	Aberdeen	FFAEM	Fellow of the Faculty of Accident and Emergency Medicine
ARHA	Associate of the Royal Hibernian Academy	FFCM	Fellow of the Faculty of Community Medicine
ATICS	Anaesthesia, Theatre and Intensive Care (Directorate)	FFCMI	Fellow of the Faculty of Community Medicine in Ireland
BA	Bachelor of Arts	FFD	Fellow of the Faculty of Dentistry
Bart.	Baronet	FFPath. RCPI	Fellow of the Faculty of Pathology of the Royal College of Physicians of Ireland
BDS	Bachelor of Dental Surgery		
BHMC	Belfast Hospitals Management Committee	FFR	Fellow of the Faculty of Radiologists
Birm	Birmingham	FFR RCSI	Fellow of the Faculty of Radiologists of the Royal College of Surgeons in Ireland
BM	Bachelor of Medicine		
BMA	British Medical Association	FKQCPI	Fellow of the King's and Queen's College of Physicians of Ireland
BPC	British Pharmaceutical Codex		
BSc	Bachelor of Science	FRCA	Fellow of the Royal College of Anaesthetists
Camb	Cambridge	FRCGP	Fellow of the Royal College of General Practitioners
CB	Companion of the Order of Bath	FRCOG	Fellow of the Royal College of Obstetricians and Gynaecologists
CBE	Commander of the Order of the British Empire		
CMG	Companion of the Order of St Michael and St George	FRC Path.	Fellow of the Royal College of Pathologists
CSSD	Central Sterile Supplies Department	FRC Psych	Fellow of the Royal College of Psychiatrists
CT	Computed Tomography	FRCP Edin	Fellow of the Royal College of Physicians of Edinburgh
DA	Diploma in Anaesthetics	FRCP Glas	Fellow of the Royal College of Physicians of Glasgow
DA Eng	Diploma in Anaesthetics of the Royal College of Physicians of London and the Royal College of Surgeons of England	FRCP Lond	Fellow of the Royal College of Physicians, London
		FRCPI	Fellow of the Royal College of Physicians of Ireland
DAO	District Administrative Officer	FRCPS Glas	Fellow of the Royal College of Physicians and Surgeons of Glasgow
DAMO	District Administrative Medical Officer		
DANO	District Administrative Nursing Officer	FRCR	Fellow of the Royal College of Radiologists
DCH	Diploma in Child Health	FRCS Edin	Fellow of the Royal College of Surgeons of Edinburgh
DDS	Doctor of Dental Surgery	FRCS Glas	Fellow of the Royal College of Surgeons of Glasgow
DIH	Diploma in Industrial Health	FRCSC	Fellow of the Royal College of Surgeons of Canada
DL	Deputy Lieutenant	FRCSE	Fellow of the Royal College of Surgeons of England
DM	Doctor of Medicine	FRCSI	Fellow of the Royal College of Surgeons of Ireland
DMRE	Diploma in Medical Radiology and Electrolysis	FRIBA	Fellow the Royal Institute of British Architects
DMS	Doctor of Medicine and Surgery	FRS	Fellow of the Royal Society
DO	Diploma in Ophthalmology	Glas	Glasgow
DPH	Diploma in Public Health	GMAC	Group Medical Advisory Committee
DPM	Department of Physical Medicine	Guy's	Guy's Hospital, London
DPM	Diploma in Psychological Medicine	Hons	Honours
DRCOG	Diploma of the Royal College of Obstetricians and Gynaecologists	JP	Justice of the Peace
		KCB	Knight Commander of the Order of Bath
DSc	Doctor of Science	KCH Lond	King's College Hospital, London
DSO	Distinguished Service Order	KCVO	Knight Commander of the Royal Victorian Order
DTM&H	Diploma in Tropical Medicine & Hygiene	KQCPI	King's and Queen's College of Physicians of Ireland
ECG	Electrocardiograph	LAH	Licentiate of the Apothecaries Hall, Dublin
Edin	Edinburgh	LDS	Licentiate in Dental Surgery
EEG	Electroencephalograph	Liverp	Liverpool
EENT	Eye, ear, nose and throat	LKQCPI	Licentiate of the King's and Queen's College of Physicians of Ireland
EHSSB	Eastern Health and Social Services Board		
EMI	Electrical and Musical Industries	LL D	Doctor of Laws
ENT	Ear, nose and throat	LM	Licentiate in Midwifery
FACS	Fellow of the American College of Surgery	Lond	London
FCO	Fellow of the College of Ophthalmologists	Lond Hosp	London Hospital
FDS	Fellow in Dental Surgery	LPSI	Licentiate of the Pharmaceutical Society of Ireland
FFA RCSE	Fellow of the Faculty of Anaesthetists of the Royal College of Surgeons of England	LRCP	Licentiate of the Royal College of Physicians
		LRCPI	Licentiate of the Royal College of Physicians of Ireland
FFA RCSI	Fellow of the Faculty of Anaesthetists of the Royal College of Surgeons in Ireland	LRCS	Licentiate of the Royal College of Surgeons
		LRCSI	Licentiate of the Royal College of Surgeons in Ireland

LSA	Licentiate of the Society of Apothecaries (London)	OBE	Officer of the Order of the British Empire
MA	Master of Arts	Oxf	Oxford
Manch	Manchester	PCA	Patient-controlled Analgesia
MAO	Master of the Art of Obstetrics	Ph.C.	Pharmaceutical Chemist
MB	Bachelor of Medicine	PhD	Doctor of Philosophy
MBA	Master of Business Administration	PTS	Preliminary Training School
MBE	Member of the Order of the British Empire	QUB	Queen's University Belfast
MC	Military Cross	QUI	Queen's University of Ireland
MCh	Master of Surgery	RAMC	Royal Army Medical Corps
MCSP	Member of the Chartered Society of Physiotherapists	RCPI	Royal College of Physicians of Ireland
MD	Doctor of Medicine	RCPS Glas	Royal College of Physicians and Surgeons of Glasgow
MDS	Master of Dental Surgery	RCPSI	Royal College of Physicians and Surgeons in Ireland
MFCMI	Member of the Faculty of Community Medicine in Ireland	RCSI	Royal College of Surgeons in Ireland
		RFU	Respiratory Failure Unit
M Med Sci	Master of Medical Science	RICU	Respiratory/Regional Intensive Care Unit
MP	Member of Parliament	RN	Royal Navy
MPhil	Master of Philosophy	RNVR	Royal Navy Volunteer Reserve
MRC	Medical Research Council	RUI	Royal University of Ireland
MRC Path.	Member of the Royal College of Pathologists	RVH	Royal Victoria Hospital
MRC Psych	Member of the Royal College of Psychiatrists	St And.	St Andrews University
MRCGP	Member of the Royal College of General Practitioners	St Bart's	St Bartholomew's Hospital, London
MRCOG	Member of the Royal College of Obstetricians and Gynaecologists	St Mary's	St Mary's Hospital, London
		St Thom	St Thomas's Hospital, London
MRCP	Member of the Royal College of Physicians	Sheff	Sheffield
MRCP UK	Member of the Royal Colleges of Physicians of the UK	SMAC	Sequential Multiple Autoanalyser with Computer
MRCPI	Member of the Royal College of Physicians of Ireland	TCD	Trinity College Dublin
MRCS	Member of the Royal College of Surgeons	TD	Territorial Decoration
MRCSE	Member of the Royal College of Surgeons of England	UCD	University College Dublin
MRI	Magnetic Resonance Imaging	UCH	University College Hospital, London
MS	Master of Surgery	UU	University of Ulster
MSc	Master of Science	UVF	Ulster Volunteer Force
NHS	National Health Service	VRD	Volunteer Reserve Decoration
NUI	National University of Ireland (Cork, Dublin or Galway)	Westm	Westminster Hospital, London

CHRONOLOGY

1774   The Poor House with its infirmary opens to the north of Belfast.

1792   The Belfast dispensary opens.

1797   The Belfast Dispensary and Fever Hospital opens in a house in Factory Row, but is forced to close after a few months because of lack of funds.

1799   The Belfast Dispensary and Fever Hospital reopens in three houses in West Street.

1817   The Belfast Dispensary and Fever Hospital moves to a new, purpose-built hospital building in Frederick Street.

1829   Belfast Lunatic Asylum opens to the west of the town on the Falls Road.

1841   The Workhouse and Union Hospital or Infirmary (later to become the Belfast City Hospital) opens to the south of Belfast.

1846   A new fever hospital, known as the Union Fever Hospital, opens in the grounds of the Workhouse.

1847   The Belfast Fever Hospital on Frederick Street is refurbished and enlarged and renamed the Belfast General Hospital.

1874   The Throne Hospital opens on the northeast outskirts of Belfast to cater for long-stay children and, in 1877, adults. A consumptive unit is opened there in 1885.

1875   The Belfast General Hospital is granted a royal charter and is renamed the Belfast Royal Hospital.

1896   The Forster Green Hospital opens on the southern outskirts of Belfast to cater for tuberculosis patients.

1899   The Belfast Royal Hospital is renamed the Royal Victoria Hospital.

1903   The Royal Victoria Hospital moves from Frederick Street to the Grosvenor Road.

1906   Purdysburn Hospital opens, replacing the Belfast Lunatic Asylum, which nevertheless continues to be used until about 1920.

1931   The Belfast Hospital for Sick Children opens beside the Royal Victoria Hospital on the site of the old Lunatic Asylum.

1933   The Royal Maternity Hospital opens beside the Royal Victoria Hospital.

1948   The Royal Victoria Hospital and its associated hospitals become part of the National Health Service. The Belfast Hospital for Sick Children changes its name to the Royal Belfast Hospital for Sick Children.

1993   The Royal Victoria Hospital becomes part of the Royal Group of Hospitals and Dental Hospital Health and Social Services Trust.

1997   Work starts on rebuilding the Royal Victoria Hospital.

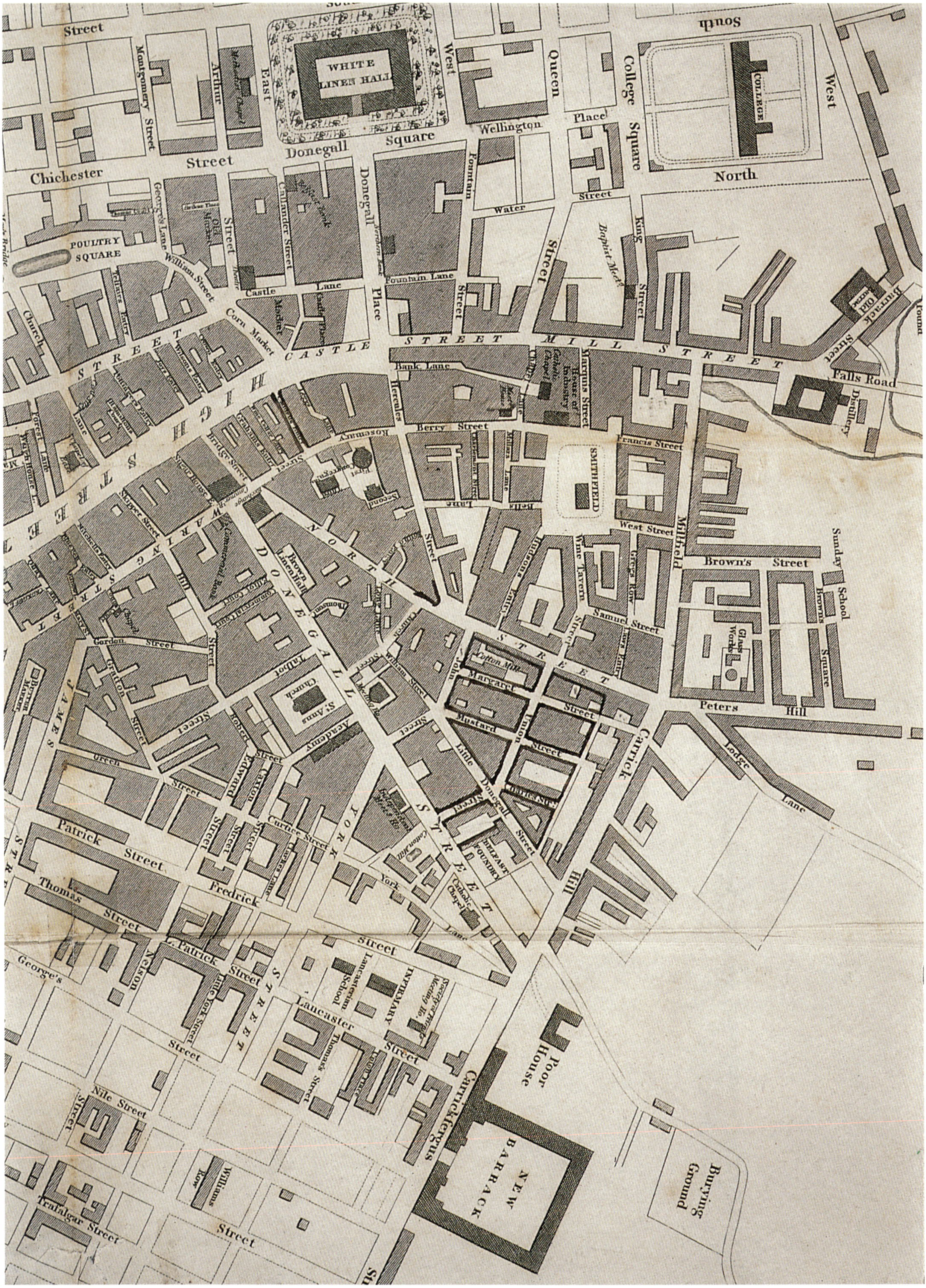
WHITE LINEN HALL
South
West
Montgomery Street
Arthur
East
Queen
College Square
COLLEGE
North
Wellington Place
Donegall Square
Chichester Street
Fountain
Water Street
POULTRY SQUARE
William Street
Callender Street
Castle Lane
Fountain Lane
Corn Market
Castle Place
King Street
CASTLE STREET
MILL STREET
Bank Lane
Hercules
Berry Street
Marquis Street
Barrack
Falls Road
Distillery
Francis Street
SMITHFIELD
Rosemary
HIGH STREET
WARING STREET
NORTH STREET
DONEGALL STREET
West Street
Millfield
Brown's Street
Sunday School
Browns Square
Samuel Street
Glass Works
Peters Hill
Carrick Hill
Lodge Lane
St. Anns Church
Academy
Talbot
Gordon Street
Margaret Street
Mustard Street
Union Street
Little Donegall Street
BELFAST FOUNDRY
YORK STREET
James Street
Green Street
Edward Street
Patrick Street
Fredrick Street
Thomas Street
Nelson Street
George's Street
Little York Street
Lancaster Street
Lancasterian School
INFIRMARY
Thomas's Street
Carrickfergus Street
Poor House
NEW BARRACK
Burying Ground
Nile Street
Williams Row
Trafalgar Street

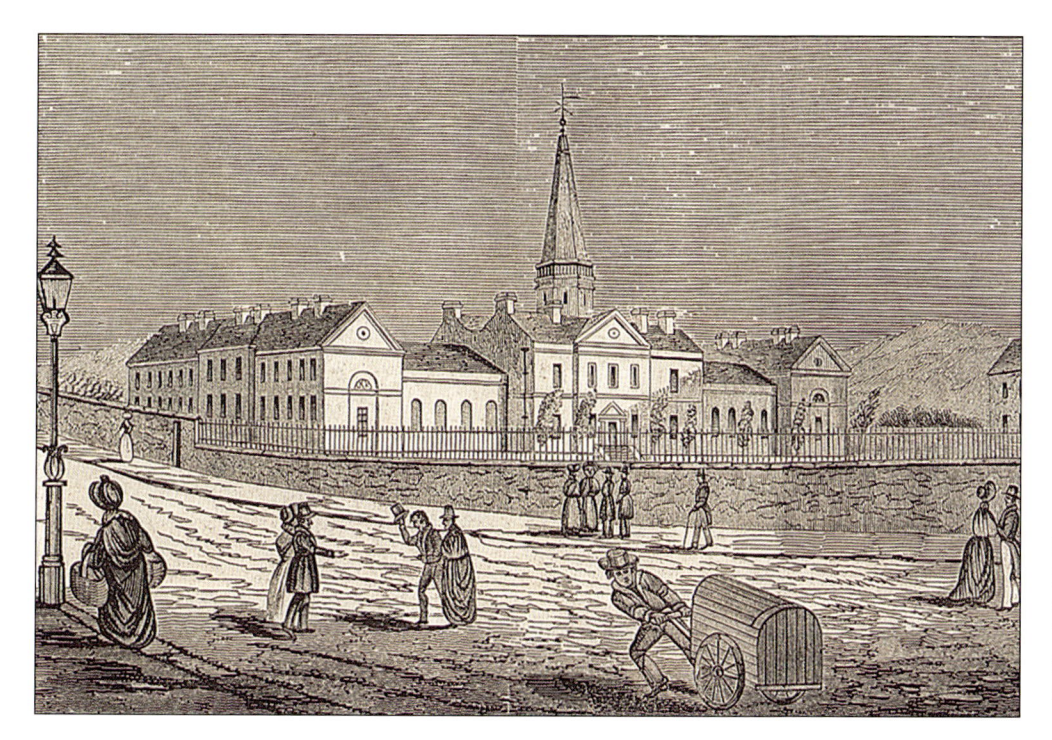

Engraving of the Poor House (now known as Clifton House), dating from 1774; from *Twenty-one Views in Belfast and its Neighbourhood*, Dublin, 1836
LINEN HALL LIBRARY

1
A GENERAL HOSPITAL FOR BELFAST

CARE OF THE SICK IN EIGHTEENTH-CENTURY IRELAND took place essentially at home, being mainly provided by the family; but if the patient could afford it, untrained help with nursing could easily be found. Indeed, at home the patient received better care than in any institution and was not exposed to the infections prevalent in all hospitals. There had, of course, been old monastic hospitals for the sick poor, but few of them survived the sixteenth-century dissolution of the monasteries. Throughout the British Isles in the eighteenth century it became obvious, however, that residential care for the

Opposite:
Map of Belfast, 1822, by J. Thomson. It shows Berry Street (formerly Factory Row) and West Street adjoining Smithfield, the Poor House, the Fever Hospital ('Infirmary') in Frederick Street and Inst. ('College') in the centre of College Square; from G. Benn, *History of Belfast,* 1823 edition.
LINEN HALL LIBRARY

1

destitute was badly needed. Dublin opened a hospital in Cook Street (forerunner of the Jervis Street Hospital) in 1718. Then came Dr Steevens' Hospital in 1720 and Cork's North Charitable Infirmary in 1721, which has been described as the most ancient provincial hospital in the British Empire. The Meath Hospital in Dublin opened in 1753. Belfast was slower in starting hospital care, but we should remember that it was still a small town in the mid-eighteenth century with a population of only 8,500, which rose to 13,000 by 1780. Dublin's population had reached 170,000 by this time, and even Limerick had 45,000. It was not until the nineteenth century with the growth in Belfast of shipbuilding and the textile mills that pressures of population and poverty began to build up.

Still, by the middle of the eighteenth century there were the beginnings of philanthropic thought in Belfast and on 28 August 1752 several local merchants met in the George Inn to form the Belfast Charitable Society and to discuss how to raise money to build a poorhouse and hospital. They came up with the idea of a lottery but, unlike more recent schemes, it collapsed within a year. The merchants then turned to more reliable sources of funds and appealed to the principal ground landlord of the city, the 5th Earl of Donegall. He was sympathetic and in 1768 promised a suitable site for a poorhouse to the north of the city (in what is now North Queen Street) and in 1771 the foundation stone of the Poor House and Infirmary was laid. It was opened by the Belfast Charitable Society in 1774 and a nursekeeper was appointed to combine nursing with general housekeeping. In the first instance the Poor House was to accommodate about fifty persons sleeping in twenty-two beds. The Poor House is one of the few remaining Georgian buildings in Belfast and, although it was mainly designed by an amateur architect, the locally born Robert Joy, it is one of the city's most beautiful buildings. Not only did it provide sleeping accommodation, but it had a dining room, board room, offices, space for teaching skills to the unemployed, separate space for children and a dispensary (outpatients' section) to treat the sick poor of the town. It was noted in the society's minutes that the physicians and surgeons of the city had generously resolved to attend the sick patients *gratis*, as was the custom in similar voluntary institutions at the time.

There was, in fact, only a thin line between the distressed poor and those who were actually sick, since poverty was so often accompanied by malnutrition, poor housing, infestations and the resultant disease. It was therefore logical to have one organisation covering both requirements. It seems that there were eight beds in this first infirmary block. The physicians and surgeons were asked to recommend equipment; this consisted of bedclothes (underblankets, sheets, upper blankets, cover and pillows), two close chairs (commodes) for the great ward and one each for the small wards, one chamberpot per bed, one pewter bedpan, chairs, tables, candlesticks, saucepans, tins, cups and spoons. Not only was provision made to see outpatients, but the sick were also visited in their own homes.

Records exist of the medical and surgical patients treated in the Infirmary and the minutes of the Poor House are well preserved. For instance, in August 1785 there were four cases in the infirmary under the surgeon Mr John Clarke: Ann Corran, with 'running sores & contractions in her limbs which I believe to be incurable', Patt Laverty with 'ulcers in his legs, recovering', Eliz. Crawford with 'an ulcer in her leg, recovering', and Jane Hunter with 'a scorbutic humour [scurvy] & inflammation in her leg & bad habit of body, recovering'. Other conditions recorded included fractures, a man with cancer in his cheek, lunacy, asthma and drunkenness; these were drawn not simply from Belfast, but from the surroundings and even from sailors arriving in the port.

Over the years the Poor House ran almost all the public services of Belfast, including the water supply and graveyard as well as the hospital, but it seems to have been ready to relinquish these one by one as a more appropriate body was formed.

THE BELFAST DISPENSARY AND FEVER HOSPITAL

Gradually the need for a separate dispensary to provide medical attention and medicines for outpatients and a hospital for those who were sick but not destitute was felt, and a subscription list was opened in 1792. However, a split over the proposals developed among Belfast's various philanthropists so that in July 1793 a motion 'that the two institutions [the Poor House and the Dispensary and Fever Hospital] are mutually calculated to support each other' was rejected. The Dispensary, with accommodation for patients, apothecary and medical officers, had opened in July 1792 in a house which they obtained free of expense. Over the next eighteen months, 733 patients were seen, and the medical officers also made home visits in the various Dispensary Districts. By 27 April 1797 the hospital planning committee was able to open a hospital in a house in Factory Row (now Berry Street). The new institution was known as the Belfast Dispensary and Fever Hospital and may be regarded as the first independent hospital in Belfast. It is the direct ancestor of today's Royal Victoria Hospital, being the parent of the Belfast Fever Hospital built in Frederick Street in 1817, which changed its name in 1847 to the Belfast General Hospital and in 1875 to the Belfast Royal Hospital. This in turn became the Royal Victoria Hospital in 1899 and moved to the Grosvenor Road site in 1903.

Dr Andrew Malcolm in his *History of the General Hospital, Belfast . . .* (1851) records considerable detail of its early funding and the staff associated with it. The house, which would replace the outpatient dispensary as well as being a hospital, was rented from a Mr Pollard for one year at £20. Funding was to be by donations, charity sermons and the recruitment of 'life governors', who were each prepared to pay a lump sum of ten guineas. In return for this a life governor could attend the quarterly meetings of the charity and had the privilege of admitting up to two patients at once.

The hospital was opened with six beds, a nurse was appointed, and the physicians and surgeons of the Dispensary were asked to provide attendance. But for all the planning and optimism, the hospital could hardly have been founded at a worse time. Over the first few months of its existence, sixty patients were treated with only one death, and yet it was nearly bankrupt. The initial appeal had raised only £58; £53 of this was quickly spent, and it seems that by the end of the year the Dispensary and Fever Hospital had fallen into complete neglect and closed. The reason for this lay partly in the turmoil that beset Belfast at that time. The Society of United Irishmen had been formed in Belfast in 1791 with the objectives of uniting Irishmen of all classes and creeds under a parliament freed from English domination. Its aims included such revolutionary topics as Catholic Emancipation, a much wider franchise, and the right to trade free of restrictions designed to help English manufacturers, and soon brought its members into conflict with the government. Large numbers of arrests were being made of known United Irishmen or those suspected of sympathy with them, and this latter group included many of the professional people and intelligentsia of the town. In addition, because of the war with France the poor suffered when commodities were scarce and prices high and to crown all the Belfast Charitable Society and the infirm poor were put out of the Poor House by the army in June 1798. Another reason for closing the hospital for a short period, according to a contemporary letter (Simms, 1932), was an epidemic of fever which laid low Dr James McDonnell, as well as the housekeeper, the apothecary, the surgeon and another doctor. Fortunately they all recovered, suggesting that it was trench fever rather than the much more dangerous typhus.

In spite of these difficulties, though, the need for a hospital was clear and on 31 October 1799 the Belfast Dispensary and Fever Hospital managed to open three houses in West Street, close to Smithfield. The funds were derived principally from a sermon preached by the Reverend William Bristow, the Vicar of Belfast (and previously Sovereign, or mayor, of the town) which raised £113. He stands out as one of the early pillars of the hospital and indeed as a pillar of many other worthy causes in the town until his death in 1809.

THE EARLY PHYSICIANS AND SURGEONS

Inevitably there was an overlap between the roles of the Poor House with its infirmary and the Dispensary and Fever Hospital, and while some doctors worked in both institutions, most confined themselves to the latter. As in other voluntary hospitals, the doctors were all unpaid in the early years (Attending and Consulting staff remained unpaid right up until 1948). Only the most dedicated maintained their attachment throughout their career.

On the other hand, they could practise freely outside hospital as general practitioners, for there was no distinction between general and specialist doctors. Indeed holding a hospital appointment often enhanced a practitioner's reputation with patients and thereby increased his income. Doctors could also practise as apothecaries, but their hospital post enabled them to make money by selling medicines to patients, and for this reason combining the two professions was later banned. (The Royal College of Surgeons in Ireland still requires its fellows to take an oath stating that they will not practise as an apothecary.)

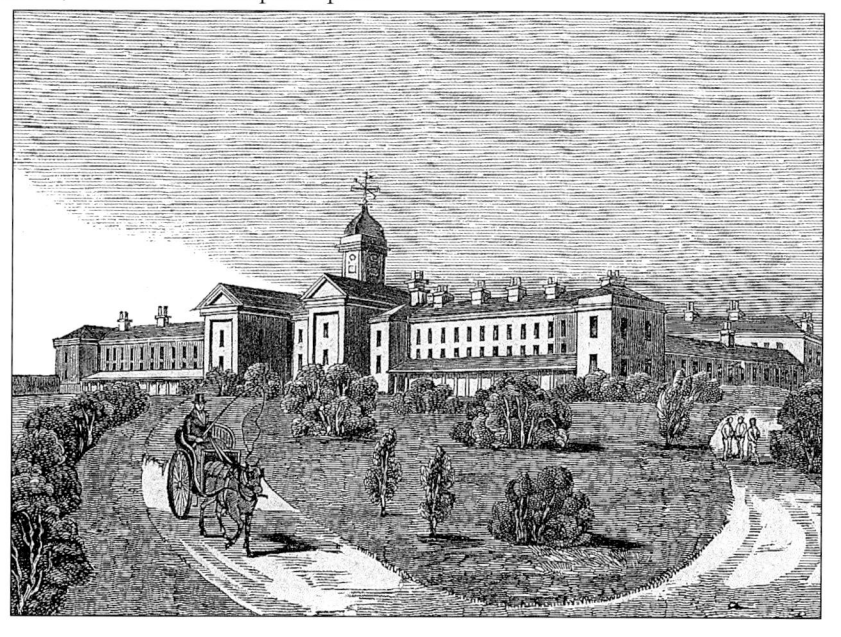

The first meeting held to plan the hospital, on 16 May 1792, appointed as Consulting Physicians Dr Alexander Henry Halliday and Dr John Mattear. These were senior physicians who presumably were not involved in the day-to-day dispensary work. Dr Halliday is well documented. In 1751 he had corresponded on medical matters with the celebrated Dr William Cullen who had founded the medical school in Glasgow, in 1771 he had tried to save agrarian insurgents of the Hearts of Steel from the wrath of the army, and we know that in 1790 he was secretary of the Northern Whig Club. Subsequently he was the first president of the Belfast Reading Society (later the Linen Hall Library), from 1792 to 1798.

Engraving of the District Lunatic Asylum, dating from 1829 and now demolished; from *Twenty-one Views in Belfast and its Neighbourhood*, Dublin, 1836
LINEN HALL LIBRARY

Less is known about Dr John Mattear, even though he was a brother of Samuel McTier (spelling was erratic in those days) and brother-in-law to Mrs Martha McTier who was secretary to the Lying-in Hospital (see page 54). Mrs McTier is known in a wider context as the writer of so many descriptive and incisive letters to her brother Dr William C. Drennan (published as *The Drennan Letters*). These not only reflect the sympathies of the group with the United Irishmen, but give perceptive comments on their medical and other friends. Both Dr Halliday and Dr Mattear are buried in Clifton Street graveyard.

Attending Physicians to the Dispensary were Dr James McDonnell and a Dr White. Dr McDonnell was at the peak of his profession and was one who promoted the Dispensary and Fever Hospital rather than the Poor

House. Dr Malcolm regarded him 'to have represented then and throughout his active life all the energy and zeal which animated and cherished this charitable movement'. He only resigned from its staff (because of ill health) in 1837. Even allowing for the flowery language of the time, references to his 'loftiest benevolence' and 'working in the Districts like a very slave or toiling in the wards for hours' must be believed. They are the more credible in that Malcolm does admit that 'on several occasions he became estranged from his brethren', a clue that McDonnell had the sort of powerful and dominating personality calculated to get a great institution off the ground. His fellow Attending Physician, Dr White, appears to have been an apothecary and physician; his name occurs periodically in the Poor House minutes of the 1770s and in the early Dispensary minutes, but not thereafter.

Much less is known about the early surgeons. Mr Bartholomew Fuller, a surgeon to the Forty-ninth Regiment, and Mr Richard McClelland, an ex-naval surgeon, were appointed Attending Surgeons in 1792. Bartholomew Fuller died on 1 January 1800, and Richard McClelland, who attended both the Poor House and the Dispensary as surgeon and apothecary, died on 17 September 1807; both of these were surgeons to the Dispensary Districts rather than the hospital. Other early surgeons included Mr Robert McCluney, a founder member of the Belfast Medical Society in 1806, who up until his death in 1837 was for many years surgeon to the hospital. These early surgeons, like many other practitioners at the time, had neither medical degree nor fellowship of any college of surgeons, but had probably attended medical classes and anatomy dissecting rooms. Their training was unregulated and they learned by an apprenticeship system, relying on the approbation of their peers for success in their careers.

An early physician was Dr Samuel Stephenson, alias the Reverend Samuel Martin Stephenson. He had been Presbyterian minister of Greyabbey, County Down, but resigned after refusing to subscribe to the Westminster Confession of Faith. He had studied medicine in Dublin and Edinburgh (MD 1776) and gave up his ministry in 1785 to become a celebrated physician in Belfast. He was involved in both the Poor House and the Belfast Dispensary and Fever Hospital and we find his name in the records of medical care of both institutions over the next twenty years. His religious affiliations are an extreme example of the wave of independent thought which was sweeping through the Presbyterian Church in Ulster. It was known as the New Light, and in many congregations the Non-Subscribers, as they became known, were in the majority and were able to retain the old church (for example Belfast First Congregation and Rademon near Crossgar). The Non-Subscribers had an influence far beyond their numbers and were leaders in such projects as the formation of the Poor House, the Dispensary and Fever Hospital, the Academical

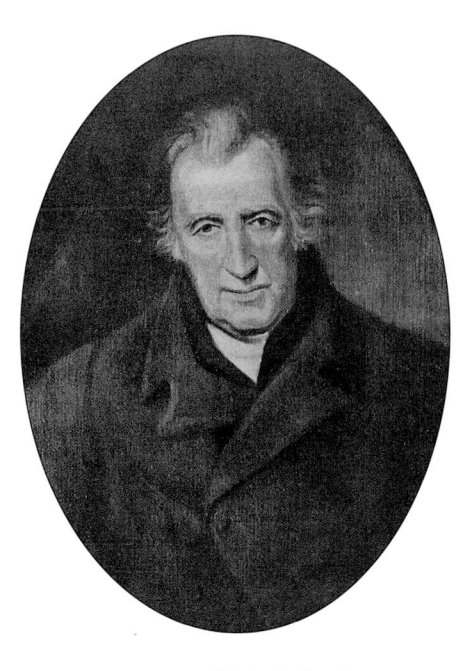

Dr Samuel Martin Stephenson, Attending Physician, 1800–1809
ROYAL VICTORIA HOSPITAL

Institution, the Linen Hall Library and, most controversial of all, the United Irishmen.

On 11 January 1801 Dr Samuel Smith Thomson was appointed Physician to the Dispensary and in 1810 he became Physician to the Fever Hospital. His career followed a similar pattern to that of the other first doctors at the Belfast Dispensary and Fever Hospital; he had been a founder of the Anacreontic Society (now the Belfast Philharmonic Society), a member of the First Presbyterian Congregation, and first president of the Belfast Medical Society. He had studied medicine in Edinburgh and obtained his MD in 1800 for a thesis on measles. He worked hard during the fever epidemic of 1816–17 but resigned with Dr Lawson Drummond in 1818 over the question of remuneration by the hospital for their work. However, he returned to the Fever Hospital and continued in practice, being appointed a Visiting Physician to the Belfast Lunatic Asylum in 1830. When he died in 1849, he too was buried in the Clifton Street graveyard behind the Poor House, where his memorial is still fixed to the graveyard wall.

A surgeon in the early years of the hospital was Dr Andrew Marshall who was unusual in having a medical qualification – having in 1804 gained the LRCP of Edinburgh, where he had already studied for two years before qualifying as assistant surgeon in the Royal Navy. In Belfast he lived at 3 Wellington Place and was in partnership with his brother-in-law James Drummond, an apothecary, in High Street. This combination of interests was obviously profitable.

The most notable apothecary perhaps ever in the hospital was Mr James Murray, who was elected to the post in 1807 at the early age of nineteen, though he resigned in the following year to set up as a surgeon and apothecary in High Street. The turning point in his career came in about 1829 when he used his fluid magnesia preparation to cure a sudden ailment which affected the Marquess of Anglesey, Lord Lieutenant of Ireland (the famous 'Peg Leg' who lost a leg at Waterloo), when visiting the Marquess of Donegall. The treatment was so successful that Murray was appointed resident physician to the Lord Lieutenant and moved to Dublin, where he had a brilliant career. He obtained the MD of Edinburgh in 1829 and the MD of Trinity College Dublin in 1832; he received a knighthood for his services to the Lord Lieutenant. His most enduring contributions to posterity were as the inventor of milk of magnesia and as the builder in 1828 of a fine set of houses in Belfast known as Murray's Terrace, which gave their name to the present Murray Street.

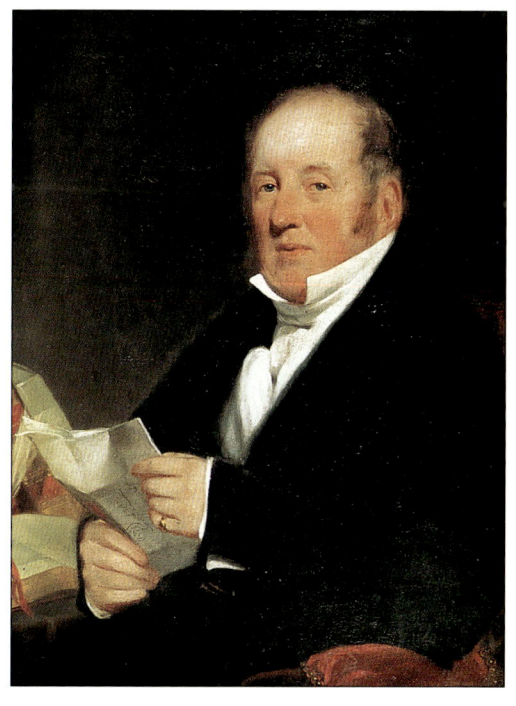

Dr Samuel Smith Thomson,
Attending Physician, 1810–30
ROYAL VICTORIA HOSPITAL

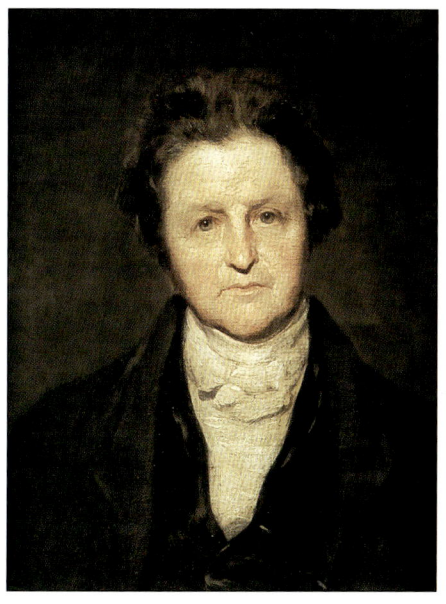

Dr Andrew Marshall,
Attending Physician, 1807–28
ROYAL VICTORIA HOSPITAL

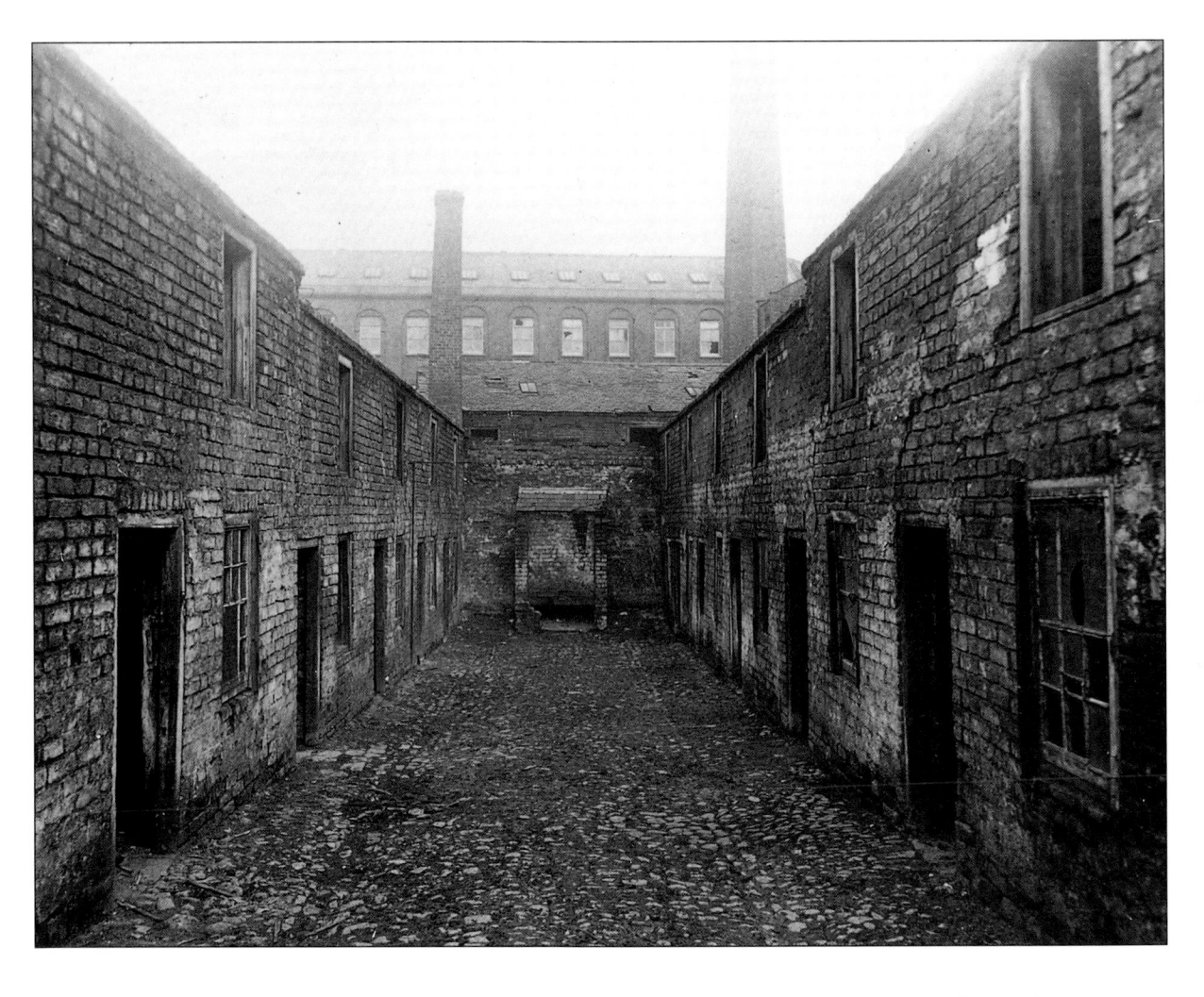

Early-nineteenth-century houses in Millfield, Belfast: the houses had no yards and all used the common privy seen at the end of the street. Earlier still there had been cess pits and piles of domestic waste and excrement in the streets; photograph by A.R. Hogg.
ULSTER MUSEUM

THE BELFAST DISPENSARY AND FEVER HOSPITAL AND THE 'FEVER'

The early years of the Belfast Dispensary and Fever Hospital were marked by recurrent epidemics of fever and a continuous shortage of funds. These epidemics were a feature of most cities of the world, with their overcrowding, poverty, polluted water supply, malnutrition and absence of efficient sanitation. Industrialisation made things worse, bringing large numbers of workers into Belfast from the country to work in damp or dusty conditions in the mills. These workers were financially unable to take time off when they became ill, and thus spread infectious diseases from one to another; they often went to hospital only when near death. When fever raged, its victims tended to fill general beds, unless the hospital could isolate them in a fever block. Between epidemics, however, it was accepted that general medical and surgical cases could again be freely admitted to hospital. Fortunately the hospital's finances were helped to some extent by an act of Parliament of 1805 empowering grand juries to grant sums towards the maintenance of public dispensaries and fever hospitals. This act and subsequent amendments gave great heart to all those concerned with the Belfast Dispensary and Fever Hospital, and over the next few years plans for a more permanent home were discussed. By 1810 a site had been selected in Frederick Street and a building fund was started. This grew only slowly, by legacies, donations and collections at charity sermons, but in 1815 the foundation stone of the new Belfast Dispensary and Fever Hospital was laid by the Marquess of Donegall.

The intention was that the new hospital would accommodate 70 medical and surgical patients and 30 fever patients. However, the following two years saw a memorable epidemic which stretched the West Street hospital to capacity and excluded all but fever cases. Under this pressure the new building was rapidly completed and on 1 August 1817, while the plaster was still wet, patients were transferred from the old hospital to the new. The final cost was calculated at £5,000.

The fever epidemic of 1816–18 finally ran its course; 212 was the peak number of inpatients at any one time in a hospital designed to hold 100 beds, and a total of 3,527 patients were treated for fever. The Poor House, the House of Industry, the Clothing Society, soup kitchens and relief committees all played their part at a time when there was no official mechanism for coping with disasters.

The term 'fever', like the previously used 'Black Death' and 'plague', is rather vague in strict medical usage. However, there is little doubt that it was a combination of typhus and relapsing fevers, both very rare in Europe today. Typhus is an infection caused by a micro-organism of the rickettsia family which is carried by the louse. It was endemic at times, though exactly why typhus occurred in the past in recurrent waves is uncertain. It was clearly associated with poverty, dirt and starvation and, even then, many people realised that cleansing of houses and isolation of victims of the fever would limit the spread of infection.

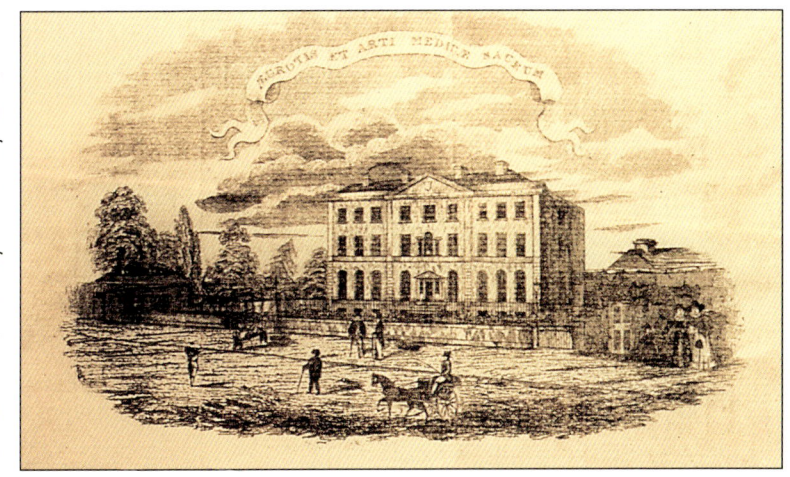

The Belfast Dispensary and Fever Hospital as built in 1817
ROYAL VICTORIA HOSPITAL

The main features of typhus fever were congestion of the blood vessels of the skin, giving the patient a dark colour, as well as a rash and gangrene of the extremities. The sufferer's temperature rose, causing convulsions and delirium – the latter so severe that patients would sometimes jump out of windows or throw themselves in the river. There was abdominal pain and vomiting, though not the acute diarrhoea of typhoid and cholera. Finally there was an intense and unpleasant smell which even the most devoted attendants found nauseating and intolerable.

Relapsing fever is also transmitted by lice and is caused by a different group of micro-organisms, spirochaetes of the genus *Borrelia*. It is characterised by fever, vomiting and exhaustion which recur every few days, hence its name. It also causes a break-up of the red blood cells and jaundice, and the Irish-language term for it means 'yellow fever'.

DISPENSARY AND DISTRICTS

The physicians and surgeons appointed in the earliest days of the Belfast Dispensary and Fever Hospital project, from 1792 to 1797, at first attended the Dispensary and Districts only, though from 1797 most of them were also appointed to attend at the hospital. There were six Dispensary Districts by 1822 and their boundaries and the medical staff responsible for them are listed in the table. The work was, as we have seen, unpaid, and over the first fifty years there were frequent arguments about the possibility of remuneration. A stimulus to this was the fact that the work on the Districts seems to have been hard and unattractive – general practice in the slums, and involving much unpaid travel – and it was not always easy to find doctors to take it up. Dr S.S. Thomson worked hard for the welfare of the patients, but was also the leading proponent of remuneration, so much so that in 1834 thirty-seven of his colleagues presented him with a gold snuff box, suitably inscribed. At all events the remuneration cause was unsuccessful in the 1830s, and the temporary solution adopted was to appoint all new physicians to work in the Districts for two years before starting work

THE DISPENSARY DISTRICTS OF BELFAST IN 1822
AND THE DOCTOR RESPONSIBLE FOR EACH

No. 1   Bounded by York Street, Donegall Street, Waring Street, Donegall Quay and George's Street, in charge of Dr Stephenson.

No. 2   Bounded by York Street, George's Street, Carrick Hill, Peter's Hill, North Street, Exchange Street and Donegall Street, in charge of Dr Robert Stephenson.

No. 3   Bounded by North Street, Peter's Hill, Brown's Square, Millfield, Francis Street, Berry Street and Rosemary Street, in charge of Surgeon Moore.

No. 4   Bounded by Donegall Place, Bank Buildings, Dalzell's Row, Berry Street, Francis Street, through Millfield to Barrack Street and Sandy Row, in charge of Dr Forcade.

No. 5   Bounded by Donegall Place, Dalzell's Row, Rosemary Street, Skippers' Street, Church Lane and Cromack Street, in charge of Dr McDonnell and Surgeon McCluney.

No. 6   Bounded by Cromack Street, Church Lane, Skippers' Street, Waring Street, Lime-Kiln Dock, Hanover Quay and May's Bridge, in charge of Surgeon Arrott.

Source: 1822 Annual Report of the Belfast Dispensary and Fever Hospital, p. 5

in the hospital. This was done and even when responsibility for the Districts was taken away from the hospital in 1846, most doctors on the staff continued to take up an outpatient appointment prior to being appointed Attending Physician or Surgeon on the wards.

Before that, the remuneration issue came up again, in 1845, with further pressure from the doctors working in the Districts, but this time they resigned from their posts (though they still continued to work) in order to push the inhabitants of the city to take action. The Dispensary as such had no funds and the hospital was unwilling to support the huge drain on its funds of medical salaries. On 26 March 1846 a plan was adopted, however, to have two additional dispensaries as well as the one in the hospital, all funded by the town. The six Dispensary Districts were each given their own doctor at £50 per year and an apothecary at not less than £60 per year. This system worked for many years and at least enabled the hospital to confine its care to its own premises.

THE ASIATIC CHOLERA AND OTHER EPIDEMICS

After the fever of 1816–18, the next epidemic to hit Belfast was the 'Asiatic' cholera in 1832. Its course from Russia across Europe during 1831 had been followed in the newspapers, and the first case hit Belfast on 29 February 1832. This was before the celebrated demonstration by John Snow who, faced with an epidemic of cholera in London and noting that the distribution of cases was clustered round the pump in Broad Street (Soho), removed the handle of the pump. In a few days it was evident that no new cases were occurring, an observation providing strong evidence of the waterborne transmission of the disease. In 1832, however, isolation of patients was still seen as vital, and a cholera block was built behind the Fever Hospital to provide for fifty patients (and sometimes more). Additional accommodation was rented in Lancaster Street for isolation of those in contact with the cholera patients. Finally a type of ambulance service was started, given the exotic name 'palanquins' by Dr Malcolm.

The features of cholera are very simply those of extreme dehydration, for from the outset the patient has intense nausea, vomiting and diarrhoea ('rice water stools'). These are followed by weakness and cramps, cold and clammy skin, sunken eyes, intense thirst, exhaustion, and death often within twenty-four hours. Treatment varied widely, reflecting all the ideas popular at the time, and fierce battles raged between physicians advocating different regimens. Opiates and astringents and fluids were generally recognised as effective, but even such a disastrous idea as bleeding had its supporters. In the end it is surprising that the mortality quoted by Malcolm was only 16 per cent out of 2,870 cases in one year.

During this epidemic, as at all times, the regular fevers continued; indeed, influenza was also recognised as an endemic infectious fever. There

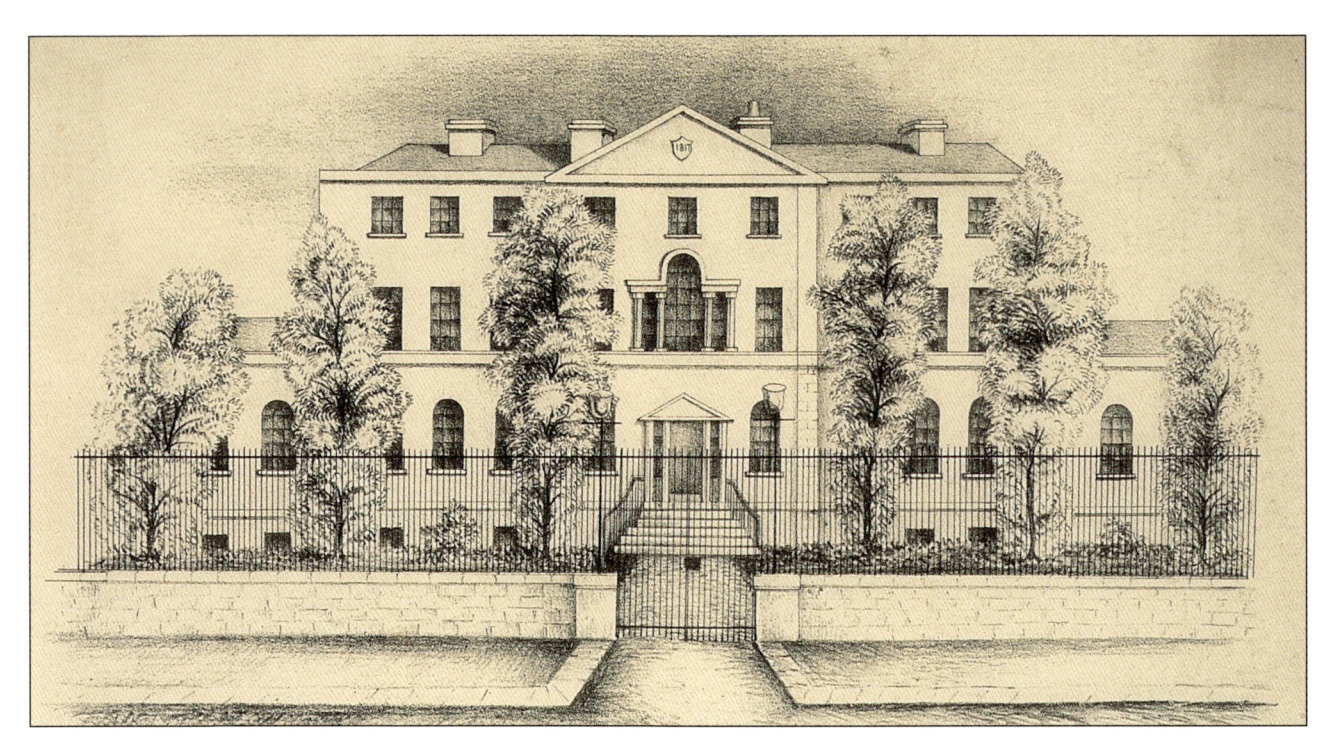

The General Hospital after Sir Charles Lanyon's additions of 1847, engraving by W. and G. Agnew; from Dr Andrew George Malcolm's *A History of the General Hospital*

was a renewed outbreak of fever in 1836–37 during which a total of about four thousand patients were admitted to the hospital. Further epidemics of fever continued into the 1840s. The old remedy of emergency beds was employed, this time in a 'fever shed' in the grounds of the Belfast Dispensary and Fever Hospital, but eventually the Workhouse and the Union Hospital or Infirmary, with six beds for the destitute sick, was opened in 1841, funded by ratepayers, as a result of the extension of the Poor Laws to Ireland (in due course this became the Belfast City Hospital). The accommodation in the Union Hospital was inevitably too small, and since the administering Board of Guardians were only allowed to use their funds in the Union's own institutions, just five years later a new hospital specifically to treat fever patients, the Union Fever Hospital, was opened in the Workhouse grounds.

The recurring crises of fever and cholera left little room or time for the Belfast Dispensary and Fever Hospital on Frederick Street to accommodate other medical and surgical problems. Charitable funds also were all channelled in the same direction. A move was made, in 1843, however, to stimulate the rich and powerful of the city into setting up a fund for a new general hospital. Within a few weeks £3,000 was collected; indeed the fund went on accumulating, though with some raids on it, over the next three years.

By now the Workhouse and with it the new Union Fever Hospital had been opened. The new fever hospital would take away the fever patients from the old building in Frederick Street. It was logical therefore not to build a new hospital but to rename the old Belfast Dispensary and Fever Hospital the Belfast General Hospital and to use the funds collected to refurbish and make some additions to the old building. At last the hospital could concentrate on illnesses other than fever. The changes are well described in the annual report of 1848–49 and can be seen clearly by comparing prints of the hospital in the 1830s and in the 1850s. They consisted in the addition of two low blocks on either side of the central part which were designed by Charles Lanyon (later Sir), architect of so much of Belfast and Ulster. They contained 'a suitable Operating and Lecture Theatre, several accident and fever wards and a suite of bathrooms, besides many other conveniences'. The main emphasis, as can be seen from the plan (on page 25), was on education and services rather than ward space.

At this point, however, the country was overwhelmed by a new disaster, the Great Famine of 1845–49. This had a less disastrous effect on the north of Ireland than on many other parts of the country, partly because the people in the north traditionally ate meal in addition to potatoes and perhaps because the strain of potato planted there was more blight-resistant. Nevertheless there was great destitution and poverty, which reached a peak between mid-July 1846 and mid-July 1847; starving country dwellers took refuge at Belfast bringing with them the diseases of starvation. One episode in particular highlights the problem. The *Swatara* sailed from Liverpool in March 1847 with several hundred Irish emigrants bound for America. Bad weather forced the ship to put in first at Belfast, then at Derry, and again at Belfast; on each occasion passengers sick with fever were taken off. Malcolm noted that the landings in Belfast were associated with peaks in the numbers of fever admissions to hospital.

During the famine Belfast had several hospitals taking fever patients: the new Union Fever Hospital, the General Hospital with the old cholera building behind it, the College Hospital in Barrack Street (see page 21), and a vacant house made available by the town council. In addition the Poor House looked after many of its own sick and the Workhouse erected tents to accommodate seven hundred convalescent patients. We have many first-hand accounts of conditions in Belfast during the famine, and with fifty new cases a day in May 1847, it is not hard to visualise the distress: many patients had to wait for hours at the gates in Frederick Street until beds became available in consequence of the death or discharge of other patients. On 20 July 1847 the *Belfast News-Letter* gave this report:

> The hospitals are crowded, and every new building erected for patients is filled to overflowing as soon as completed. Yet hundreds – for whom there remains no provision – are daily exposed in the delirium of this frightful malady, on the streets, or left to die in their filthy and ill-ventilated hovels … It is now a thing of daily occurrence to see haggard, sallow and emaciated beings, stricken down by fever or debility from actual want, stretched prostrate upon the footways of our streets and bridges, unable to proceed further than the spot where they had fallen down.

Throughout the famine most of the deaths were the result of disease, rather than starvation alone. These diseases included the familiar typhus and relapsing fever, the mild trench fever, and what was probably typhoid fever. There was no true cholera in Belfast at the time, though many patients died of some form of diarrhoea. The notorious Asiatic cholera returned in 1849 with disastrous effects on the weakened population; again it caused chaos in the hospitals. It affected a smaller proportion of the population, however – perhaps 2 per cent rather than the 5 per cent of 1832. Against that, the mortality, at 33 per cent, was more than double the previous figure.

SURGERY BEFORE THE ADVENT OF ANAESTHESIA

The annual reports of the Belfast Dispensary and Fever Hospital and its successors have survived complete from 1818. The first of these make little mention of conditions other than fever, and not until 1823 do we find non-fever patients being accounted a major expense:

> Accident patients were admitted into the hospital gratis with the least possible delay, and formed the principal expense of the surgical department. Many of these were cases of fracture which would remain some weeks in the establishment ... some of these were cases of cancer, which were all extirpated successfully with the exception of one, that had been of long standing. Besides a considerable number of surgical patients have been benefited by being daily attended at the Dispensary.

From 1824, a definitive surgical report was included in each annual report and when one considers that all these surgical patients were treated before the advent of anaesthesia, recoveries bear tribute to the stoicism of the patients and to the skill of the surgeons. In the year 1823/24 (from 1 May 1823 to 30 April 1824), there were 39 injuries of some sort, though only one of these was treated surgically (amputation). There were 8 patients with cancers, 2 of whom died, and the remainder were described as having been operated on successfully. Out of 5 patients with cataracts, 3 had them successfully removed. One femoral aneurysm was successfully treated as was a strangulated hernia. A few years later, particular stress was laid on the need for early admission and surgery if such hernia patients were to recover. Most of the trauma cases among these admissions were the result of industrial accidents: the numbers employed in the cotton mills grew steadily throughout the first half of the century. By this time linen was well established, with family businesses such as John Barbour of Hilden and Andrew Mulholland of York Street which had expanded their flax spinning and weaving throughout the 1830s and 1840s. The harbour and the shipbuilding industry (with such names as Ritchie and McLaine) expanded throughout the first half of the century and produced many injuries; some injured sailors were admitted from ships arriving in the busy port of Belfast. Each year there were several cases of severe burns, both domestic and industrial, and a high proportion of these patients died. They included a climbing boy (chimney sweep) in 1834 'who was literally scorched to death in an overheated chimney'. This was a common occurrence at the time, which Charles Kingsley successfully campaigned against in his fantasy *The Water-Babies*.

The number of accidents continued to grow in the 1830s, and in 1836 Mr Robert Coffey, a Senior Surgeon, reported 114 very severe accidents in less than a year. According to Coffey, such high accident rates often necessitated too early discharge of patients or even their accommodation two to a bed, 'a practice disreputable to a well regulated Hospital'. He commented also on the need for a suitable operating theatre. 'At present operations must be performed in a room, on a storey higher than the surgical wards, to which the patients are generally obliged to be carried, at great suffering and much risk.' Their situation was not helped by the presence of up to thirty pupils witnessing the operations. And though a high proportion of accidents in this period were probably industrial, there is no evidence that the factory owners either paid anything towards the costs of patient management or gave compensation to the victims. Wealthy merchants did of course contribute annually to the hospital, but rarely more than one guinea each.

Unfortunately, in spite of the good intentions of the medical staff, the system used to classify cases varied from decade to decade, which makes it difficult to establish trends. For some reason syphilis and gonorrhoea were always classified as surgical, and in 1829 some 57 of these cases are recorded, with 40 apparent recoveries, but many such patients remained in hospital for a long time. In 1839, Mr David Moore entered the following record:

> … next to accidents the most numerous class of patients is that of syphilis, all of them female. They are kept by themselves in the lock-ward … and after being cured some return to their friends, others are received into the Penitentiary, where they are usefully employed and taught habits of regularity and industry.

In case anyone should think that men were immune from this scourge he added, 'If the hospital could afford accommodation it would be highly useful to establish a lock-ward for males …!' In other cities it was the practice to refuse all such patients admission or at least to treat them harshly as a sign of social disapproval. In Belfast, however, it was always the practice to set aside space for them, but with segregation 'from the virtuous part of their sex', and in 1828 a separate female lock-ward was opened. It was never comfortable – it had no heating and sometimes had ten patients for seven beds – but at least it provided isolation and some care. However, during and after the next outbreak of cholera the ward was taken over for victims of the epidemic, and gradually patients with syphilis were accepted into the surgical wards, though never in numbers that met the real need. In 1841 a lock-ward was provided in the new Union Hospital.

Inflammation and infection generally figured high among the problems classified as surgical, but were not usually treated by surgery. The large numbers of ulcers recorded in all years were presumably benign and related to varicose veins. Certainly in 1834 Mr Coffey comments that they are 'tedious in recovery and very expensive on the funds of the Institution'. The problem did not subsequently go away.

In general, fever patients always had priority, and surgical emergencies, though few in number, were admitted before venereal or general medical patients. There seems therefore to have been surprisingly little conflict among doctors over admission rights.

There were no striking changes in the pattern of surgery before the advent of anaesthesia. It is not easy to calculate how many operations were performed each year – probably no more than twenty. It is clear, however, from the 1834/35 annual report's mention of successful 'excision of the elbow-joint' by Dr James Sanders (see page 18) that increasingly complicated surgery was being undertaken. Another procedure, not without risks even today, was the creation in 1845 of an 'artificial anus' in a man with a strangulation. It was later closed up and he was discharged in six weeks. Another example of the diversity of practice in this era is two cases of tetanus (following one injury to the head and one to the toes) included in the 1845 report, both of whom died.

THE SECOND GENERATION OF PHYSICIANS AND SURGEONS

Dr James Lawson Drummond had the varied career that was still possible for a medical man in the early nineteenth century. He was born in the Larne area of County Antrim, the son of William Drummond, Surgeon RN, was educated at Belfast Academy (later Belfast Royal Academy), and joined the Royal Navy as a 'surgeon's mate' in 1807. He attended examinations at the Royal College of Surgeons in London from 1806 to 1809 and was personally judged to be fit to practise although he did not have a licentiate or fellowship. He left the navy in 1813, was awarded an MD by Edinburgh University for a thesis on the comparative anatomy of the eye in 1814, and began private practice in Belfast in the same year. He was appointed Physician (not Surgeon) to the Dispensary and to the Belfast Fever Hospital in 1814, but resigned in 1818. He was the instigator and first occupant, in 1818, of a chair in Anatomy and Medical Physiology at the Academical Institution's new medical school (see pages 20–22), a post he held until the collegiate department of the Academical Institution (known from 1831 as the Royal Belfast Academical

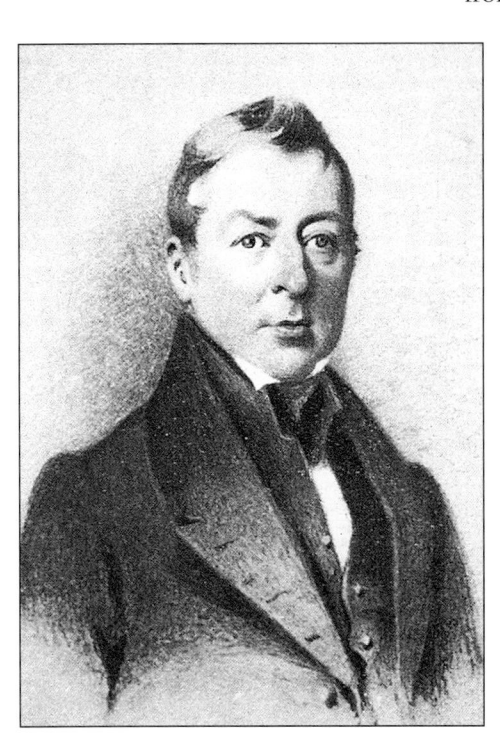

Professor James Lawson Drummond, Attending Physician to the Fever Hospital, 1814–18, and Professor of Anatomy and Physiology in the collegiate department of the Academical Institution, 1818–49
ULSTER MEDICAL SOCIETY

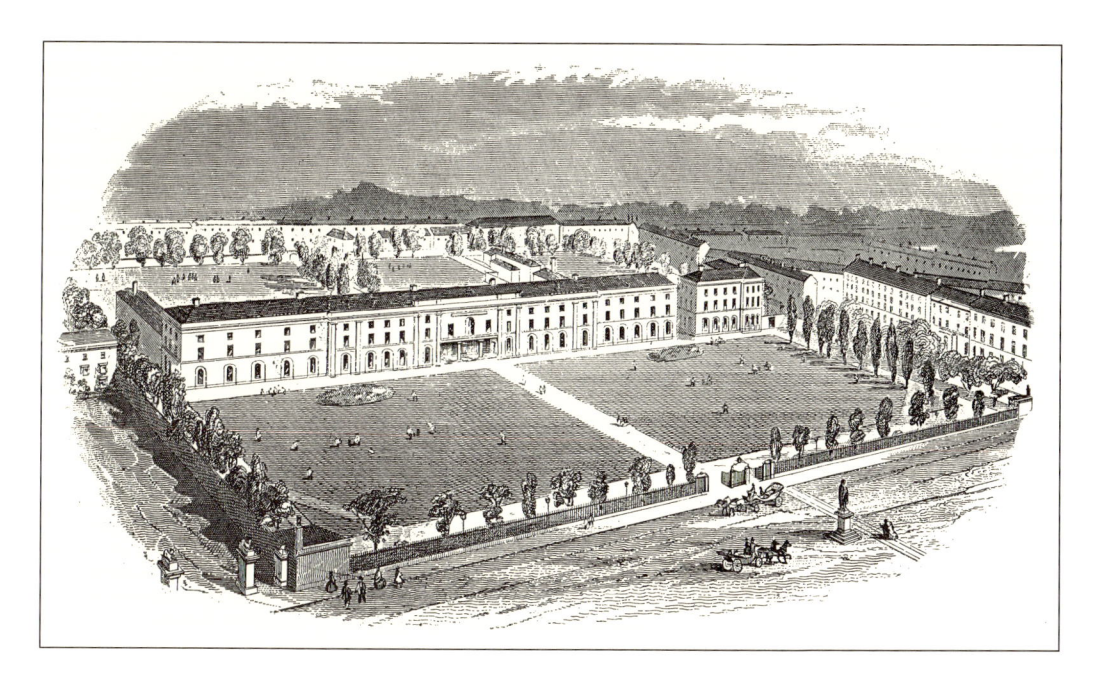

Institution and still usually referred to as Inst.) was merged into the new Queen's College in 1849.

Drummond is perhaps best known as president of the Belfast Literary Society from 1815 to 1816, as one of the leading enthusiasts who brought about the opening of a botanic garden in Belfast in 1820, and as the founder and first president of the Belfast Natural History Society in 1821. His interests in natural history and medicine were combined when he held the chair of Botany at Inst., from 1835 to 1836, and was for several years president of its Faculty of Medicine. He died close to the Belfast Museum of Natural History and Inst., at 6 College Square, Belfast, on 17 May 1853.

Dr Robert Stephenson, a physician (son of Dr S.M. Stephenson page 6 – and not to be confused with Mr Robert Stevenson, surgeon to the Poor House), was elected Attending Physician to the Belfast Dispensary and Fever Hospital in 1818 and again in 1826. Dr Henry Forcade, who had been an army surgeon and had served with distinction under Wellington in the Peninsular War, was appointed Attending Physician to both Dispensary and hospital in 1820. He was one of those who helped revive the Belfast Medical Society, which had almost faded out in 1814 as a result of discord among the hospital doctors. In 1822, however, doctors Forcade and McDonnell and Mr Moore RN had revived it, and Dr Forcade served as its treasurer until his death in 1835.

From the 1820s onward the pace of appointments quickened and only the more notable will be mentioned in these pages. Dr Thomas McCabe MD was appointed Attending Physician in 1827 but he died in 1828 at the age of thirty-seven (cause unknown). Dr Benjamin Thompson was appointed in October 1826 and died the following month, on 14 November 1826, of typhus fever. These are only two of the many young doctors who died probably from infections caught during their work, before the days of antibiotics.

The Belfast Academical Institution (Inst.), *c.* 1850: the school was opened in 1814, followed by the collegiate department in 1818 (Arts) and 1835 (Medicine). The collegiate department was superseded by Queen's College in 1849.
ROYAL BELFAST ACADEMICAL INSTITUTION

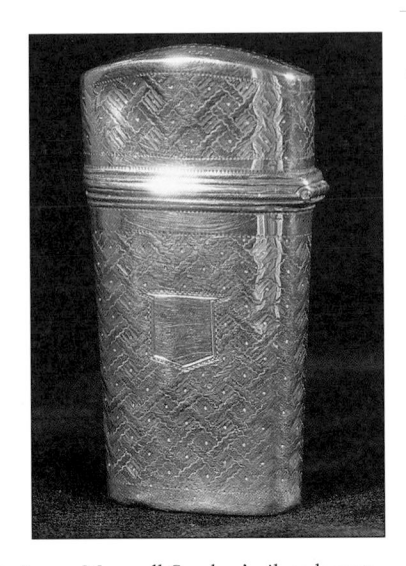

Dr James Maxwell Sanders's silver lancet case (approximately 6 cm in height): it was made to contain six lancets, that is, little knives for opening abscesses or releasing fluid from cavities, and so forth. It was presented to the Royal Victoria Hospital by Mr Ronald Cohen, dental surgeon, of Warwick.
ROYAL VICTORIA HOSPITAL

Dr James Maxwell Sanders, Attending Surgeon from 1838 until his early death in 1846
ULSTER MEDICAL SOCIETY

Dr Henry MacCormac is one of those eccentric physicians who is better known for his general activities – which included an appearance at the Belfast Police Court charged with breaking a patient's window with his umbrella to ensure a flow of fresh air – than for his work in the hospital. He was educated at Dublin, Paris and Edinburgh, obtaining the MD from the last of these in 1824. He then made visits to West Africa, the USA and Canada before settling down in general practice in Belfast. He was appointed Physician to the Fifth District in 1828 and Attending Physician to the Belfast Dispensary and Fever Hospital in 1831, so he was eminently qualified by experience and energy to take charge of the management of the cholera epidemic when it reached Belfast in 1832. He gets the credit for setting aside the small building behind the hospital as an isolation block, for the quarantine house in Lancaster Street, and indeed for the low death rate from that epidemic. He was elected Professor of Physic (Medicine) in the Medical School at Inst. in 1836 and was dean of the faculty from 1840 to 1845, but was not appointed when this was replaced by Queen's College in 1849. He was Consulting Physician to the Belfast Dispensary and Fever Hospital from 1836 and was appointed Physician to the Belfast Lunatic Asylum in 1849. He was very active as a writer on medical and other topics but was somewhat isolated by his eccentric views, such as refusal to accept Robert Koch's discovery of the role of the tubercle bacillus. On the other hand his emphasis on the value of fresh air for tuberculosis and public health generally was well ahead of his time, even if his description of his young son sleeping below a wide-open window on a snowy winter's night verges on the extreme. His fame is complemented by the success of his son, the surgeon Sir William MacCormac (see pages 49–50).

A physician who receives a special eulogy from his medical contemporary Dr Malcolm is Dr James Maxwell Sanders. Orphaned early in life and brought up by an uncle and aunt, Sanders was educated at Inst., Dublin, Glasgow and Edinburgh. He was awarded the MD by Edinburgh University for a thesis on delirium tremens in 1835, was appointed Attending Surgeon to the Belfast Districts in 1836 and Attending Surgeon to the Belfast Dispensary and Fever Hospital in 1838. He died, probably of pulmonary tuberculosis, on 26 July 1846 at the early age of thirty-two and is buried in Clifton Street graveyard. According to Malcolm, 'none probably, at his early age, ever before enjoyed so high a place in the public mind'.

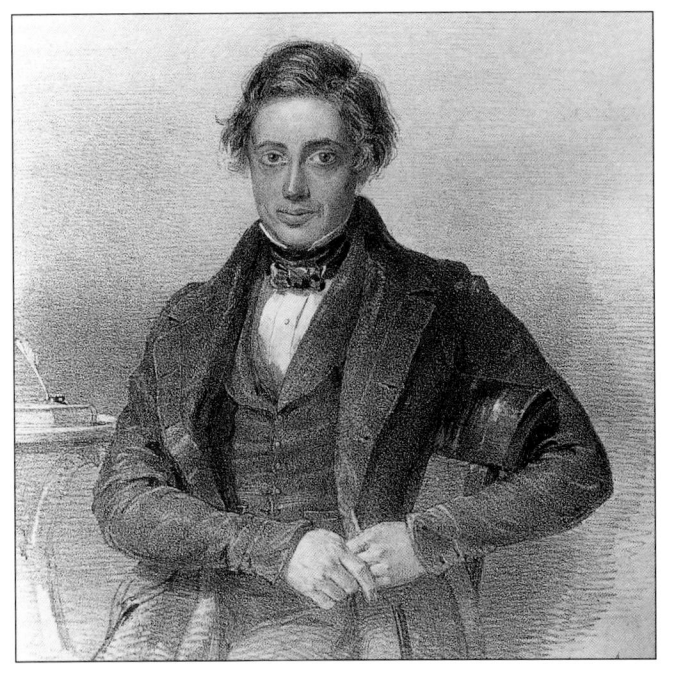

One of the surgeons of this era who is well documented is Dr Thomas Henry Purdon MB (TCD), FRCSI (at this time surgeons who had a medical qualification seem to have been known as 'Dr'). He was a member of a remarkable medical dynasty, having a father, grandfather (Dr Henry Purdon) and two brothers doctors before him, and a doctor son and three nephews to follow him. The Purdons came originally from Cumberland, in England, but had settled in Ireland, in County Westmeath, in Elizabethan times, and later married into two Huguenot families, Crommelin and De La Cherois, of the Lisburn area. Thomas Purdon entered Trinity College Dublin at the age of thirteen and was only twenty-one when he was appointed Physician to one of the Dispensary Districts of the Belfast Fever Hospital (1827); he became an Attending Surgeon in 1834. His district was Number Four, bounded by Donegall Place, Berry Street, Millfield, Barrack Street and Sandy Row and, with the cholera epidemic of 1832, we can well imagine the difficult and exhausting time he had before he achieved his staff appointment and general fame. In the surgical field he was the first in Ireland to employ the operation of tracheostomy (1840) for laryngeal obstruction. He was still working in retirement in 1873 and he died in 1886; he is buried in Lisburn.

Perhaps the most distinguished member of the hospital staff in this period was Dr Thomas Andrews, one of the Comber family of flour millers and linen weavers. He was born in Belfast and graduated with an MD at Edinburgh University in 1835. He was immediately appointed Professor of Chemistry at Inst., at the age of just twenty-two, became Physician to the Dispensary Districts in 1837, and in the following year was appointed Attending Physician to the Belfast Dispensary and Fever Hospital. He was Consulting Physician at the hospital from 1846, vice-president of the newly formed Queen's College from 1845, and Professor of Chemistry there from 1849. In 1849 also he was elected a fellow of the Royal Society – in fact he was the only member of the hospital staff ever to have been an FRS. Although he was a physician, it is for his work on thermodynamics that he is best known.

In 1851, the year in which this first chapter ends, Dr Andrew Malcolm's *History* was first published. Its full title is *The History of the General Hospital, Belfast, and the other Medical Institutions of the Town; with Chronological Notes & Biographical Reminiscences Connected with its Rise & Progress*, and this truly indicates its scope. Andrew Malcolm himself was born in Newry, County Down, in 1818; the family subsequently moved to Belfast, and he was educated at Inst., in both the school and the collegiate section, from 1829 to 1836. He went on to study medicine at Edinburgh University and obtained the LRCS of Edinburgh in 1842. He returned to Belfast, and at the beginning of 1843 he was elected surgeon to Dispensary District Number One of the Belfast Dispensary and Fever Hospital. Only three years later he was elected Attending Physician to the hospital.

Malcolm took a special interest in the health of Belfast's factory workers. Indeed this interest appears constantly in his book, and he comes across as a devoted social reformer and tireless worker for the Belfast Working

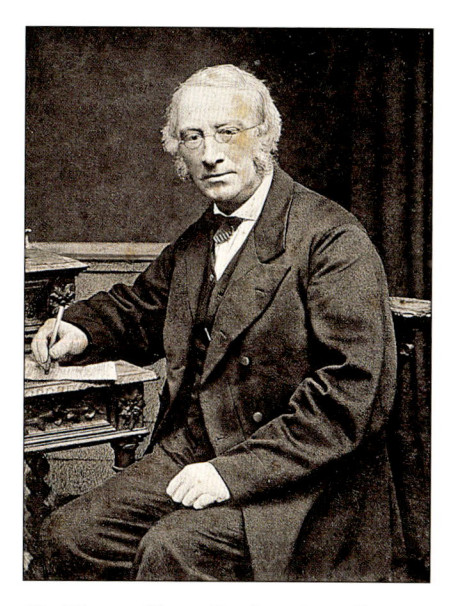

Dr Thomas Henry Purdon, Attending Surgeon to the Belfast Dispensary and Fever Hospital, 1834–51
ULSTER MEDICAL SOCIETY

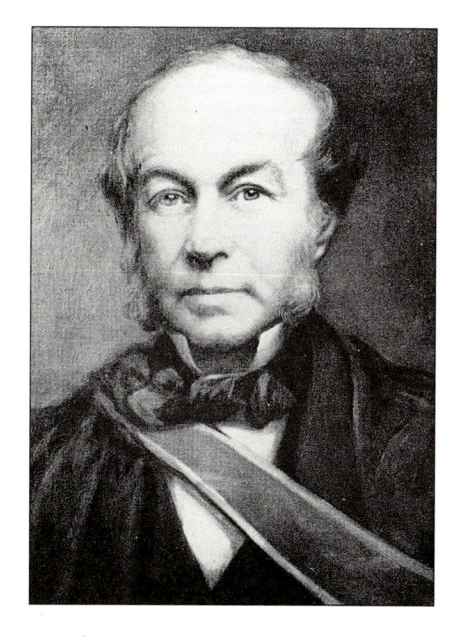

Dr Thomas Andrews, Professor of Chemistry in the collegiate department of the Academical Institution, 1835–47, and at Queen's College, 1849–79, and Attending Physician to the Belfast Dispensary and Fever Hospital, 1838–46
QUEEN'S UNIVERSITY BELFAST

Classes' Association (founded in 1847) which published the *Belfast People's Magazine*, and for the Amelioration Society. Malcolm's wife was Maria Glenny Home, also of Newry, another philanthropist and the moving spirit in founding the Domestic Mission to the Poor of Belfast in 1853. Tragically, Andrew died of some type of heart failure on 19 September 1856, aged only thirty-seven. His only child died of meningitis a few months later but his widow lived on until 1906. All three are buried in the Non-Subscribing Presbyterian churchyard in Dunmurry, near Belfast. Soon after his death a memorial fund was set up, and he is still commemorated in the Malcolm Exhibition and Prize for final-year medical students at the hospital.

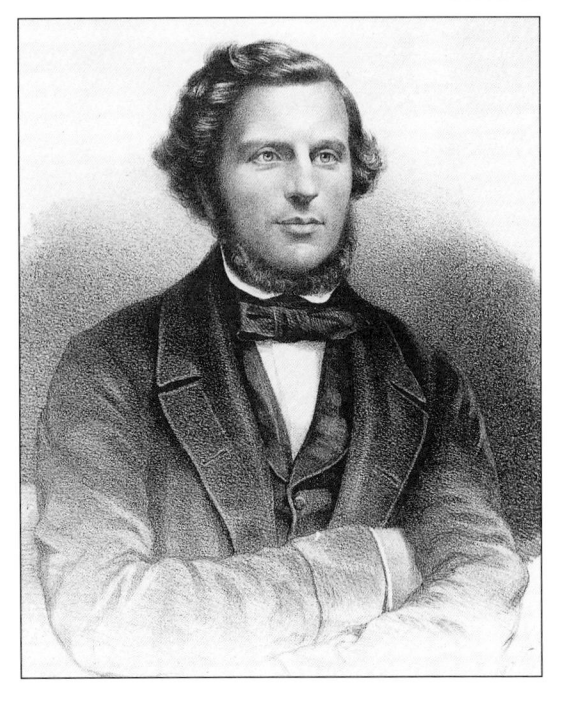

Dr Andrew George Malcolm, Attending Physician from 1846 until his early death in 1856; from a painting by Richard Hooke
ROYAL VICTORIA HOSPITAL

Title page of Dr Andrew George Malcolm's *History of the General Hospital, Belfast . . .* (1851)

THE BEGINNINGS OF MEDICAL TEACHING

In the eighteenth and the early nineteenth century most Belfast physicians graduated from Glasgow or Edinburgh. Indeed, in all fields of study there was a steady flow of Presbyterians and Catholics to Scotland since Trinity College Dublin had only recently opened its doors to them and they were still discriminated against in eligibility for prizes, et cetera. It was the deficiency of cheap and undenominational education that led to the founding in 1814 of the Belfast Academical Institution with its 'school' and 'college' sections. The founders intended to establish a medical school, but it was not until 1818 that James Lawson Drummond was appointed to a chair in Anatomy and Medical Physiology. His classes were attended mainly by medical students but also by apothecaries, apprentices and even students for the Presbyterian ministry. Accommodation was cramped; Professor Drummond shared a room in rotation with four other teachers, had no dissecting room and only a small communal museum. The dissecting room had to wait until the Medical School block was built in 1835.

By January 1820 the Belfast Dispensary and Fever Hospital was sufficiently well established for the Committee of Management to resolve that it should admit pupils for instruction. Each pupil was to be introduced by one medical attendant who would be responsible for his conduct; the pupil would look after the patients of that physician or surgeon only. In the following year the first registered pupil, a Mr W. Bingham, entered the hospital and in due course he became a general practitioner in Downpatrick, County Down; he died in 1848. By 1826 it was noted that 'a few pupils … are found very useful to the surgeons as dressers, and it was, of course, advantageous to the pupils to have close contact with the surgeons'. These dressers dressed accidental and surgical wounds and performed other necessary tasks to assist the surgeon.

The next stage was the beginning of systematic teaching and this was eventually arranged by 3 June 1827 when Dr James McDonnell gave the first clinical lecture. This lecture is regarded as the forerunner of the still-continuing annual oration, now given every October. Teaching was not, of course, free, and pupils at this time paid one guinea a year to the hospital for the provision of books, et cetera. (The role of collecting this fee for the costs of clinical teaching was later taken over by the University Faculty of Medicine which in turn passed on remunerations to the hospital staff – this remuneration has now been discontinued.)

Not long after McDonnell's first lecture, in 1829, a meeting of the medical staff of the hospital and a deputation from the Belfast Academical Institution discussed 'the expediency of the establishment of a Medical school'. Professor Drummond was already lecturing at Inst., and judging by a letter of 1 November 1826 published in the *Belfast News-Letter*, was the moving spirit behind the formation of the Belfast medical school. Initially he had wanted a direct and exclusive connection between Inst. and the Belfast Dispensary and Fever Hospital, but after James McDonnell's lecture of 1827 the separate roles of both bodies became clearer.

It was not until 1835 that a medical department was properly set up at Inst. with chairs of Anatomy and Physiology, Theory of Physic, Surgery, Practice of Physic, Chemistry, Materia Medica and Pharmacy, Midwifery, and Botany. Three chairs were held by Drummond who took on Botany as well as Anatomy and Physiology, Thomas Andrews held the chair of Chemistry, James D. Marshall took on Materia Medica and Pharmacy, Robert Little took on Midwifery, and John McDonnell (son of Dr James McDonnell) took the chair of Surgery. Drummond was elected 'president' (equivalent to Dean). All these men except John McDonnell were present or future members of the staff of the Belfast Dispensary and Fever Hospital, but perhaps because of this the board of Inst. did not want the hospital to have undue influence in the Faculty of Medicine generally. The board also wanted to ensure that its professors had access to patients and could not be turned out by a change in hospital policy. In 1836, therefore, the board bought a disused cavalry barracks in Barrack Street (now a Christian Brothers school) to use as an accessory building to the hospital; this became known as the College Hospital. The building did provide much-needed hospital beds for Belfast but it was disastrous both for general teaching, since it held mainly fever patients, and in using up the scarce resources of Inst. John McDonnell retired from the chair of Surgery in 1836, and was replaced for a few months by Thomas Farrar, and then by Robert Coffey.

The collegiate part of Inst. was always in the centre of religious controversy since from the outset it favoured liberality of thought and a Non-Subscribing doctrine generally. In 1839 the Synod of Ulster withdrew recognition of Inst. for the training of ministers and the Faculty of Arts closed in 1841. The building of the new Union and Union Fever hospitals in the 1840s threatened the College Hospital and it finally closed at the end of 1847; meanwhile the concept of a 'northern college' of the new Queen's University in Ireland threatened the collegiate part of Inst. Gradually the Medical Faculty faded; it was dissolved in 1849 and replaced by the new Faculty of Medicine at Queen's College Belfast.

NURSING BEFORE FLORENCE NIGHTINGALE

Nursing in the first half of the nineteenth century was regarded as a form of domestic service which required no real teaching – only firm discipline to ensure that the work was carried out thoroughly and without waste.[1] The fact that it was in the end caring and helpful is a tribute to the nurses themselves and to the example of the head nurse.

The first Belfast Dispensary and Fever Hospital, in Factory Row, employed one nurse, and even though it moved to larger premises, over the first twenty years there were rarely more than ten nurses covering up to two hundred patients. The numbers fluctuated, however, and between epidemics nurses were paid off to save money (nothing changes!). The core of female nurses was helped by washerwomen, kitchen maids and male nurses (mainly there to restrain violent patients). In the early years of the nineteenth century, nurses were responsible to the housekeeper – Mrs Dobbin from 1822 to 1832 – but when she retired it was decided to appoint a head nurse for the entire hospital. In all medical matters nurses were responsible to the resident house surgeon, who could fine or dismiss them for neglect or impropriety of conduct.

The first Head Nurse, Ann Marshall, who had been a patient in the West Street hospital in 1810, became a domestic assistant nurse in 1812, a nurse in 1819, and Head Nurse in 1832. She retired in 1851, in which year Dr Malcolm wrote of her thus: 'after a lapse of 41 years unremitting servitude ... she may be seen by the visitor making her daily rounds amongst the wards, and with anxious solicitude and homely care, rendering her little offices to comfort the distressed and the forsaken'. She remained active at the hospital until her death in 1860 at the age of sixty-five and gave all her savings in various forms to the hospital. After her death a plaque was erected in her honour in the hospital.

There had already been clashes about who was boss between Ann Marshall and the Housekeeper, a Mrs Gihon, and in 1841 the Housekeeper was dismissed until she made an abject apology. After Ann Marshall's retirement it seems that Mrs Gihon took over; certainly her successors in the 1850s and 1860s were called 'Matron and Housekeeper'.

The only requirements of a nursing applicant in the early days were a good character and the ability to read and write. The nurses lived in the basement of the hospital, though from the plan of the 1850s it is hard to see where, between the dead room, the kitchen, the stores and the baths.

---

1. Any history of nursing in the Royal Victoria Hospital and its predecessors must be indebted to Peggy Donaldson's *Yes, Matron* (1988); her picture of the nurse's life and work should be read to give a fuller view.

Food was dull and pay was low, though it rose from 6 pence a week in the 1820s to 6 shillings a week in the 1870s. This last sum was the amount paid to a nurse in charge of a department and was no higher than the wages of a parlourmaid, even though parlourmaids did not have to be able to read or write. Night nurses were paid more than day nurses and lock-ward nurses were the most poorly paid of all. Nurses in fever wards were more highly paid than others and received bonuses after epidemics. Several of the General Hospital's doctors died of fevers during the first half of the nineteenth century, as we have seen, and it can be imagined that the death rate among the nurses, given their closer contact with patients, was higher. Indeed, nurses frequently died from tuberculosis well into the twentieth century.

In the early nineteenth century the work of the nurses was largely domestic – scrubbing floors and stairs daily and carrying out 'slops' before the introduction of flush toilets in 1834. The new toilets improved conditions in the hospital and enabled the management committee to save on the salaries of two nurses, but toilet paper was an invention still in the future and blockages of the system, when too much tow (cotton waste from the mills) was flushed down, were frequent. Coal for heating still had to be carried by the nurses to the wards, and oil lamps had to be refilled and maintained by them daily until gas lighting was introduced in 1840.

The nurses also carried out basic patient care, of course, washing the patients and changing sheets and straw mattresses. The more experienced nurses were responsible for giving out medicines and applying poultices. Responsibility for surgical dressings came late in the nineteenth century when doctors realised that nurses were better at bandaging than doctors were. Nurses worked long hours by today's standards – from 6 or 7 a.m. to 10 p.m., working only until 2 p.m. on their two half days (Sunday and Tuesday or Thursday). Only in 1836 had nurses' hours been thus changed to allow them to attend Sunday worship, largely in an attempt to improve moral standards.

Nurses could be dismissed for many misdemeanours. Drunkenness was rare in spite of the picture that Dickens gave us of Sarah Gamp. The main offences seem to have been having visitors in their rooms (even close family were not allowed), absence without leave, inefficiency in the wards, waste of materials, and harshness to patients. The full rules and regulations for nurses' conduct in 1832 have survived and although they seem harsh in terms of hours and working conditions, they do present an ideal of ward management and patient care that would still be accepted today. For example:

> To see as accurately as possible that wine [widely used at that time], nourishment and medicine have been delivered to the patient as ordered.

And this:

> When the night nurse comes on duty, at ten o'clock, [the day nurse] will take her round the wards, and point out to her each particular case, and give those directions and instructions which may tend for the comfort and welfare of the patients during the night.

This was forty years before Florence Nightingale's reforms, and one hopes that the routine practice lived up to the ideals, especially when wards were overcrowded and nurses' numbers had been reduced.

THE HOSPITAL IN MID-CENTURY

The Belfast General Hospital of 1850 was a much more compact institution than the old hospital, shorn of its role as a Dispensary and of the District work and with the care of fevers and the destitute in the hands of a separate institution. It was run by a Committee of Management (replaced in 1853 by a General Committee), with the Marquess of Donegall as president and the shipowner Gustavus Heyn as honorary treasurer. The committee had about twenty other members, who retired in rotation, and included a small group of doctors representing the medical staff. It met approximately weekly throughout the year but had an annual general meeting in public usually in the spring, which was fully reported in the press and in the annual report of the hospital. The annual reports also include medical and surgical reports; they list in detail the donations to the funds and present an overall statement of accounts.

Committee minutes, which have survived from 1822, chronicle the day-to-day events of the hospital, such as the annual whitewashing of the wards, changes in staff, purchases of opium, linen, and other necessities, and the frequent shortage of funds to run the institution.

The building we see in the prints and plans of about 1850 had a central block of three storeys plus a basement, flanked by two side wings of one storey plus a basement. There were steps up to the front door, which had pillars and a pediment, above which was a triple first-floor window, also pillared. Above all this was a pediment with a plaque inscribed '1817'. It was, in short, an attractive and symmetrical Georgian building, set back from Frederick Street and surrounded by railings.

The top floor had wards for female patients, the floor below held male patients, while beds specifically allocated for accident, ophthalmic, private and further medical patients were on the ground floor. Officially there were 81 surgical beds, 45 medical beds and 2 private beds, but there were one or more buildings at the back for fever and isolation patients, which increased the total to approximately 270 patients. The wing on the west side held the operating theatre and the library of the Belfast Medical Society, and the wing on the east side had two wards. Despite the apparently large number of beds, it would appear that the bed occupancy rate was low and, in the absence of epidemics, largely confined to the main block. The average number of patients in 1850 was between 70 and 80 and did not change much over the next decade, though the numbers were partly kept down by shortage of funds.

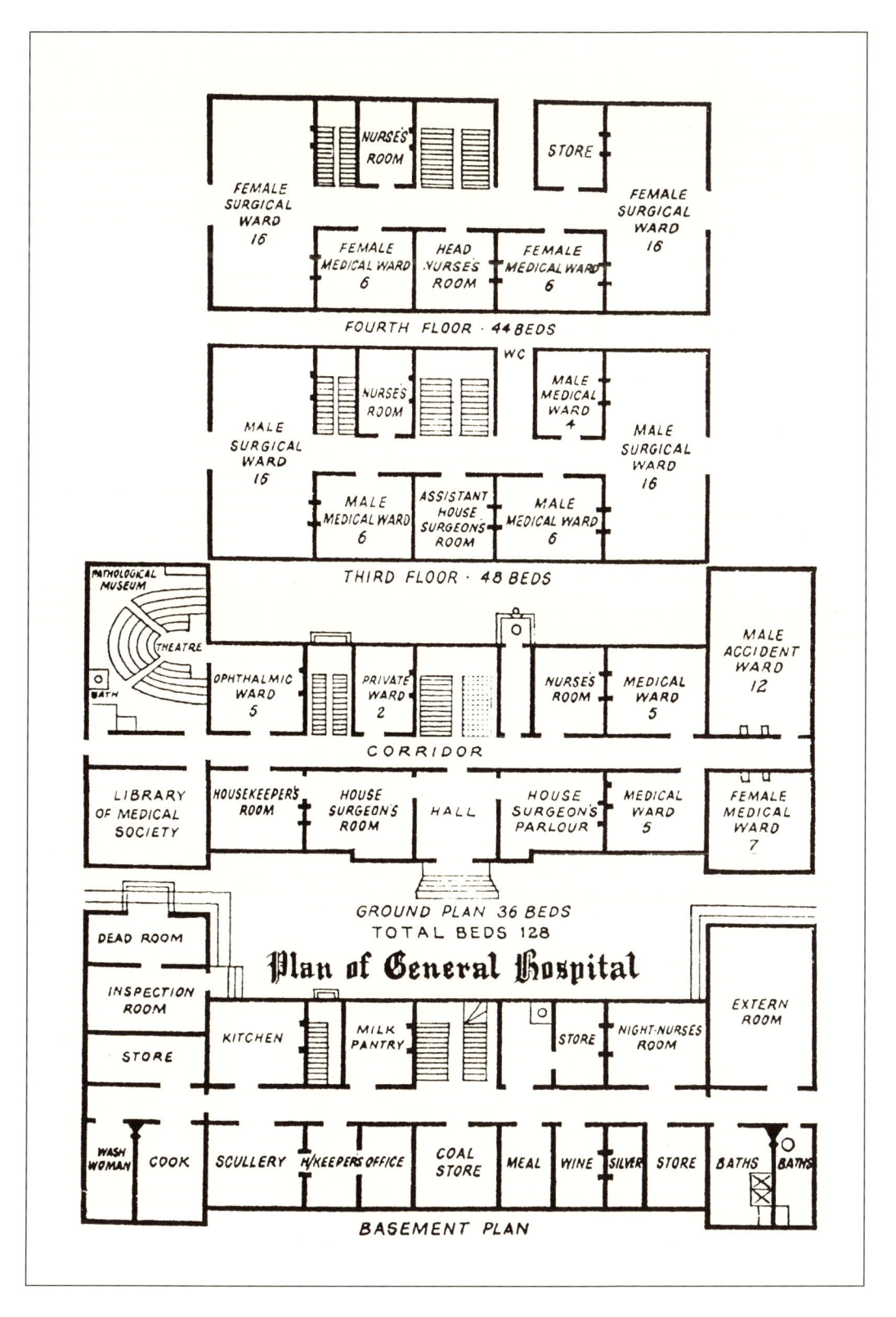

Ground plan of the various floors of the Belfast General Hospital, c. 1851; from Dr Andrew George Malcolm's *History of the General Hospital, Belfast*

Physicians and surgeons to the Belfast General Hospital, as in most voluntary hospitals in the British Isles, were elected by the Committee of Management on a short-term basis, one of each retiring annually, but eligible for re-election. The system of regular elections created difficulties, however, and only in 1865, when it was apparent that most other hospitals appointed for the doctor's full working life (to age sixty-five), was the system regularised to give permanent appointments. During the first half of the century, the first post to which a doctor was normally elected was physician or surgeon for the Dispensary Districts, but with no standing in the wards until elected to Attending status. After 1847, however, suitably qualified doctors were appointed directly as Attending Physicians and Surgeons to the wards, until the intermediate post of Assistant was created in 1879 and 1880. Finally, if they had held Attending status for at least five years, they could retire with the title Consulting Physician or Surgeon. In 1850 the working staff consisted of four Attending Physicians and four Attending Surgeons, together with a resident house surgeon who remained in post for one or two years, and an apothecary. After 1851 there was an assistant house surgeon in place of the apothecary.

In the first half-century of its existence the hospital had already achieved much. It had looked after the sick poor of Belfast through terrible epidemics of disease and one of the worst famines recorded – all at a time when the normal living standards of the poor left no safety margin. The hospital had done this with a very small resident staff by modern standards, but with some very enthusiastic senior figures giving a lead. They had managed to erect a fine building which, now that it was relieved of the wildly fluctuating burden of fever victims, could accommodate a planned intake of patients and steadily expand. From this firm base, physicians would be able to practise better-informed medicine, and surgeons helped by anaesthesia could move into an era of constructive and enterprising surgery.

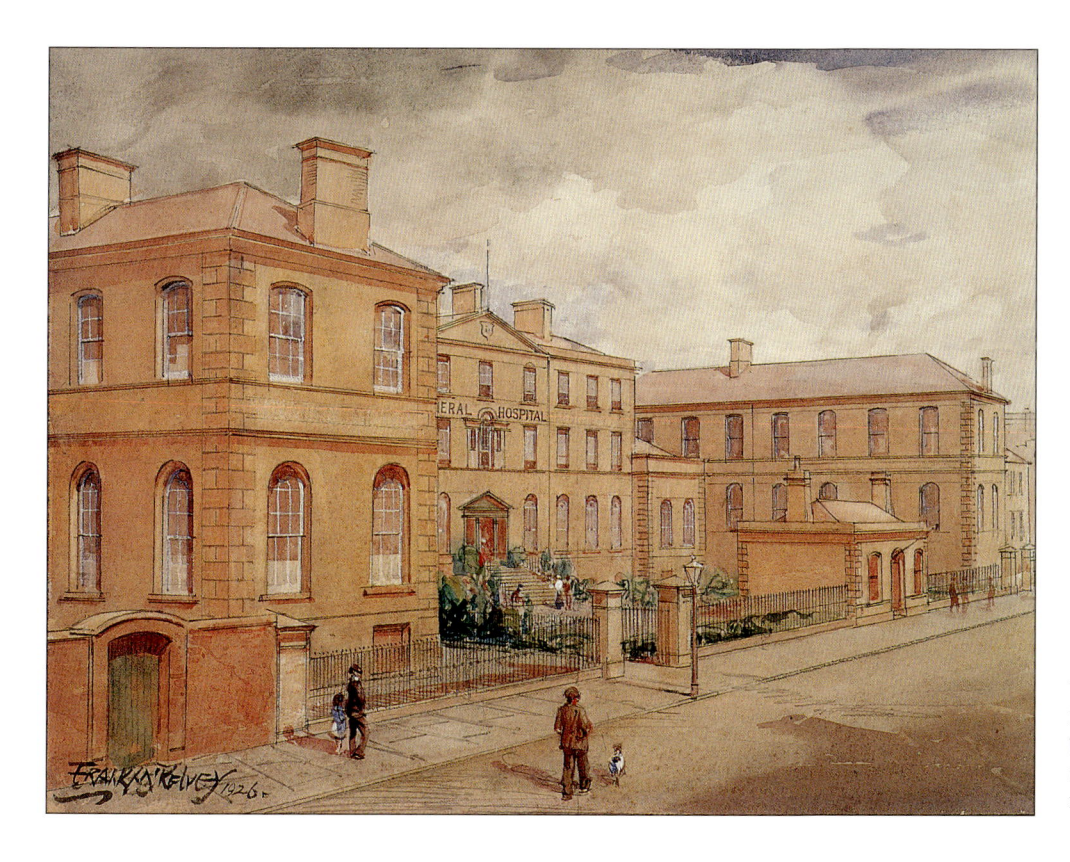

The old Royal Hospital in Frederick Street; watercolour by Frank McKelvey (1926)
ULSTER MUSEUM, COPYRIGHT ROBERT McKELVEY, ESQ.

2

THE BELFAST GENERAL HOSPITAL
AND BELFAST ROYAL HOSPITAL
1850–1903

By the middle of the nineteenth century the Belfast General Hospital still had not achieved a steady financial basis. Poor Law funds went to the new Workhouse and Union Hospital and Union Fever Hospital. In addition the new dispensaries, with their paid medical staff, channelled off the sick poor and public funding for them. The General Hospital still had no regular income and donations depended on the whim or goodwill of an individual or organisation, influenced by the frequent appeals made at the hospital's annual general meetings. The main sources of income were voluntary subscriptions; collectors were appointed to go round on a house-to-house basis so that the amounts subscribed by each citizen of Belfast could be listed street by street in the annual report. These lists are a valuable record, and were certainly a way of putting pressure on donors. Individual subscriptions in 1850 ranged from two shillings and six pence to twenty pounds (the latter from the mill owners A. Mulholland and Sons). Such large donations as this were rare, however, and in the previous year the hospital had only been saved from closure by the donation of £300 by Queen Victoria, who visited Belfast in that year. Large donations and bequests formed an increasingly important part of hospital funding as the nineteenth century progressed, helped by the increasing affluence of the city, as well as by the greater professionalism of the honorary treasurer. Casual donations came in from passengers on the steamers to and from England, and from the merchant ships which frequently used the services of the hospital for their injured sailors.

The medical profession usually contributed generously. One episode of medical generosity which should be mentioned is the gift of Surgeon-Major Allen Bryson who died on 8 March 1874 'bequeathing to the hospital the savings of a lifetime' (according to the memorial tablet in the Royal Victoria Hospital main corridor). Born in Carrickfergus in 1832, Bryson was a student in the Belfast General Hospital and graduated with an MD from Glasgow. He joined the British Army in 1854 and served as a regimental medical officer in the Crimea, being promoted to staff surgeon in 1865 with the rank of Surgeon-Major (equivalent to Lieutenant-Colonel). In the will he made in 1873, he left money amounting to £2,975 to the hospital 'to be expended as the Board saw fit', the largest bequest received by the hospital in the nineteenth century. Allen Bryson died on the steamship *Indus* on his passage home from India aged only forty-two, and was buried at sea; he is commemorated in the old graveyard in Kilroot in County Antrim.

The Mulholland and Charters families made donations in the 1860s specifically for building new wings (see page 52). Among the other generous benefactors of the General Hospital from the 1850s were the Sinclair family, prominent merchants of Tomb Street, Belfast. When Thomas Sinclair JP, of Hopefield House, died in 1867, a public subscription in his honour raised £2,287 which was given to the hospital as the Sinclair Memorial Fund. As a result, the first accident ward in the General Hospital was renamed with a tablet bearing the words '1869 Sinclair Memorial Ward', followed by a list of forty subscribers. The Sinclair family continued to support the old hospital, and in 1882 it was recorded in the board minutes 'that the best thanks of the Board of Management are due and are hereby tendered to the members of the Sinclair family for the excellent work they have done in completely renovating and supplying with all modern requirements the Sinclair Memorial Ward'. Another Thomas Sinclair of the same family was the second Professor of Surgery at Queen's University Belfast. The JP Thomas Sinclair's grandson, Mr T. Sinclair Kirk, was a surgeon in the hospital from 1897 to 1934 (see Chapter 4 for both surgeons).

The church contributions were usually in the form of an annual collection taken on or near the last Sunday of the year, also referred to as a 'charity sermon'. These collections were supported by appeals from all the church leaders, though the amounts raised varied widely (see table below). They rose steadily over the 1850s and 1860s but by the end of the nineteenth century, although the number of churches had grown, individual collections had largely fallen.

COLLECTIONS TAKEN UP IN BELFAST'S HOUSES OF WORSHIP 1850–51

	£	s.	d.
Third Presbyterian Congregation, Rosemary Street	10	6	8
Fisherwick Place (Sept. 1850)	30	0	5
Alfred Street	4	2	6
York Street	13	17	6
Trinity Church	2	0	0
College Square Meeting House	3	5	0
First Presbyterian Congregation	24	7	10
Roman Catholic Chapel, per Dr Denvir	35	0	0
St Ann's Church	40	19	2
Fisherwick Place (July 1851)	20	3	10
Mrs Owens, per Dr. Ferguson 21s:			
from Newtownards £1	2	1	0
Ballysillan Presbyterian Church	1	10	0
	£187	13	11

Source: Annual Report of Belfast General Hospital, 1851

Minor sources of income included court fines, which were often donated to the hospital in the 1850s and 1860s. There were also tuition fees from medical students, and contributions from paying patients. This latter group seems to have included any patients whom the committee considered capable of paying for their own costs. Investment income, amounting to only £117 in 1855, was another minor source of funds.

Many efforts were made in the 1850s to ensure the regularity of the income but in practice it was almost impossible without abandoning the status of a voluntary hospital. A scheme introduced in 1854, however, was the creation of a General Committee of not only the vice-presidents and life governors (subscribers of ten guineas in one sum), but also sixty subscribers of one guinea or more, with the right of some to sit on the

General Committee, in rotation. Twelve of these subscribers were specially charged with soliciting subscriptions in particular wards of the city, and due credit was given to them by listing the amounts raised. The General Committee met quarterly and from its number formed a Board of Management, meeting weekly. In 1863 the life governors scheme was boosted greatly by inviting 'noblemen and gentlemen' to subscribe £50 in one sum, with the same privileges as before. The scheme continued throughout the nineteenth century, and was further expanded for the funding of the new Royal Victoria Hospital.

Increasing emphasis was also placed on raising subscriptions from the working men of the city, stimulated by generous contributions from the mill owners. It was indeed a matter of pride that the workers in factories should be able to support their voluntary hospital and be taken to it rather than as paupers to the Union Hospital. The mill owners' involvement took the form of a published promise from twenty-eight mill owners of Belfast (note the number) to give ten shillings annually per 100 spindles and five shillings per week for each of their workers who was in the hospital on their recommendation.

The hospital was well served by its honorary treasurers: Gustavus Heyn (1849–54), James Girdwood (1854–73), and W.F. MacElheran (1881–98) were the key figures. Gustavus Heyn had to resign after five years because of pressure of work in the family shipowning business; he had kept the hospital going through difficult financial times and remained a trustee for another twenty years.

In the main corridor of the present Royal Victoria Hospital is a tablet to James Girdwood which was transferred from the old Frederick Street hospital. The tablet reads as follows:

> This memorial is erected by the late Mr Girdwood's numerous friends who have deeply mourned his removal from their midst, to record their high estimation of him as a citizen and his sterling worth as a friend. Also to testify their admiration for his indefatigable energy and invaluable services on behalf of this Institution for a period of eighteen years.

James Girdwood was born on 23 January 1823 and owned a carpet, damask and wallpaper warehouse at 44 High Street, Belfast. He must have had the business well organised when he was only thirty-one, to be able to give himself time for the demanding and unpaid task of hospital treasurer. Again and again it was said in annual reports that the hospital's growing prosperity was due to his farseeing and shrewd handling of the finances. Girdwood died, still in post and leaving a young family, on 14 September 1873; he is buried in Knockbreda parish graveyard, Belfast. A bust by S.F. Lynn ARHA and C.B. Birch was completed in 1876 and erected in the Board Room of the General Hospital; under it was the inscription 'So long as the Hospital exists his name will never cease to be associated with it.' The bust is now in the King Edward Building of the Royal Victoria Hospital.

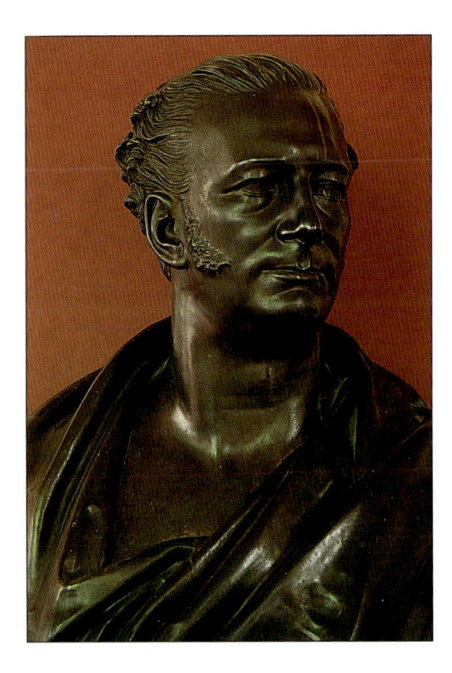

Bust of Mr James Girdwood, honorary treasurer of the hospital from 1854 until his death in 1873
ROYAL VICTORIA HOSPITAL

W.F. MacElheran was a branch inspector of the Belfast Bank when he was elected honorary treasurer in 1881; he too gave devoted service until his death, seventeen years later. Again, it is difficult to realise how anyone could spend a great deal of time managing the whole finances of a large and precarious hospital, while employed elsewhere on an effectively full-time basis.

HOSPITAL EXPENDITURE

The largest item on the table of expenditure for 1850 was food for the patients at £512; of this sum, most seems to have been spent on beef and bread. Surprisingly £135 2s. 5d. was spent on bread compared with only 15s. 6d. on potatoes and even less on other vegetables (but this was only a few years after the Great Famine). Alcoholic beverages cost £25 8s. 0d. and included 6 gallons of whisky bought for only £1 16s. 0d., some of which may have been used for anaesthetic purposes. Alcohol generally was cheap throughout the century and its widespread use (even in hospital) meant that alcoholism and delirium tremens were scourges of the poor. The bill for coal, gas, soap and starch was about £112, which does not seem excessive to cover all cooking, heating and laundry. Salaries were not a prominent expense in 1850; even if the house surgeon was paid £90 a year, the head nurse only received £10 and the cook £6, and the entire paid staff was fewer than twenty in number. Sundries included twenty-six single and eight double trusses – the standard treatment for hernias until well into the twentieth century. Gardening implements bought included a rake, pitchfork and hook, and there was an item for plants and gardener's wages, so we must envisage the General Hospital surrounded by a lawn and flowerbeds, though these are not usually shown in the plans. There was, however, insufficient space to grow vegetables.

Mr W.F. MacElheran, honorary treasurer of the hospital from 1881 until his death in 1898
BELFAST HEALTH JOURNAL, 1893

The expenditure on stationery was only £2 18s. 0d., including 4s. 9d. for quill pens. However, an additional sum of approximately £16 went on printing and advertising: even in 1850 one could not raise money without some outlay for publicity.

The need for economy over the years resulted in some savings, and by 1855 the General Committee was able to report a saving of £50, compared with the previous year, on the consumption of coal, gas and soap. By 1863 the cost per patient per day was brought down from 1s. 6d. to 11¼d., while the average stay in hospital had fallen from twenty-six days to twenty-five. On the whole, in spite of the regular lamentations in annual reports, the ratio of hospital income to expenditure improved steadily over the third quarter of the nineteenth century.

GENERAL MEDICINE

The Great Famine and its aftermath of fever marked the end of an era in medical care in the Frederick Street hospital. No longer were there recurring epidemics of fever which overwhelmed beds and facilities to the exclusion of all other types of cases. Nevertheless, there were still slums of the worst type in the Hercules Street area, which were only cleared in 1878 when they were replaced by Royal Avenue. As a result of this and infection from the marshy areas round the Farset and other rivers, sporadic cases of typhus, typhoid, influenza and trench fever, still persisted. Indeed, medical admissions, which were running at about 300 per year in the early 1850s, rose to 767 by 1875 – a reflection of increased finance to fund beds and greater patient confidence in the hospital. In spite of this confidence, the mortality for medical patients remained at 8–10 per cent over this period. It was certain to remain high so long as treatment for fever was limited to tepid sponging and ice packs, a bland diet, milk (3–4 pints daily) and opiates by mouth. Intravenous fluids were still to come, and intestinal perforation by an ulcer was usually fatal, with or without surgery.

Conditions other than 'fever' are noted in the annual reports; there was a steady flow of smallpox cases, explained by the absence of compulsory vaccination in Ireland. The death rate from smallpox was only about 14 per cent, however, and even patients with severe confluent rash frequently recovered. There were also small numbers of pneumonia admissions (which are much less common nowadays with early antibiotic therapy) and for these too the death rate in the 1850s and 1860s was only about 16 per cent. The term 'bronchitis' is loosely used in annual reports and probably includes many cases of pulmonary tuberculosis and lung cancer. Belfast's atmospheric pollution, a major cause of lung complaints, was very heavy as a result of increasing numbers of coal-fired mills, and this pollution continued for another century until there was effective clean air legislation. Until the discovery of the tubercle bacillus by Koch in 1882 the infectious nature of tuberculosis was not really understood and such patients were still nursed with others in open wards. Even when the cause was known there was much dread of the disease until specific drugs became available after World War Two.

Diagnosis was becoming more precise and in the 1850s and 1860s we meet terms such as chorea (known from medieval times as St Vitus's dance), sciatica, infantile croup, scurvy, gout, and ulcer of the stomach. The stethoscope had been in use since 1819 but the ophthalmoscope was not introduced until 1851 and the clinical thermometer not until 1869. Treatment could not be directed at the causes of symptoms since these were rarely known, but instead was largely directed at the outward signs of disease, based often on the use of plant extracts or simple inorganic chemicals. These were made up into elegant prescriptions as described below, and indeed the end of the nineteenth century has been termed 'the golden age of the prescriber'. In fact the benefit of the medical consultation was a medical package with the imposing physician in the frock coat and gold chain, the Latin prescription, the highly coloured and flavoured mixture, and drugs that had either no effect or an effect that was often quite irrelevant to the disease. In the absence of specific drugs, the whole procedure at least made the patient feel that something was being done, and indeed he frequently got better afterwards.

The complete physician had to be able to grind solids with a pestle and mortar and compound them into pills, powders or liquid mixtures. The prescription had to contain a superscription (the letter *R*), inscription (the names and quantities of the drugs), the subscription (directions to the pharmacist in Latin) and the signature (directions to the patient in Latin or English). The drugs used fell into such groups as narcotics (morphine), sedatives (bromides), expectorants (tincture of ipecacuanha), purgatives (jalap or colocynth) and tonics (digitalis for the heart, strychnine for the nervous system, gentian for the stomach). All this is detailed in William Whitla's *Elements of Pharmacy, Materia Medica and Therapeutics*, first published in 1882 and subsequently in his *Dictionary of Treatment*, first published in 1892 (see page 44). The difference in medical practice then from that of today can be seen by the nine pages that the *Dictionary of Treatment* devotes to constipation, a condition scarcely considered worthy of discussion nowadays. In addition pulmonary tuberculosis (phthisis) receives twenty-five pages, most of which we would now consider quite irrelevant to the patient's comfort or survival. Similarly among the drugs used, arsenic receives two pages covering treatment of a wide range of conditions including chorea, 'gastric neuralgia', malaria, pernicious anaemia, phthisis and syphilis. Mercury was also given freely in many treatments (including syphilis). Both arsenic and mercury were prescribed even though the severe toxic effects of both were well known.

Other types of treatment were widely used. Linseed poultices were used for bronchitis and pneumonia. Leeches were used mainly for reduction of localised swellings, and blood-letting by lancet was at least confined to relief of pulmonary engorgement. In the days before the relatively short-acting sedatives, the calming of patients with delirium tremens and similar conditions was a problem. It is notable that Sir William Whitla felt that the straitjacket 'should be rightly regarded by every physician with disfavour'. He favoured the commonsense use of alcohol in the management of delirium tremens, at least for older patients, in addition to appropriate restraint, but warned of the dangers of sedation with opium. Paraldehyde was then, and well into the twentieth century, the safest sedative available. The great prescriber could be human,

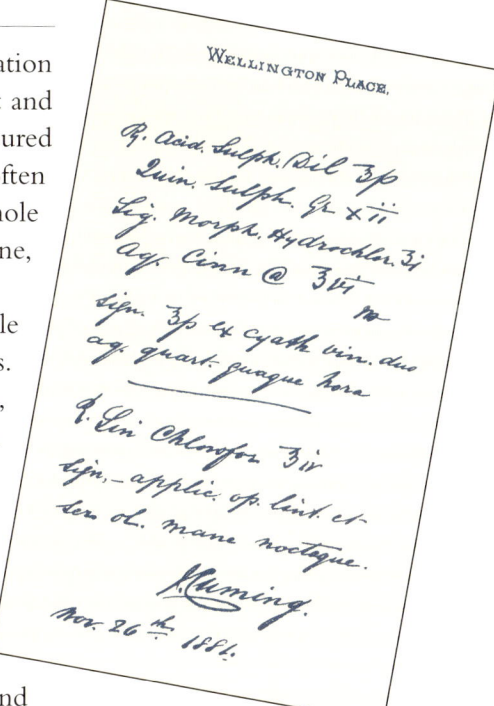

Two prescriptions of Professor James Cuming with full transcription and translation; from William Whitla's *Elements of Pharmacy, Materia Medica and Therapeutics,* 1882
ROYAL VICTORIA HOSPITAL

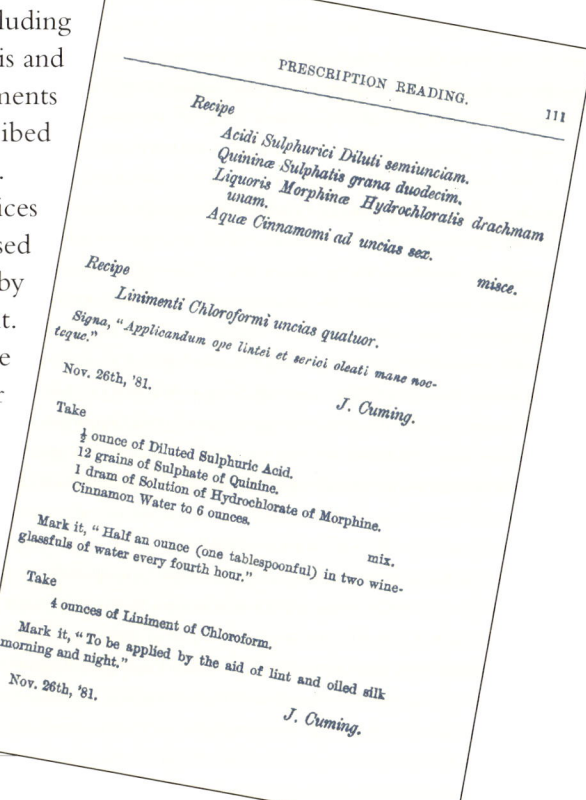

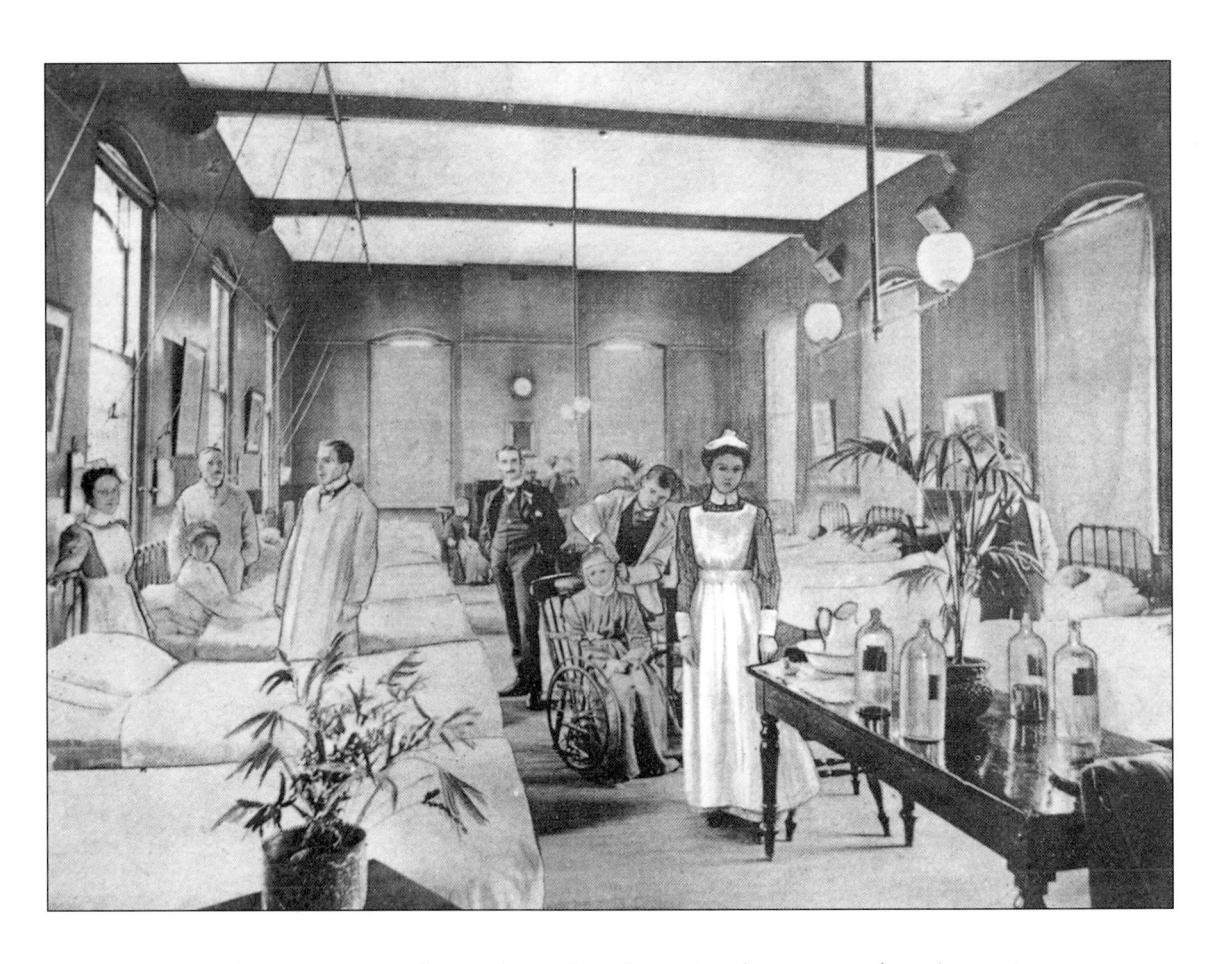

A ward in the Belfast Royal Hospital: the gentleman in morning clothes standing in the middle of the ward is the pharmacist, Mr 'Matt' Cole, and the tall figure, wearing a white coat and a bow tie, by the bedside is that of Dr T.S. Logan, House Surgeon
ROYAL VICTORIA HOSPITAL

however, as when, discussing hysteria, he states that 'sometimes a tumblerful of cold water thrown forcibly against the face acts like magic'.

Certain diseases were untreatable in the absence of specific knowledge. In particular, diabetes mellitus was associated with sugar in the urine and this could be measured, but the withholding of sugar was a very poor substitute for insulin medication. Uraemia was treated by induced sweating in the knowledge that sweat contains urea and so sweating can be used as an excretory route, although it is a very inefficient one. A form of acupuncture, with multiple incisions in the legs, was used to treat oedema.

Cardiac disease, on the other hand, has had two excellent lines of medical management for many years. Rheumatic fever was common in the nineteenth century, and the benefits of salicylic acid (the forerunner of aspirin) in controlling pyrexia (raised temperature) and joint pains have been known since 1875. Similarly, the value of digitalis preparations for cardiac failure has been known for many years; indeed, digitalis was one of the few really effective drugs employed before the twentieth century.

THE BEGINNINGS OF ANAESTHESIA

The use of general anaesthesia spread rapidly from the first demonstration with ether in Boston, USA, in October 1846 to its use in London in December 1846 and in Dublin in January 1847. There is no record of the early use of ether in the General Hospital, and the first mention of anaesthesia is in the surgical part in the annual report covering 1 April 1849 to 31 March 1850:

> 42 surgical operations have been performed, several of them under the influence of chloroform. The facts in reference to this agent are not yet sufficiently numerous to enable us to recommend or condemn its general use. It is perhaps, however, only right that we should take this opportunity of stating that it requires great caution and considerable experience to render its administration safe.

Chloroform had been introduced in Scotland and England by James Young Simpson in 1847, and it was found to be more easily administered and pleasanter for the patient than ether. It is not surprising, therefore, that it had been taken up in Belfast by 1849, even though there had already been a fatality (Hannah Greener) in England in January 1848.

The annual reports of the General Hospital became increasingly positive about the use of chloroform. The 1851 report states: 'The use of chloroform, which tends so much to allay the sufferings of the patient during an operation, has been more generally adopted than formerly, and with decided success, no injurious effects having, in any case, resulted from its employment in this establishment.' This was the first year that an annual report included under 'Expenditure (sundries)' a figure for chloroform: £1 4s. 0d. (£2 13s. 0d. was spent on leeches!). These figures covered the seventeen months ending 5 September 1851. In 1852 the annual report stated:

> Chloroform, we may remark, has continued to be used in almost every case of surgical operation, with the happiest effect in the alleviation of human suffering, and it is very satisfactory to report that in no case has the least unpleasant result followed its use.

Altogether, 85 operations were performed, the largest group being amputations. In 1852 the annual expenditure statement (for the eleven months 1 September 1851 to 4 August 1852) records 6s. 2d. for chloroform. In 1853 the report stated:

> Chloroform has been administered to the patients, when practicable, and with the most gratifying results in alleviating both mental dread and physical pain; and it is our duty to put it on record, that, during the several years it has been exhibited in this institution, no accident whatever or evil has followed its administration.

The cost for thirteen months' supply was £2 0s. 6d.

In 1854, 1855, 1856, 1857 and 1858 again the comments were favourable and 'No untoward symptom was manifest.' In view of the fact that patients did not fast for a period prior to anaesthesia, nor were they sedated, and with the subsequent record of chloroform for causing cardiac

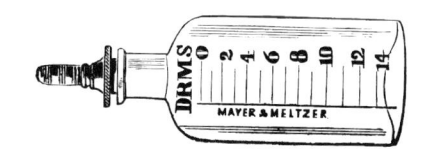

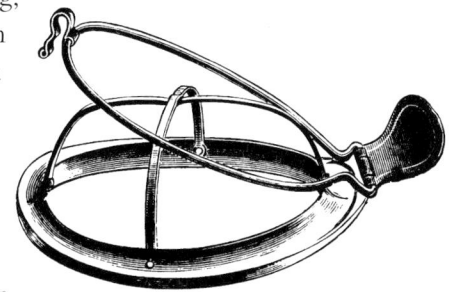

A wire mask, used in conjunction with cloth or gamgee to absorb ether or chloroform dropped from a bottle: this type of mask was introduced soon after 1850 and remained in use until after World War Two.
MAYER AND PHELPS CATALOGUE, 1931

arrest during anaesthesia and liver failure afterwards, the early anaesthetists must have been very lucky or simply had no follow-up procedures to detect problems.

The number of operations performed annually rose steadily, passing one hundred in the year covered by the 1858 report, with five deaths. One of the advantages of anaesthesia was that it reduced the sense of urgency of the surgeon, permitting a more careful dissection or preparation of the amputation stump. It was also felt that anaesthesia reduced the risks to the patient by 'lessening the severity of the shock to the system'. This view is hard to prove and some took the opposite view, namely that the pain of surgery was actually beneficial in helping patients to recover from the operation.

By 1859 the surgical report refers to the use of chloroform as 'so long established in this hospital' and the annual bill had risen to £5 2s. 0d. (though in that year it was unusually high). The 1866 report stated that 'the ether spray, as recommended by Dr Richardson' had been fully tried as a local anaesthetic in several of the minor operations, another innovation. This comment presumably refers to the use of ether to numb the perception of pain in the skin, a role for which ethyl chloride was later used. In subsequent years both chloroform and ether continued to be bought by the hospital, and the expenditure is often added together, but exactly what the ether was used for is uncertain.

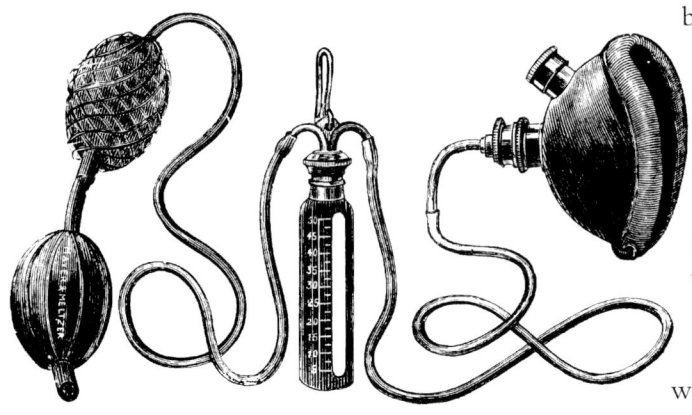

Chloroform is specifically mentioned as being used in about 70 per cent of the surgical operations during the early 1880s; it was administered 100 times during the year 1880 alone. Later there were changes, with methylene first mentioned in 1884, the ACE mixture (alcohol, chloroform, ether) in 1885, and nitrous oxide in 1888. We have figures for each year, which show that the choice of anaesthetics was very conservative; chloroform was still used for 420 out of 543 surgical operations in 1900.

Junker's inhaler, dating from 1867, with bellows for blowing air in a regulated manner through a glass bottle and onwards into a face mask
MAYER AND PHELPS CATALOGUE, 1931

Until the end of the nineteenth century, the method of administration of these anaesthetics was mainly by the open drop technique. This consists of a single metal frame containing layers of gauze which was held over the mouth and nose and onto which the liquid anaesthetic was dropped. The method worked well in skilled hands, and the anaesthetic could easily be discontinued if the pulse became weak or irregular, or if respiration slowed, or if the patient began to vomit. During the fifty years to 1900, death on the operating table attributed to anaesthetic is recorded in only two instances, though this figure is almost certainly an underestimate. Many deaths must have been blamed on the disease or injury rather than the anaesthetic. We do not know who administered the anaesthetics but it was probably the resident house surgeons; the first honorary Anaesthetists were only appointed in 1900. Joseph Lister had written in Holmes's *System of Surgery* in 1861 and again in 1870 and 1882 that the action of chloroform on the heart was unimportant and 'The appointment of a special chloroform giver to a hospital is not only entirely unnecessary, but has the great disadvantage of investing the administration of chloroform with an air of needless mystery.'

GENERAL SURGERY

The surgical emphasis was still very much on accidents and, reflecting this, cases of drowning or 'submersion' were also admitted to the surgical wards. In his surgical report for 1848–49, Dr Horatio Stewart expressed his colleagues' gratification at 'the spacious and well-ventilated wards of the front building' and at the infrequency, since the move to better wards, of post-operative erysipelas (a widespread inflammation in the skin) and phlebitis (inflammation of the veins often leading to clotting). The number of patients with burns from the bursting of boilers or contact with molten metal continued to be high though the number of industrial injuries had remained the same as earlier in the century, in spite of the steady growth of mills and factories. This may reflect some benefit from the Factory Inspectorate. On the other hand the number of injured sailors was growing as Belfast's shipping trade expanded. The type of injuries resulting from these accidents included fractures (simple and compound), dislocations, concussion, contusions (bruises) and wounds, and many of the fractures required amputation to avoid tetanus and gas gangrene. Children were widely employed in spite of prohibitions, and many of them lost fingers in cutting and die stamping machinery. In addition, drunkenness in parents led to large numbers of child patients injured either by brutality or by neglect. Just as abuse of children is not new, neither too are street accidents: the phrase 'furious driving of car owners' was applied to bread carts, ginger beer sellers, and other vehicles. Drunkenness played its part in street accidents too, and also in the number of fights that resulted in admissions. The view was sometimes expressed that such patients 'should not be put in with respectable artisans and others who contribute in part to the hospital but should be treated in the Workhouse Hospital'. Clearly, however, such a view could not be maintained.

Although the dispensaries were no longer administered by the hospital, an extern department was opened in December 1848 to see medical and surgical outpatients. The pioneers were Dr Andrew Malcolm and Dr James Moore and, even though drugs were not supplied but had to be obtained from the dispensaries, the department proved widely popular. With Andrew Malcolm's death in 1856, patient numbers fell, but they increased again as a result of the surgical efforts of Mr William MacCormac in 1858.

The annual report for that year recorded 118 surgical operations, including 2 tracheostomies, presumably for diphtheria. The growth in numbers of outpatients continued during the 1860s and 1870s until in the year 1873/74 there were 6,769 attendances. Syphilis and gonorrhoea continued to be common, and whilst 20–30 patients a year were admitted, many more were treated as outpatients.

One group of patients that will certainly strike a chord is those injured in the riots of August 1864. The middle years of the century were, in fact, punctuated by riots, including the famous episode of Dolly's Brae in July 1849, those following a sermon to Orangemen by Thomas Drew in July 1857, and those of August 1864. The last originated in the erection of a memorial in Dublin to Daniel O'Connell, champion of Catholic Emancipation, which was accompanied by a counter-demonstration in Belfast and several days of anti-Catholic violence. A report of all casualties was compiled by Mr Henry Murney, with the co-operation of the general practitioners. These casualties amounted to 238, of whom 5 were under fifteen years of age, 27 were aged fifteen to twenty, and the rest were older. There were 98 gunshot injuries and it is probably a reflection of the types of weapon used (swords and bayonets, sticks and bottles), rather than of the medical care, that only 11 patients died. As in the riots of the 1970s, many of the public appear to have had an exaggerated idea of the number of casualties from the violence.

There were no dramatic changes in surgery after the introduction of anaesthesia until the advent of Lister's doctrine of antisepsis – the use of a carbolic acid spray to drench the wound. Joseph Lister (later Lord Lister) first propounded the idea in a paper to the *Lancet* in 1867, but of course it followed on Pasteur's discovery of micro-organisms in liquids undergoing fermentation. For some time surgeons had blamed post-operative sepsis on overcrowding and lack of ventilation in surgical wards, but Lister's paper identified a more specific cause. In Belfast, William MacCormac took up the topic of carbolic acid use in a paper of 1869 dealing with antiseptic treatment of wounds. The Franco-Prussian war of 1870–71 was probably required to concentrate surgeons' minds on the cause-and-effect relationship between bacteria and sepsis. At all events the mortality from 'capital' or major amputations at Belfast General Hospital fell from about 35 per cent in the mid-1860s to 10 per cent in the mid-1870s and the annual expenditure on carbolic acid and carbolic dressings rose correspondingly.

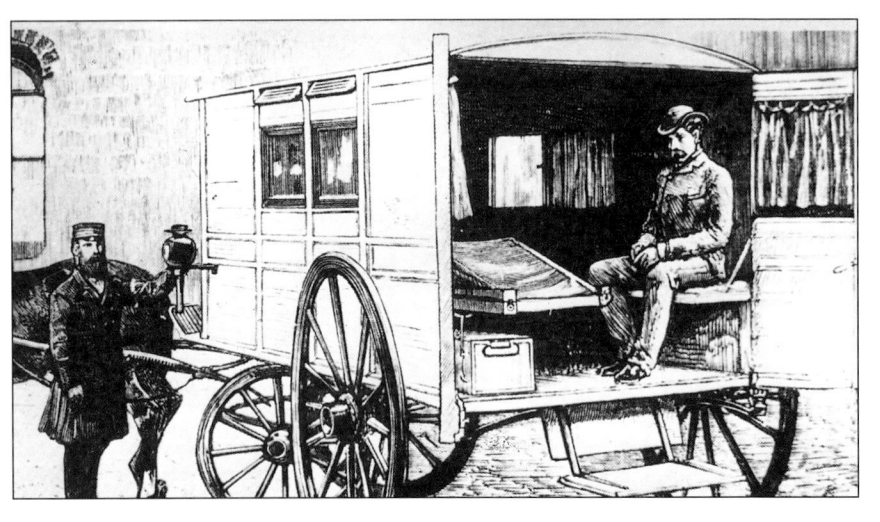

A horse ambulance of 1886, as used in London
RADIO TIMES HULTON PICTURE LIBRARY

The measures advocated in this period included spraying carbolic acid into the air, using dressings soaked in carbolic acid, clean clothing to be worn by those in contact with the patient, and isolation of infected patients. By this time some lessons had been learnt from the Crimean War, and Florence Nightingale's nursing reforms, with their emphasis on cleanliness, were reaching Belfast. Erysipelas, involving infection of skin as well as underlying tissues, was a particular scourge of surgical wards, and it was realised at about the same time that cases of erysipelas should be isolated in a separate building (see ground plan on page 52). However, it was not until the implementation of the Infectious Disease Acts in the last years of the nineteenth century, that it was made compulsorily notifiable (1889) and an offence (1899) to treat patients with erysipelas in open wards.

A late-nineteenth-century wooden operating table: it was discovered lying in the basement of the Royal Victoria Hospital in the late 1940s.
ROYAL VICTORIA HOSPITAL

The nature of general surgery changed only slowly with the introduction of antiseptics. Even in the 1880s bites, burns, fractures, dislocations and lacerations formed the largest part of surgical practice. Tapping of the abdomen to drain off excess fluid and of the bladder in prostatic obstruction was carried out, but no intra-abdominal, intra-cranial or thoracic surgery was done. In the 1870s, however, planned orthopaedic surgery for tuberculous joints began under Dr John Fagan and, in spite of the risks, was preferable to amputation.

If the 1870s was the decade of antisepsis, the 1880s was the era of asepsis. Surgeons like Lawson Tait in Birmingham flushed out the abdominal cavity with boiled water, and Spencer Wells (now known for his forceps) adopted strict asepsis including the wearing of sterile rubber gloves. Sir William Macewen of Glasgow, Lister's most brilliant pupil, would never

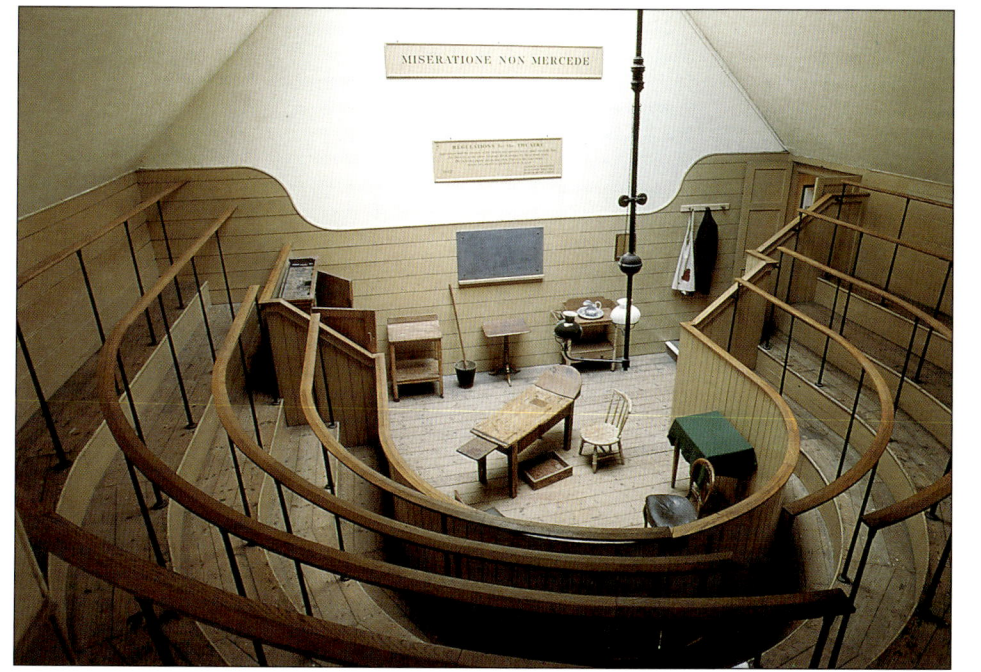

A typical contemporary operating theatre at old St Thomas's Hospital, Southwark, London: the theatre was in use from 1822 until 1861 and then hidden from view until 1957, when it was discovered and restored.
LORD BROCK MEMORIAL TRUST

have been able to advance orthopaedic surgery in the 1880s had he not adopted aseptic methods, and these soon came to Belfast. The first abdominal procedures to be tackled systematically were hernias but they were usually strangulated, where peritonitis had developed and the mortality was high. By 1889–91 things had changed and a 'radical cure' operation for hernia could be safely performed (8 were performed in three years at the Belfast General Hospital with 1 death) and colostomy was also being carried out occasionally (4 in three years with 1 death). Bladder stones were now being crushed; the fragments were either passed spontaneously later or extracted at the time. More formal abdominal surgical procedures had to wait until 1895, when three patients had operations: for relief of intestinal obstruction, a gastroenterostomy to relieve pyloric obstruction, and a cholecystectomy for an impacted gallstone in the bile duct. All three patients survived. In 1896 the first operation for acute appendicitis was carried out. All these operations were too uncommon for experience to be built up, and generally the mortality was high.

THE QUEEN'S COLLEGE BELFAST, AND ITS FACULTY OF MEDICINE

The Queen's Colleges at Belfast, Cork and Galway opened in October 1849 to prepare students for the degrees of the Queen's University in Ireland. The colleges each had their own medical school and that in Belfast, as we have seen, absorbed the former medical school at the Royal Belfast Academical Institution. However the college only allocated a lecture theatre and preparation room in the north wing, and students still attended the old dissecting room at Inst. Students had to walk even further, from the college to the General Hospital in Frederick Street, for their clinical instruction. The course then lasted four years (of which two were clinical) and the degree awarded by the QUI was the MD. Students could elect to take the LRCP and MRCS (equivalent to a medical degree) in Dublin after three years, and many who matriculated did not take the MD at all, or took it much later.

The Medical Act of 1858 defined, for the protection of the public, the question of who could call themselves a registered medical practitioner, that is, who could hold an appointment in hospital and many other rights and privileges. Essentially the categories eligible for registration were fellows, members and licentiates of the various royal colleges of physicians and surgeons and of the Society of Apothecaries in London and the Apothecaries' Hall in Dublin, as well as doctors, bachelors and licentiates of medicine or surgery of any university in the UK. The act also made eligible those practising before 1815 who did not have the above qualifications and those who held appointments as surgeons in the army or navy.

Queen's College Belfast, *c.* 1850
QUEEN'S UNIVERSITY BELFAST

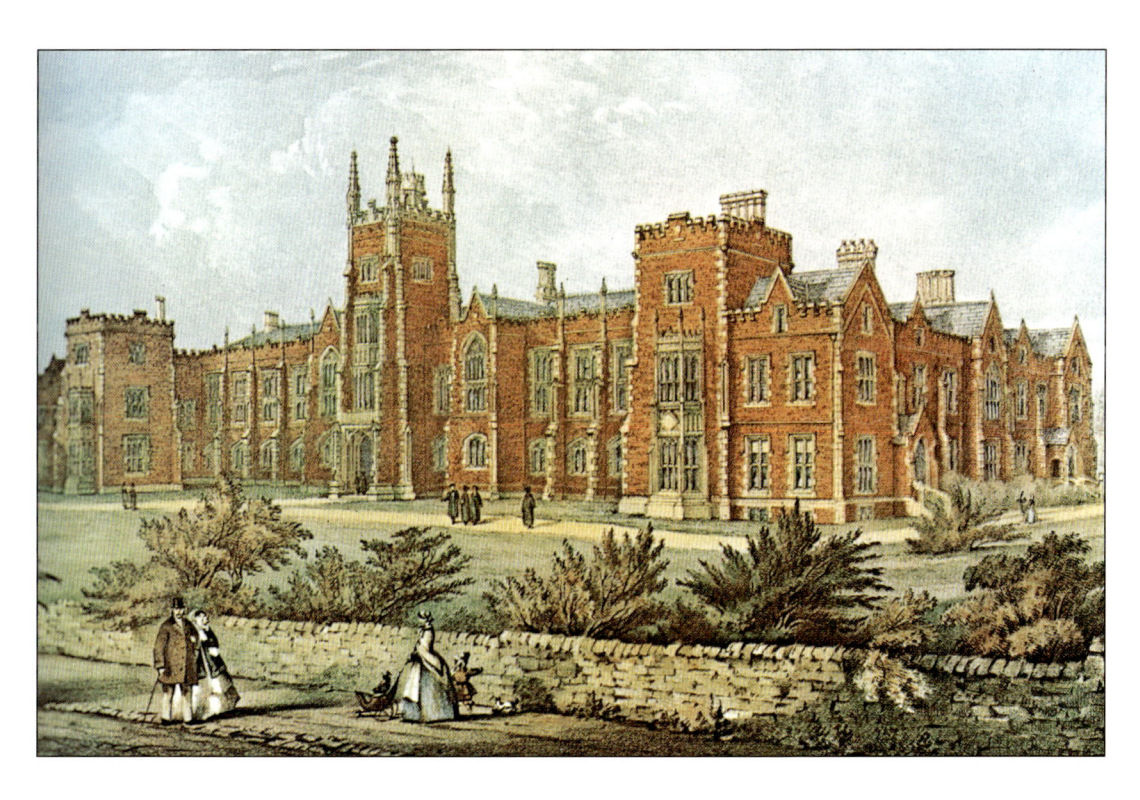

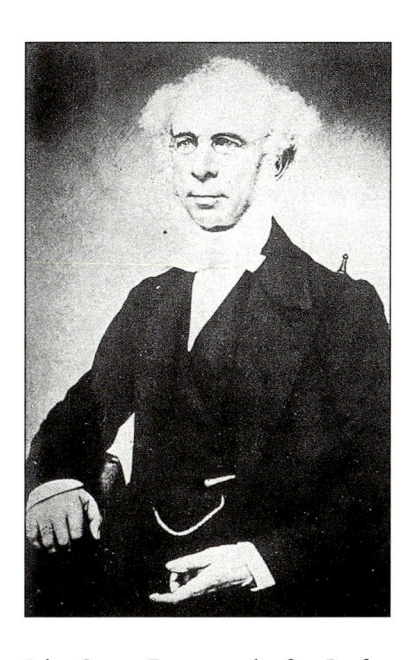

For a variety of religious–political reasons, the Queen's University in Ireland was replaced in 1882 by a Royal University of Ireland, but this body only examined and awarded the degrees. At the same time the primary medical degree became the MB as in other British universities rather than the MD, which became a postgraduate qualification. Not until 1908 did the Queen's College achieve full academic independence as the Queen's University of Belfast, conducting its own final examinations and awarding degrees.

Virtually all the professors of the medical school were members of the Visiting staff of the General Hospital and its successor hospitals. The first Professor of Medicine was John Creery Ferguson. He was born in Tandragee, County Armagh, the son of a doctor, graduated MB with gold medal at Trinity College Dublin, was for three years Professor of the Practice of Medicine there and was appointed to the chair of Medicine at Queen's College in 1849 and Attending Physician at the General Hospital in 1853. He did distinguished work in Dublin on the care of typhus and cholera patients and was the first man in the British Isles to hear the foetal heart. In Belfast he was a keen lecturer and teacher, and he was the first president of the Ulster Medical Society when it was formed in 1862 by amalgamation of the Belfast Medical Society and the Belfast Clinical and Pathological Society.

J.C. Ferguson died in 1865 and was replaced by Professor James Cuming. He also came from County Armagh – from Markethill – but graduated MD (QUI) at Queen's College in 1855, one of the first batch to train entirely at Queen's. He was a fluent linguist and travelled throughout

John Creery Ferguson, the first Professor of Medicine at Queen's College Belfast, 1849–65, and an Attending Physician to the Belfast General Hospital from 1853 until his death
ULSTER MEDICAL SOCIETY

continental Europe, studying particularly the diseases of the nervous system and attending clinical demonstrations in La Salpêtrière, Paris, by such figures as Professor Charcot, Hughlings Jackson, Brown-Sequard and Romberg. He was elected to the Attending staff of the General Hospital in 1865 and remained in this post until he died on 27 August 1899. He was celebrated for giving clear, logical and well-arranged lectures to his students but, being cautious in expressing an opinion, he gained the title 'High Priest of Philosophic Doubt'.

Dr James Alexander Lindsay was born in Fintona, County Tyrone, and like his predecessor, he was of farming stock. He was educated at Inst., Methodist College and Queen's College Belfast, from where he graduated with an MD in 1882. He was the first House Physician at the Belfast Royal Hospital, became Assistant Physician in 1883 and Attending Physician in 1888, and subsequently (1890) gained the MRCP of London. He was appointed to the Queen's College chair of Medicine in 1899 on the death of Professor Cuming, and he retired in 1921. He belonged to the school of physicians who concentrated on accurate diagnosis, and that with the aid of his own senses and acumen, but had little interest in medical treatment; he never took up such artificial aids as the electrocardiograph. This pedantic approach was crystallised in the instruction cards of technique for examination of patients that he published. His lectures also were precise and old-fashioned, delivered at dictation speed throughout, to provide notes for future reference, as was common until good textbooks became more freely available in the 1950s.

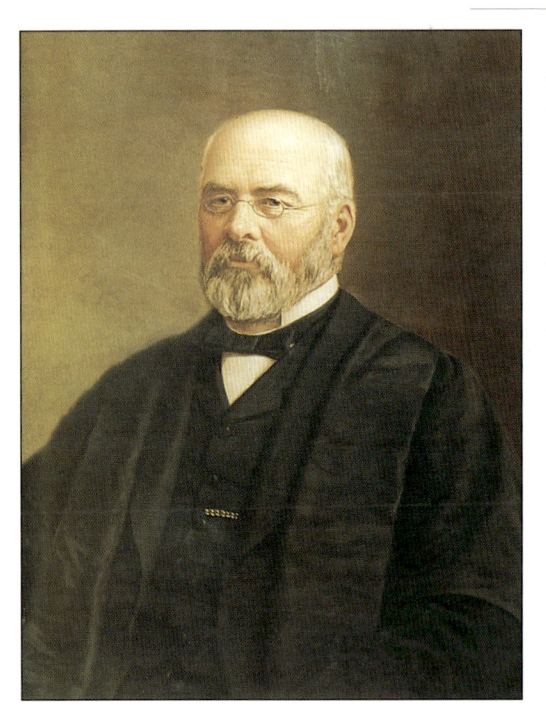

Professor James Cuming, the second Professor of Medicine at Queen's College Belfast, 1865–99, and an Attending Physician to the Belfast General Hospital and later the Belfast Royal Hospital
ROYAL VICTORIA HOSPITAL

The first Professor of Surgery at Queen's was Alexander Gordon. He was born at Saintfield, County Down, studied medicine at Inst., and graduated with an MD of Edinburgh University in 1841. He was demonstrator in Anatomy at Inst. before being appointed to the chair of Surgery in the new Queen's medical school in 1849. He was appointed Attending Surgeon to the General Hospital in 1845, and always took a particular interest in fractures and their management. Sir William Whitla commented in his usual flowery language that Gordon 'transformed the treatment of fractures from being a stagnant pool into being a clear crystal spring'. Gordon was noted as a great personality: untidy, rough in speech, careless in dress, but beloved by his students (to whom he was 'old Alick') and his patients. One of the best-known stories about Gordon describes how Dr T.H. Purdon called to collect him one day because the Earl of Shaftesbury had requested a consultation. Gordon came rushing out with his usual disreputable old cap. Seeing this, Dr Purdon suggested that, as they were going to the house of a member of the aristocracy, he might take a better hat. 'Hold on,' Gordon said, and going back into the hall he

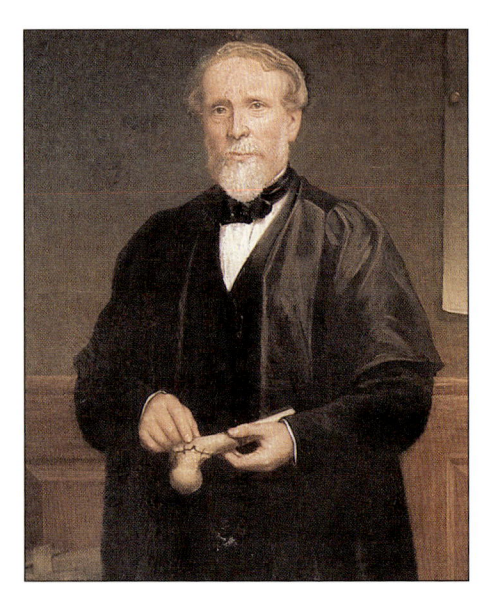

Professor Alexander Gordon, the first Professor of Surgery at Queen's College Belfast, 1849–86, and an Attending Surgeon to the Belfast General Hospital
QUEEN'S UNIVERSITY BELFAST

handed Dr Purdon one of his best top hats saying, 'If it is a hat you want, here is one.' Then, closing the door, he left Dr Purdon and the hat outside.

Gordon filled the chair of Surgery for thirty-seven years and was succeeded by his favourite pupil, Thomas Sinclair, then aged twenty-seven. Sinclair was unusual in Belfast at this time in having the FRCS of London, and was appointed assistant surgeon to the General Hospital in 1885 and professor at Queen's College in 1886. He was the opposite to Alexander Gordon, being a dapper, shy bachelor who always wore a dark pinstripe suit and a waistcoat with a white lining. He published an account in 1894 of the first gastroenterostomy performed in Ireland. At the outbreak of World War One he was appointed Colonel in the RAMC and when the German air ace Baron von Richthofen was shot down, Sinclair was asked to perform the postmortem specifically to decide the controversial point of whether the baron was shot in the air or after capture. In the event he was able to show from the track of the bullet that it had come from below, that is, while the plane was in the air, though inevitably the Germans were not convinced and published a libellous version as recently as 1985. On retirement Sinclair was elected a member of the Senate of Queen's University, pro-chancellor, and Unionist MP for the University seat. He had a large private practice which he maintained by charging large fees appropriate to his status.

Another important chair was that of Materia Medica. Its first holder was Dr Horatio Agnew Stewart, who had been an Attending Surgeon at the General Hospital from 1847 and was appointed Professor in 1849. He died in 1857 at the early age of thirty-six and was succeeded in that year by Dr James Seaton Reid. Reid was part of a family dynasty, many of whom were nineteenth-century Presbyterian ministers. He came from Ramelton in Donegal and, after graduating with an MD from Edinburgh in 1833 with a thesis on the effects of ergot (a fungus found on rye which causes spasms and gangrene), he started to practise in Londonderry. In 1840 he was appointed Attending Physician to the General Hospital, and in 1847 he was appointed as one of the first physicians to the new Belfast Union Hospital. As his portrait shows, he was strongly built, of a florid complexion, and with an abundance of snow-white hair. When Dr Reid retired from the chair in 1890 he was replaced by the truly notable figure of Sir William Whitla.

William Whitla was born in Monaghan and started his working life at the age of fifteen, as an apprentice to his brother James, a pharmaceutical chemist. After a period with chemists in Belfast, he decided to train as a doctor, obtaining first his licentiates and later, in 1877, the MD with gold medal. In that year he was appointed Assistant Physician to the Belfast Charitable Institute, and in 1882 he became Attending Physician to the Belfast Royal Hospital. He had maintained his expertise in pharmacy and in the same year he produced the first edition of his book *Elements of*

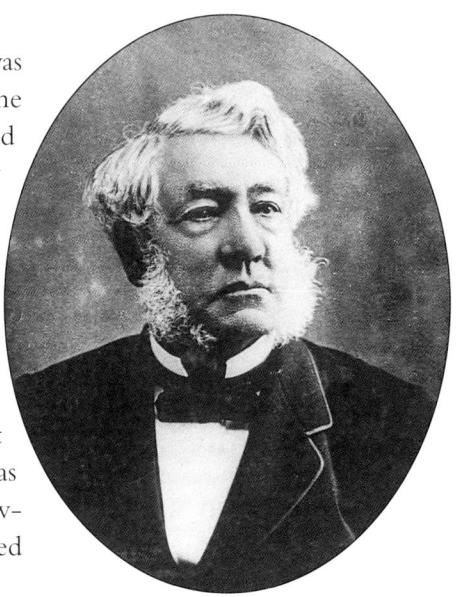

Professor James Seaton Reid, the second Professor of Materia Medica at Queen's College Belfast, 1857–90, an Attending and Consulting Physician to the Royal Victoria Hospital, and also medical officer at the Belfast Union Fever Hospital, 1846–90
ULSTER MEDICAL SOCIETY

Pharmacy, Materia Medica and Therapeutics, which ran to thirteen editions. At the same time he was becoming a more successful physician, and he moved his practice from Great Victoria Street to 8 College Gardens.

In 1890 Dr William Whitla was appointed to the chair of Materia Medica, and in 1902 he was knighted (unusually, for medical distinction alone). In 1918 he retired from his hospital post, and in 1919 he retired from his professorship. His distinctions were numerous – he was twice president of the Ulster Medical Society, president of the BMA, MP for the University, and pro-chancellor of the university. Whitla's 1892 *Dictionary of Treatment*, like the *Materia Medica*, went into many editions, the last as recently as 1957. Whitla was certainly a distinguished physician, but he is remembered now for his exceptional generosity to the citizens of Belfast. He first built the Medical Institute in College Square North (now demolished) for the Ulster Medical Society. He gave the much-loved Good Samaritan window to the Belfast Royal Hospital in 1886 (the window was removed in 1903 to the extern hall of the new Royal Victoria Hospital and is currently in the long corridor of the hospital). He bequeathed £10,000 to Methodist College which was used to build its Whitla Hall, and the residue went to Queen's University along with his house at Lennoxvale, now used as the vice-chancellor's residence. In the university he is commemorated by the practical and impressive Whitla Hall, by the Whitla Chair of Therapeutics and Pharmacology, and by the Whitla Medical Building which now houses the Ulster Medical Society on the ground floor.

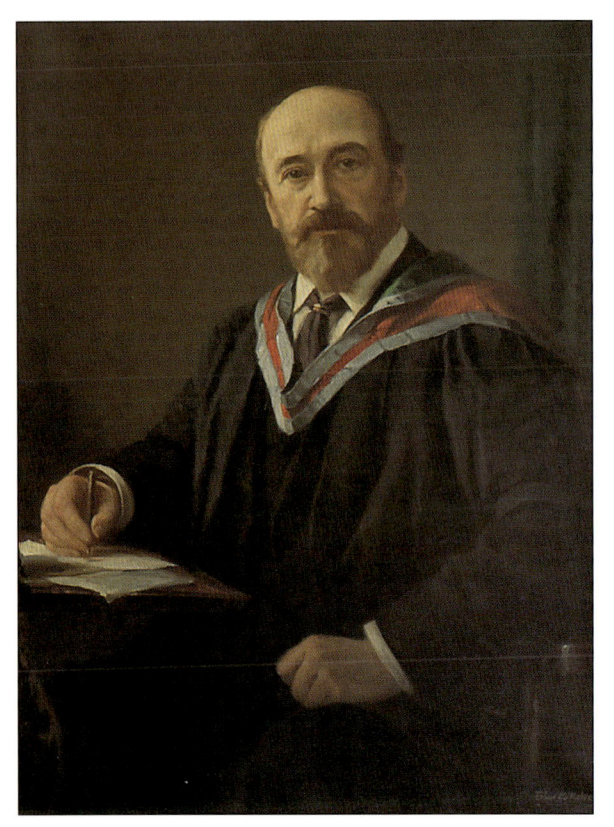

Professor Sir William Whitla, third Professor of Materia Medica at Queen's College Belfast, 1890–1919, an Attending and Consulting Physician to the Belfast Royal Hospital and later the Royal Victoria Hospital, and a generous benefactor to many institutions in Belfast; portrait by Frank McKelvey
ULSTER MEDICAL SOCIETY

MEDICAL STUDENTS AND HOSPITAL TEACHING

By the 1850s teaching at the Belfast General Hospital had fallen into a pattern not dissimilar to that of one hundred years later. There were medical and surgical teaching ward rounds and there was opportunity to use the stethoscope. There were lectures by the Attending Physicians and Surgeons. Pupils also attended operations, saw accident cases brought in, visited the extern department and received instruction in the use of the microscope. The whole field of clinical pathology in the nineteenth century was limited to simple tests carried out in the side wards. The student would also attend lectures at Queen's College and have instruction in the specialist hospitals that opened one by one in Belfast in the latter half of the century.

As mentioned on page 21, the first annual address to students, or Annual Oration, was given by Dr James McDonnell in 1827 on the topic

The opening page of the register of medical students attending the Belfast General Hospital in 1866, the first entry being John Walton Browne
ROYAL VICTORIA HOSPITAL

'Systematic medicine'. Over the next fifty years various Attending Physicians have been identified as having given the opening address of the winter term, but this may well have been simply the first clinical lecture. Not until 1883 was it formally proposed by Dr Whitla, and recorded by Dr Byers, that 'an introductory address' be given annually. Dr John Moore, senior Attending Surgeon, gave the oration in that year, and apart from a few interruptions when the chosen speaker declined, the tradition has been continued almost without break since then. In 1884 it was proposed that lecturers should not be appointed simply on the basis of seniority but instead an appropriate speaker should be selected and invited six months in advance. The earliest address of which we have a copy is that of Dr Malcolm in 1852 but this is exceptional and until the 1930s we rarely have even the title. From that period onward, however, the text has usually been published in full in the *Ulster Medical Journal*.

Clinical clerks and dressers were 'selected from the most deserving pupils' and would have had a more specific attachment than other students to a particular ward, with defined duties. These included seeing and examining (or 'clerking') the new patients, following their treatment, and dressing the wounds of the surgical patients. From 1858 three resident pupils were elected, who paid for their board and had a more rigorous, apprenticeship-type instruction than other students. All students paid a fee for their clinical instruction, which was divided among their teachers, though this charge was offset over the years by competitive exhibitions and prizes such as the Malcolm Exhibition. Another exhibition open to students was funded in 1875 as a memorial to Dr John Gordon Coulter, a former pupil of the hospital who had died in India.

In the 1850s about fifty medical students attended the hospital but their names are largely lost. The register from 1866 has survived, however, and it records each student's name, home address and fees paid, term by term. What is most striking is that the students came largely from rural areas rather than Belfast: in the first ten entries, places such as Castlederg, Banbridge, Portglenone, Newton-Limavady, Broughshane, Dungiven, Manorhamilton and Kilmore are recorded. The question of admitting women students was first discussed in 1870 and indeed supported, but only in 1882 did the new Royal University of Ireland agree to admit women students to the Faculty of Arts. The hospital Board of Management agreed to admit women students in 1889, and in that year the first three, Elizabeth and Margaret Bell from Newry, County Down, and Harriette Neill from Belfast, entered the Medical Faculty.

THE MEDICAL STAFF AFTER 1850

In 1851, the medical staff consisted of four Attending Physicians, four Attending Surgeons and two House Surgeons. However one of the latter seems to have doubled up as an apothecary until 1883 when an additional post of Pharmaceutical Chemist was created. Thereafter, numbers of resident medical staff increased, and by the end of the nineteenth century there were three House Surgeons and one House Physician. In 1879 and 1880 further expansion of the hospital's work required a grade of Assistant Physician and Assistant Surgeon – ranking between Attending and Resident medical staff – with responsibility for the extern department. In 1883, by which time specialisation was increasing, the Attending staff numbered five physicians and five surgeons, but there were six of each (plus further assistants) by 1900.

The physicians of the hospital in 1850 included Dr John Miller Pirrie who was appointed Attending Physician in 1849 and made his own contribution to the hospital before his family became noted benefactors. His father, Captain William Pirrie, had been born in Wigton in Scotland in 1780, had travelled much as a ship's captain, and had settled in Belfast in the 1820s. In 1827 he was elected to the Ballast Board, which was responsible for improving Belfast harbour by cutting across the bends at the lower end of the River Lagan, and as a Harbour Commissioner he had opened the new Victoria Channel in 1849. His son John, after graduating at Trinity College Dublin, played a large part in medicine in the General

Hospital first as physician, then as honorary secretary, and from 1865 as honorary Consulting Physician. It was he who commented in the annual report on the tragic effects of the absence of compulsory vaccination against smallpox in Ireland. He died in Liverpool on 16 July 1873 at the early age of forty-eight. By this time his nephew W.J. Pirrie was one of the partners in Harland and Wolff (see page 71).

Dr John Swanwick Drennan is best known as the son of Dr William Drennan of Newry and Dublin, one of the United Irishmen. He had graduated with a BA (1831), MB (1838) and MD (1854) of Trinity College Dublin; he obtained the LRCSI in 1834 and studied in England before returning to Belfast to become Attending Physician to the General Hospital in 1856. He retired as a Consulting Physician in 1870. He is also noted as a literary figure and a volume of *Poems and Sonnets* (1895) was published posthumously. This includes the well-known obituary to his father:

> Pure, just, benign: thus filial love would trace,
> The virtues hallowing this narrow space,
> The Emerald Isle may grant a wider claim,
> And link the Patriot's with his Country's name.

Dr John Drennan is said to have been the first person to refer to Ireland as the 'Emerald Isle'. He was first secretary of the old Belfast Medical Society and later president of the Ulster Medical Society, in 1866; he was therefore a strong advocate of the value of medical meetings (what would now be called continuing medical education).

The name of Dr James W. Thomas Smith is little known now; he was appointed Attending Physician in 1864 and was also Physician in the Belfast Lying-in Hospital and Belfast Hospital for Sick Children. After his death, Whitla commented that 'he was a brilliant clinical teacher … in diagnosis he was absolutely unrivalled … he was often sparkling and really lustrous'. His son Dr Robert Strafford Smith joined the staff of the Belfast Royal Hospital in 1888 as Assistant Physician; he was Attending Physician from 1895. Another Physician of the period, elected in 1865, was Dr Richard Ross, but he has left no enduring mark on the hospital records.

Dr Henry Samuel Purdon graduated with an MD at Glasgow University and was part of a long Purdon dynasty of doctors, including his uncle Thomas Henry Purdon (see page 19). From the time of qualifying he was interested in dermatology. In 1865, at the age of twenty-one, he called a public meeting at 12 Wellington Place to attract support for the establishment of a dispensary for the treatment of skin diseases. The dispensary was opened in that year, and in 1869 the Benn Hospital for Diseases of the Skin was opened beside the Benn EENT Hospital in Clifton Street, later to be replaced by a larger hospital which in turn was destroyed in an air raid in 1941. Dr Purdon was appointed Attending Physician to the

General Hospital in 1870, with an interest in dermatology though with no designated responsibility for the field. Dr Purdon resigned from the hospital staff in 1882 but unusually did not become a Consulting Physician.

Dr Henry Lawrence McKisack was born in Carrickfergus, County Antrim, studied medicine at Queen's College and graduated MB with honours in 1887, and MD in 1890. He became Assistant Physician at the Royal Victoria Hospital in 1899 and Attending Physician in 1900. He was a broadly based general physician and published two medical textbooks on medical diagnosis and the taking of case histories. He retired in 1924 and after his death in 1928 a memorial fund was set up to erect a plaque in the hospital and establish a research endowment.

Dr William Calwell was educated at Queen's College and graduated with an MD in 1883. He became the hospital's first registrar in 1894 and an Assistant Physician with an interest in consumption (from 1895 this involved responsibilities at the Throne Hospital – see page 59; he added on the field of dermatology from 1900. During World War One he developed a further interest in functional nervous diseases and took charge of shell-shocked soldiers in the UVF Hospital, Craigavon, for which he was awarded the OBE. He supported the introduction of x-ray equipment at the turn of the century and had a broadly based private practice at 6 College Gardens, Belfast. He was a shy and at times caustic man, but was popular with his younger colleagues.

At least three surgeons called Moore worked at the hospital during the middle years of the nineteenth century. Mr David Moore FRCS, who was elected Attending Surgeon in 1821, is referred to above in connection with the lock-ward (see pages 15–16), and is credited with introducing clinical teaching within the hospital. Dr James Moore was David Moore's son, and studied medicine at Edinburgh where he graduated with an MD in 1842. There he must have attracted the notice of Professor James Syme, for he provided the illustrations for Syme's *Principles of Surgery*, published in the same year; in that year also James Moore obtained the MRCSE. He subsequently studied in Dublin and Paris but settled in Belfast in 1843; he was elected Attending Surgeon to the General Hospital in 1846. He strongly promoted the outpatient facilities of the hospital and appears to have been a skilled surgeon since he attracted medical students from far outside Belfast to watch his operations. He was president of the Ulster Medical Society, 1865–66. Nevertheless, having trained with various Scottish painters, he is perhaps best known as a watercolour artist in the tradition of Andrew Nichol. The Ulster Museum has over four hundred of his drawings and paintings; like Nichol's, they are nearly all sketches of identifiable sites though few, if any, were completed to be ready for sale.

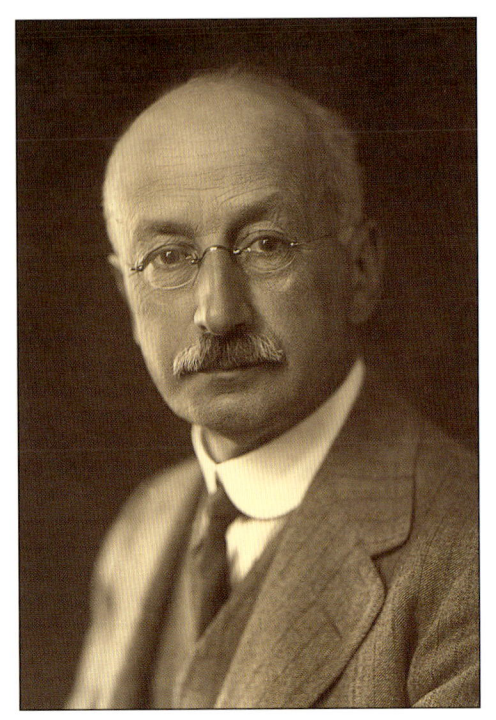

Dr Henry Lawrence McKisack, Attending Physician to the Belfast Royal Hospital and later the Royal Victoria Hospital, 1900–1924
ULSTER MEDICAL SOCIETY

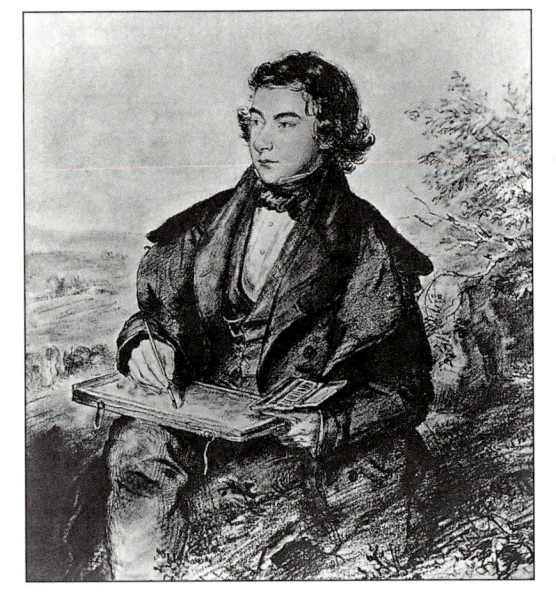

Dr James Moore, Attending Surgeon at the Belfast General Hospital, 1846–77, and a noted watercolourist; drawing by Felice Piccioni
REPRODUCED BY PERMISSION OF THE OWNER

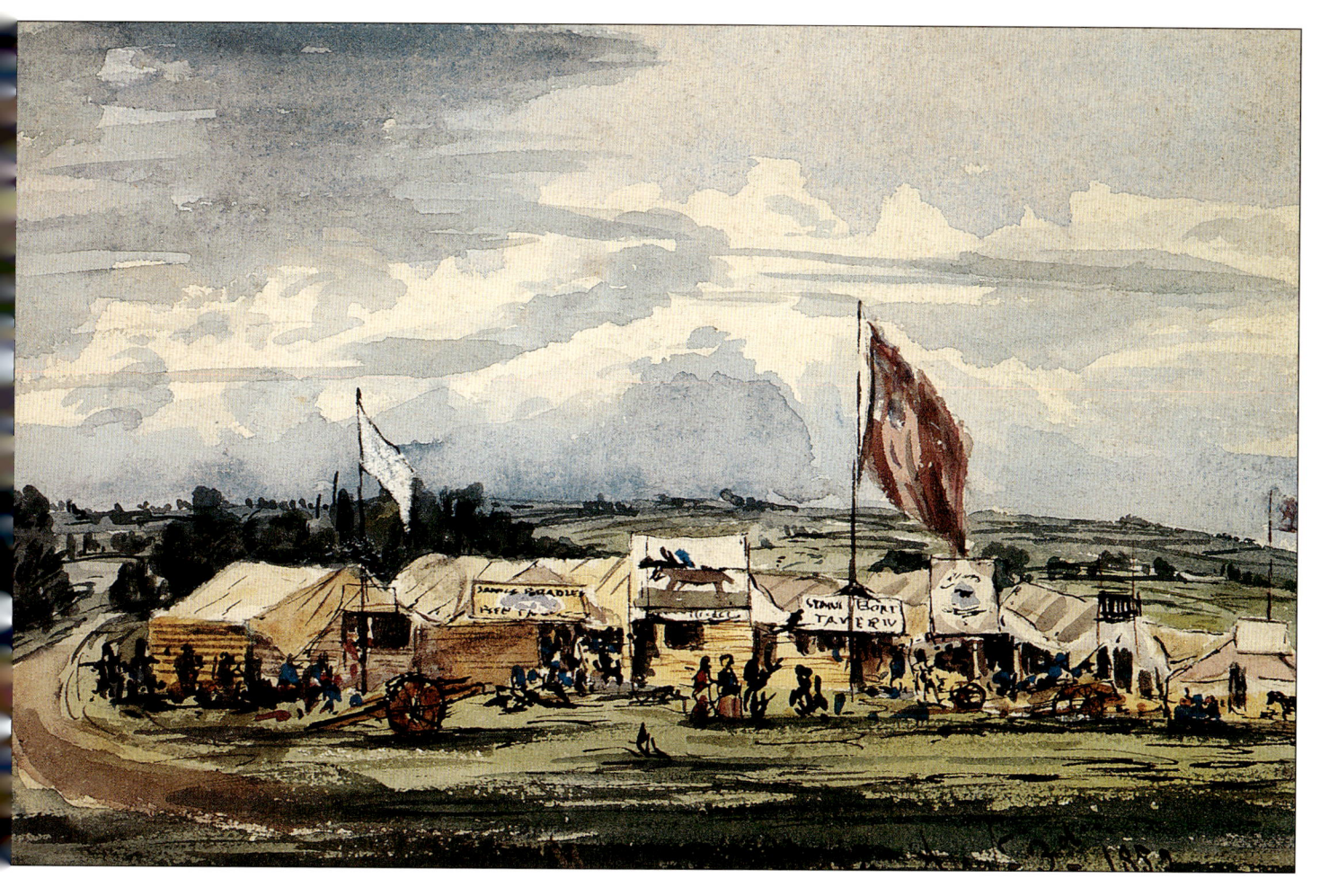

Watercolour of the Maze Racecourse, 1852, by Dr James Moore
ULSTER MUSEUM

His eminence as a surgeon was never in doubt and was recognised by Sir Charles Bell, Professor Goodsir of Edinburgh and Dr Thomas Reade of Belfast, who all left him their cases of surgical instruments.

Dr John Moore, unrelated, was one of the first to graduate with an MD (1851) in the old Queen's University in Ireland. He practised in Glenarm, County Antrim, before setting up practice in Belfast. He was appointed Attending Surgeon in 1871 and was soon president of the Ulster Medical Society (1873–74), being described as 'a man of the loftiest ideals in everything pertaining to the honour and dignity of the profession'. He published no fewer than four papers in the first volume of the *Transactions of the Ulster Medical Society*. Sadly he committed suicide while on holiday in Scotland in 1887.

Dr Henry Murney was elected Attending Surgeon in 1854 and Consulting Surgeon in 1882. He obtained his MD at Edinburgh for a thesis on tetanus but is now best known for his detailed account of the medical aspects of the 1864 riots in Belfast (see page 38). He was deeply involved in the hospital administration, and it was he who achieved security of tenure for the Visiting staff. He was one of the two hospital trustees for the extension to the hospital donated by John Charters in 1865 (see page 52).

The next notable general surgeon in the hospital was William

MacCormac. He was eldest son of the physician Henry MacCormac mentioned on page 18, and was educated at Inst. and Queen's College, taking a BA degree in 1855 before graduating with an MD in 1857. In the latter year he also obtained the MRCSE; he studied as a postgraduate in Dublin, Paris and Germany, and in 1864 he obtained the FRCSI. By this time he already had international contacts with such notable surgeons as Bilroth, von Esmarck and Langenbeck, and thus was well prepared for his appointment as Attending Surgeon. He had a large and flamboyant personality and crowned his early career by eloping with Katherine Maria Charters, daughter of the rich merchant and philanthropist John Charters. He was a pioneer of antisepsis in surgery (see page 38), and his six years in the General Hospital were filled with dynamic ideas. He was already getting restless when the Franco-Prussian War (1870–71) provided him with a wonderful opportunity to develop his skills and see life. After experiencing difficulties in being accepted by a French surgical team he joined a large American Ambulance contingent working in France under Dr Marion Sims. He was present at the surrender of Sedan with the Emperor Napoleon III. The medical staff coped with enormous numbers (about 12,000 were wounded at Sedan) but at least they had chloroform anaesthesia and Lister's carbolic acid spray. MacCormac's war experiences are eloquently described in Sir Ian Fraser's 'Father and son' lecture (1968), whose subject is the careers of William MacCormac and his father.

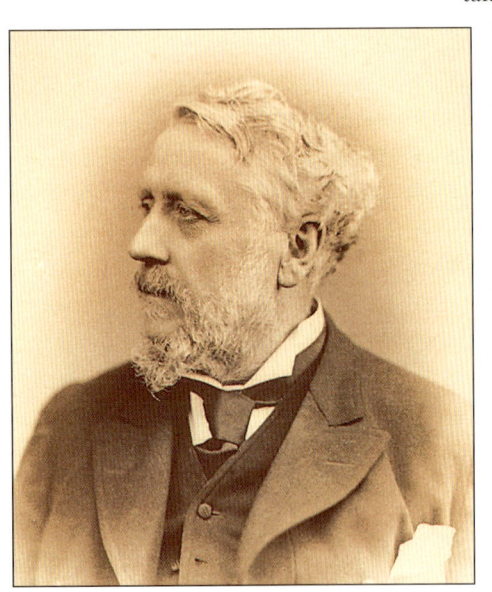

Sir William MacCormac Bart., Attending Surgeon to the Belfast General Hospital, 1864–70, later Consulting Surgeon to the hospital, Attending Surgeon at St Thomas's Hospital, London, and president of the Royal College of Surgeons, England
ROYAL VICTORIA HOSPITAL

William MacCormac never returned to work in Belfast. He applied successfully for a surgical appointment to St Thomas's Hospital, London, and went on from strength to strength, living at 13 Harley Street, borrowing and repaying £4,700 to set himself up in practice, serving in yet another war in 1875–76, becoming president of the Royal College of Surgeons, England, and eventually Sir William MacCormac, Bart., KCB and KCVO. He never forgot Belfast, however, and remained an honorary Consulting Surgeon of the General (then Royal) Hospital until his death.

In 1875 Dr John Walton Browne joined the staff as an Ophthalmic Surgeon (see page 56), and in 1877 Dr John Fagan FRCSI was elected Attending Surgeon. He maintained William MacCormac's commitment to antisepsis and the surgery of trauma generally. His other major contributions were as a founder of the Belfast Hospital for Sick Children in 1873 and his work with bone and joint tuberculosis in children. Sadly, after a mistake in operating in 1890 he gave up surgery, and in 1897 he resigned from the hospital staff to move to Dublin to become Inspector of Reformatory and Industrial Schools in Ireland. He remained a popular and highly esteemed figure in spite of his surgical error, as is evident from the staff minutes, and he was knighted in 1910 for his wider work.

Henry O'Neill was a lineal descendant of Hugh O'Neill of Tyrone, the great Irish leader during the reign of Queen Elizabeth I. Henry O'Neill was born in Crossnacreevy, County Down, and was apprenticed to a pharmaceutical chemist before studying medicine at Queen's College, graduating with an MD in 1877. He passed through junior posts in the Belfast Royal Hospital until he was elected Attending Surgeon in 1882; in 1886 he founded and was first president of the Belfast Medical Students' Association. He not only had a busy hospital and private practice in surgery, but he worked unofficially as a pathologist and, most important of all, in 1893 started the *Belfast Health Journal*, a periodical that brought public health issues to the forefront of public awareness. This led him to seek election to the Belfast Corporation in which he became High Sheriff in 1905; it also led to effective schemes for meat inspection, a new public abattoir, purer water, eradication of bovine tuberculosis, clean air, better working hours, and improvements to the Belfast Court House. In all these ideas, he can only be compared with Andrew Malcolm as a tireless worker for the well-being of the citizens of Belfast.

Thomas Kennedy Wheeler was the son of a general practitioner in Belfast; he studied at Queen's, graduated with an MD in the Royal University of Ireland in 1879, then worked at St Bartholomew's Hospital, London, and was appointed Attending Surgeon to the Belfast Royal Hospital in 1884. He retired from the hospital as Consulting Surgeon in 1902 but lived to see a daughter and three sons become doctors; one son, Mr James R. Wheeler, became an eye, ear, nose and throat surgeon in the Royal Victoria Hospital (see pages 120–21).

Arthur Brownlow Mitchell studied medicine at Queen's, graduating in 1890, and was elected to the Visiting staff of the Belfast Royal Hospital in 1894. In *The Seeds of Time* R.S. Allison suggests that between 1894 and 1928 he did more than any other surgeon at the hospital to introduce new techniques to both orthopaedics and abdominal surgery; his interests ranged from treatment of haemorrhoids to fractures. In 1909 Mitchell reported on 28 of his cases of perforated duodenal ulcer, which had resulted in only 3 deaths in contrast to a classic study by Boas of 1901 who referred to the 'absolutely hopeless prognosis' for such cases. In 1928 he developed a crippling infection of his hand as a result of pricking his finger during an operation, with subsequent sepsis. He continued to be a very highly respected surgeon, however, and was chairman of the Royal Victoria Hospital Board of Management from 1930 until his death in 1942.

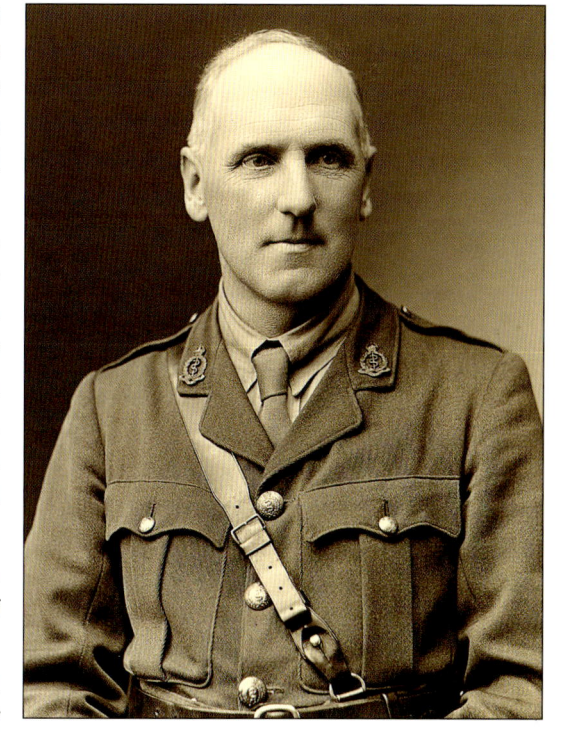

Mr Arthur Brownlow Mitchell in his RAMC uniform: he was a Visiting Surgeon to the Belfast Royal Hospital and later the Royal Victoria Hospital, 1894–1930
ROYAL VICTORIA HOSPITAL

FURTHER EXPANSION OF THE HOSPITAL

Some rebuilding had been carried out in 1847 but, in spite of the building of the Union Hospital, Belfast still required more hospital beds. In response to this need, in 1863 St Clair Kelburn Mulholland gave the committee £2,000 to build an extension to the surgical wards as a memorial to the family. The Mulhollands (later barons Dunleath) had a cotton mill in York Street but switched to linen following a fire in the mill in 1828. As a result they were very successful, employing steam power from the outset and benefiting particularly from the scarcity of cotton during the American Civil War (1861–65). St Clair Kelburn Mulholland derived his distinctive name from the noted minister of the Third Presbyterian Congregation, the Reverend St Clair Kelburn, who was imprisoned for 'seditious practices' before the 1798 United Irishmen rising. St Clair Mulholland was involved with his brother Andrew in the mill and had his own company in Durham Street, but when his only son died before him, his business was wound up. The donation in memory of his son was the largest single donation yet made to the hospital and enabled a further 30 beds to be added in a wing adjoining the operating theatre at the west end of the hospital. These beds were operational by 1865 and brought the total bed numbers up to 300.

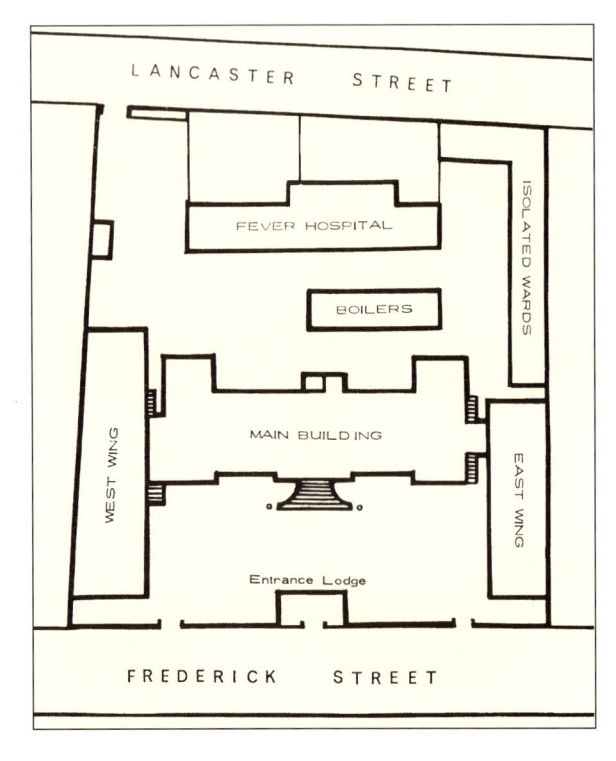

Ground plan of the Royal Hospital site, c. 1880; it shows the Mulholland Wing (west) and the Charters Wing (east), as well as the old cholera ward (here labelled 'fever hospital'), the 'isolated wards', the boiler house and the gate lodge
ROYAL VICTORIA HOSPITAL

The year in which the Mulholland Wing of the Belfast General Hospital was opened saw the announcement of a further donation, this time by John Charters, another linen merchant. He was already a life governor, and like the other mill owners he gave an annual contribution in proportion to the number of his looms and spindles, but in 1865 he decided to give another £2,000 for the building of a Charters Wing. He was also a generous donor to the Royal Belfast Academical Institution and the Belfast Charitable Institute, both of which still benefit from his generosity. Three tablets to the Mulholland family and the bust of John Charters were transferred to the Royal Victoria Hospital (wards 11 and 13) on its opening in 1903.

The Charters Wing was at the east end of the central block of the hospital and both wings now projected forward almost to Frederick Street, enclosing a front courtyard. John Charters at this stage also paid for the construction of a waiting room for visitors and the erection of new railings and entrance gates in front of the hospital. The new layout can be well seen in Frank McKelvey's painting of the hospital as it must have looked in the latter part of the nineteenth century (see page 27).

After the administrative changes that established the Belfast General Hospital in 1847, the next such development was the granting of a royal charter in 1875, creating the Belfast Royal Hospital. This did not in itself make any great change to the running of the hospital but it undoubtedly helped to encourage financial support, and it recognised the achievements

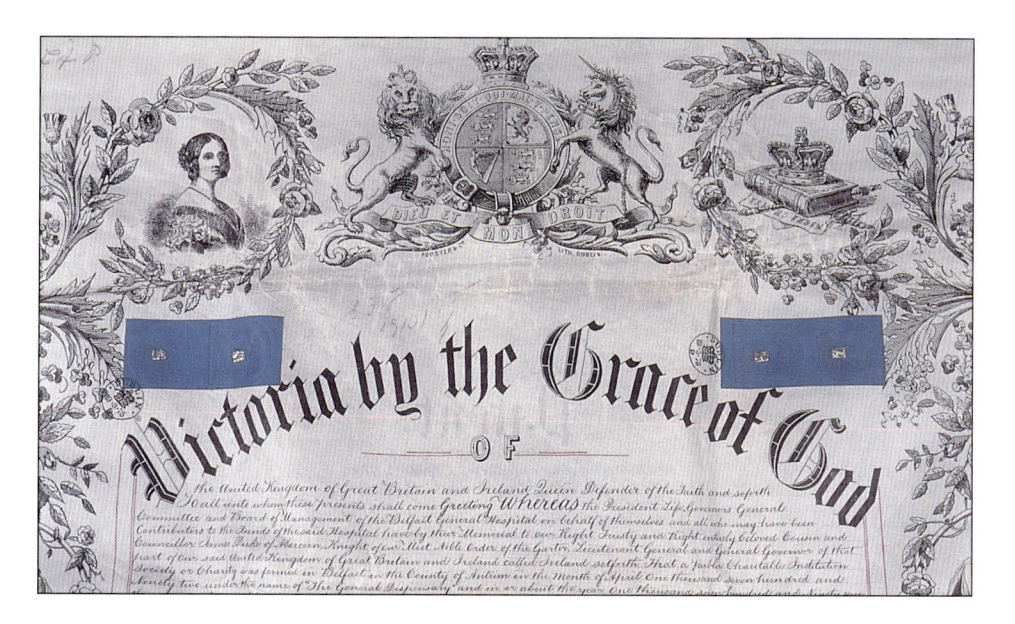

The first charter granted to the old Belfast General Hospital and naming it the Belfast Royal Hospital (1875)
ROYAL VICTORIA HOSPITAL

already completed. This was largely due to the work of the honorary treasurer, James Girdwood, and the honorary secretary, Adam J. Macrory, a local solicitor. His name appears in all the hospital annual reports from 1860 to 1879 and he was a very active force in the management of the hospital until his death, on 28 March 1881, at the age of eighty-two. As well as running the hospital, Macrory appears to have had to spend a lot of his time and energy pushing and cajoling the collectors to have their money and books ready in time for the annual meeting.

The day-to-day administration of the hospital in earlier times had been divided between the Housekeeper and the resident House Surgeon. In one of the periodic economy drives, however, in 1862 James Girdwood cut the House Surgeon's salary from £90 to £10 per year. At the same time a house steward, Mr Black, was appointed (also resident), at a salary of £80 per year, to relieve the House Surgeon of the task of ordering food and other supplies. The post of house steward increased in importance and in 1875, when the hospital was granted the royal charter, his title was changed to superintendent and his salary was increased to £200 a year. Commander F. Cox RN held the post from 1875 to 1878, Lieutenant-Colonel Clavell Blount held it from 1878 to 1880, and Colonel John Glancy MD held it from 1880 until his sudden death on 27 July 1901. Glancy was succeeded by Colonel Andrew Deane MD.

OBSTETRICS AND GYNAECOLOGY

Obstetrics in Belfast has always been managed in hospitals separate from the Belfast Dispensary and Fever Hospital and its successors, so this book is not the place for a detailed history of the field. In fact, the first maternity hospital in Belfast, the Lying-in Hospital, was a house in Donegall Street rented in January 1794, three years before the opening of the Belfast Dispensary and Fever Hospital in Factory Row. The Lying-in Hospital was run from the outset by a committee of philanthropic ladies, with Mrs Martha McTier as secretary and an untrained midwife but no regular medical attendants until 1822, when Dr Stephenson was appointed. The house was dirty, puerperal fever raged, and any food supplied was watery and miserable. In 1830 a new Lying-in Hospital (now demolished) was opened in Clifton Street on ground donated by the Belfast Charitable Society, which ran the Poor House. It housed only eighteen patients but was a great improvement on the house in Donegall Street, having such amenities as a range able to provide a constant supply of hot water. Eligible patients had to have a written recommendation from a subscriber, countersigned by a member of the committee, and a certificate stating that they were married. The unmarried were left to fend for themselves.

Dr Stephenson was succeeded in 1837 by Dr Burden who became Professor of Midwifery at the Royal Belfast Academical Institution in 1840. In 1849 he became the first Professor of Midwifery at Queen's College and by 1852 he had instituted a course of lectures and (not without opposition from the Ladies' Committee) practical instruction. Professor Burden was never on the staff of the Belfast General Hospital and retired from his professorship in 1867. He was succeeded by Dr Robert Foster Dill who had already been an Attending Physician at the Belfast General Hospital since 1856. Ironically, although Dill had been on the staff of the Lying-in Hospital, he was not re-elected in 1861 and had to act as Professor of Midwifery without access to a maternity hospital. This was apparently the result of a disagreement with the Ladies' Committee, and perhaps fits in with one description of him as 'combative and at times pugnacious, but essentially kind-hearted'. Incidentally he lost an eye in one of the riots that were common in Belfast during his working life.

Professor Dill died in 1893 and was succeeded by Dr John William Byers, son of a Presbyterian minister and Margaret Byers LL D, who was founder and first principal of Victoria College, the first secondary school for girls in Belfast, which opened in 1859. Like Dill, Byers was not on the staff of the Lying-in Hospital, though he was an Attending Physician in the Belfast Royal Hospital from 1883. During the four decades in which the Lying-in Hospital was run by a Ladies' Committee at war with the professors of Midwifery its standing gradually deteriorated. Although it accepted medical students from 1852, it did not undertake the teaching of nurse-midwives until 1879, largely on the grounds that 'it is impossible a woman could require or would be capable of receiving so much instruction'. These remarks were made not by a man and not in the days of Jane Austen, but by ladies responsible for safer midwifery in the city, and twenty years after the opening of Victoria College. It is difficult now to understand the philosophy governing the

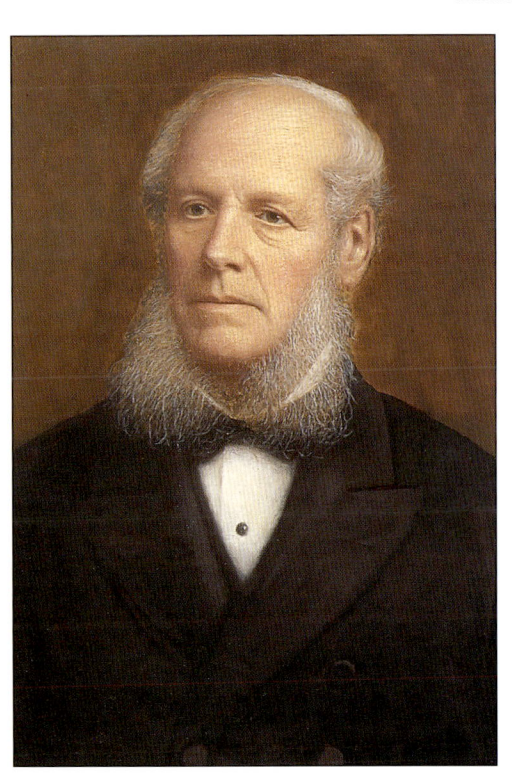

Professor Robert Foster Dill, second Professor of Midwifery at Queen's College Belfast, 1868–93, and Attending and Consulting Physician to the Belfast General Hospital, 1856–64; portrait by Richard Hooke
QUEEN'S UNIVERSITY BELFAST

running of this hospital. The Ladies' Committee appears to have never really trusted the medical profession or medical students but some doctors were necessary provided they conformed to the committee's views. The Belfast General and Royal hospitals and the Charitable Society, which were their landlords, reciprocated by making things difficult for the Lying-in Hospital. Inevitably the quality of care suffered as a result of the clashes, and the standing of Belfast midwifery only recovered in the time of Professor C.G. Lowry (see page 118).

The centenary of the Lying-in Hospital was marked by a change of name to the Belfast Maternity Hospital. In 1904 it moved to a new building in Townsend Street.

Gynaecology was not identified as a specialised field by the Belfast General Hospital, and it was not until the Royal University of Ireland came into being in 1882, with more comprehensive regulations for teaching, that pressure came to form a separate department. When Dr John Byers was appointed to the hospital in 1883 as a physician with an interest in this field, a small ward of four beds was set aside for his patients. He treated the majority of his patients in the extern clinics and, since gynaecology was a medical rather than a surgical discipline, it is hardly surprising that only six operations were performed in 1884, of which four consisted of draining large ovarian cysts with a needle. Byers was knighted in 1906 and did not retire until 1919. He died as the result of a cerebral haemorrhage in the following year. In his leisure time Sir John Byers was a noted expert on the folklore and dialects of Ulster.

EYE, EAR, NOSE AND THROAT SURGERY

In Belfast, ear, nose and throat surgery was mainly grouped with ophthalmic surgery until the end of World War Two. Blindness is mentioned in the initial prospectus for the Dispensary (1792) as one of many reasons for inoculation against smallpox, but no attempt was made to establish an ophthalmic dispensary until 1816. This failed, and it was only in 1827 that eye disorders began to be treated at the Dispensary in Chapel Lane. This closed in 1839. We hear little of eye disease in the early days of the Belfast Dispensary and Fever Hospital, however, and it was not until 1850 that Dr Samuel Browne was able to have a five-bed ward set aside there for severe eye infections. He had opened an ophthalmic dispensary in Millfield in 1845, but this ward was the first inpatient provision. The next step was the opening of a specific Ophthalmic Hospital in Great Victoria Street in 1867, to provide additional accommodation, through the munificence of Sir William and Lady Johnston. Dr Browne can therefore be regarded as the father of ophthalmic surgery in Belfast.

Samuel Browne was the son of a Presbyterian minister in Castledawson, County Londonderry. He went to school in Dublin and trained at the

Royal College of Surgeons in Ireland in order to qualify for entry to the Royal Navy as a surgeon's mate. He joined the HMS *Nelson* at Portsmouth in 1830. It was a time of peace and promotion was slow, so he was not confirmed in the rank of surgeon until 1839. Then disaster struck: in the next year, on being appointed to the HMS *Victor*, he was rather harshly court-martialled for an episode of drunkenness. He was dismissed from his ship and put on half pay, his chances of further promotion destroyed. He reacted energetically, however, and in 1851 obtained membership of the Royal College of Surgeons in London, later taking the LKQCPI (1859) and MRCPI (1881). He had kept in touch with medical affairs in Belfast and had a home address in the centre of the town throughout the 1840s. It was in this period that he developed an interest in ophthalmic problems, and from the opening of his eye dispensary (outpatients clinic) in 1845, he saw about one thousand patients yearly. About 2 per cent of these were patients with cataracts, and permanent relief by surgery was obtained in half of them. He also treated patients with other problems, so with a well-supported case for ophthalmic beds he was strongly placed for election to the post of Attending Surgeon in 1851. Dr Browne devoted himself to surgery and particularly ophthalmic surgery in the Belfast General Hospital and from 1867 in the Belfast Ophthalmic Hospital. He retired in 1875, the year after the opening of the Benn Eye, Ear and Throat Hospital. He was Lord Mayor of Belfast in 1870 and after his retirement was appointed Chief Sanitary Officer in 1876 and in 1880 the first Chief Medical Officer of Health – surely a dramatic overturning of his earlier rebuffs. He married a Miss Walton and his children included a son, John Walton Browne, who succeeded his father as Attending Surgeon to the Belfast Royal Hospital in 1875.

John Walton Browne had studied at Queen's College Belfast, and had an MD of the Queen's University in Ireland as well as a MRCSE. He undertook postgraduate studies in eye, ear and throat diseases in London and Vienna before returning to Belfast. Originally his main interest in the Belfast Royal Hospital was in ophthalmic surgery, but by 1883 he saw the chance to move towards general surgery. In 1899 he was elected chairman of the medical staff, and he gave the welcoming address to the King and Queen at the opening of the new Royal Victoria Hospital in July 1903. He retired in 1912, became Deputy Lieutenant for Belfast in 1913, and was knighted in 1921. He had always worked in the Ophthalmic Hospital and even though now retired, he worked there throughout World War One. He died in 1923, leaving his considerable fortune to the Royal Victoria Hospital.

Dr Joseph Nelson was appointed in 1883 as Attending Surgeon for the Eye, Ear, Nose and Throat (EENT) Department of the Belfast Royal Hospital when Dr Walton Browne changed to general surgery. He was

Dr Samuel Browne RN, the father of ophthalmology in Belfast and Attending Surgeon to the Belfast General Hospital, 1851–75
ROYAL VICTORIA HOSPITAL

another son of a Presbyterian minister (indeed of the nine preceding generations, eight of his forefathers were ministers). He was born in Downpatrick, County Down, where his father was the Non-Subscribing minister, and he started medicine conventionally in 1858 at Queen's College Belfast. After two years, however, he became inspired by the ideals of Giuseppe Garibaldi and set off with another student to join Garibaldi's Red Shirts at Genoa. He was commissioned as lieutenant in the famous Regimento Inglese, campaigned through Sicily, fighting in the Battle of Volturno, and received the Sword of Honour from the great patriot himself as well as medals from the new king of all Italy, Victor Emmanuel. He survived the gruelling battles, both in the open and in cities such as Palermo, without a scratch, and in late 1860 he returned to his studies, qualifying as an MD and LRCSI in 1863. After the dramatic start to his career he could not easily settle down, and he set off for India to work as surgeon on a tea plantation. He managed to combine medicine, fighting in a minor expedition and running several estates, but in particular he developed an interest in diseases of the eye. After he returned to Ireland in 1877, he studied ophthalmology in Dublin and Vienna in order to equip himself for a specialist appointment in both the Belfast Royal Hospital and the Belfast Hospital for Sick Children. As one would expect from such a career, Dr Nelson had a wide knowledge of life and was an inspiring teacher and a flamboyant host. Although he had responsibility for the whole field of EENT diseases, it was ophthalmic work that dominated his attention, though surprisingly that included very little cataract surgery. It was probably the difficulty of providing anaesthesia and the risk of a dangerous infection that delayed progress in ear, nose and throat surgery into the twentieth century. Dr Nelson retired in 1905 and was given 'a handsome service of plate' by his colleagues.

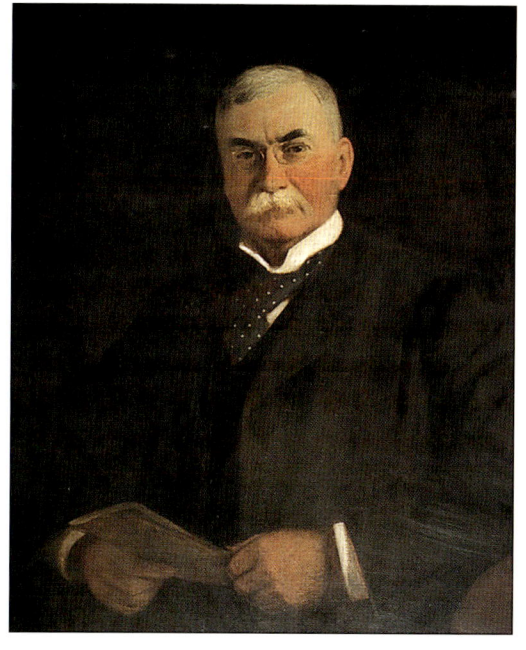

Dr Joseph Nelson, Attending Ophthalmic Surgeon to the Belfast Royal Hospital, 1883–1905
ULSTER MEDICAL SOCIETY

DENTISTRY, PATHOLOGY AND DERMATOLOGY

In 1881 John Clough Clarke LDS, RCS was appointed honorary Dentist. In that year alone, 3,900 patients received treatment in the Belfast Royal Hospital for diseases of the teeth. One of the first dentists in Belfast to hold a British dental qualification, Clarke was given the use of a room in the extern department on three mornings a week together with the initial sum of £5 to purchase dental instruments. He had a large private practice in Belfast and was noted for his advocacy of nitrous oxide anaesthesia in dental work. When he died in 1894, he was replaced as honorary Dentist by Mr George Campbell LDS, but after only two years he was asked to resign. No replacement was made until the new Royal Victoria Hospital was opened in 1903.

There were no facilities for the study of pathology in the hospital until 1884, when the medical staff took note of the problem. From this date the surgeon Dr Henry O'Neill worked unofficially as a pathologist and began teaching medical students. In 1888 it was decided to set up a pathological museum and in 1890 it was recorded that 'a pathologist's room, the first in the history of the hospital, has been fitted up'. In 1888 too the first pathologist, Dr Henry Burden, was appointed. He resigned in 1892 and died the following year; his post was left vacant until Dr James Lorrain Smith was appointed in 1895 as hospital Pathologist and lecturer in Pathology at Queen's College. In 1901 Dr Smith was appointed the first Musgrave Professor of Pathology. He held this post until 1904 when he was elected to the chair of Pathology at the Victoria University of Manchester. Until the arrival of Dr Smith very few postmortem examinations were carried out; but by gentle persuasion he was able to increase relatives' awareness of their need. His presence ensured that when the new hospital was being planned, provision was made for a special building to be set aside as a mortuary, postmortem room and laboratory.

A large number of skin complaints presented themselves for treatment in the extern clinics including psoriasis, scabies and tinea, and many of these patients required admission to hospital. Attending Physician Dr Henry Purdon, who had an interest in dermatology (see pages 47–48), resigned in 1882, leaving a vacuum in treatment, and the question of establishing a separate department was discussed in 1889–90. Only in 1900, however, was an Attending Physician given special responsibility for the Dermatological Department; he was Dr William Calwell (see page 48). He had many other interests, however, and it remained a minor speciality, largely confined to outpatients, until well into the twentieth century.

THE THRONE HOSPITAL

The figures for duration of hospital stay in the mid-nineteenth century were surprisingly high by present standards – as already noted, a mean of twenty-five days is given in the annual report for 1863. This long stay was required because on leaving hospital patients had to be reasonably fit and able to go back to often poor and ill-equipped homes. As a result, beds in the hospital would be blocked and patients with acute illnesses would have to be turned away. However, in 1872 John Martin of Shrigley, County Down, gave the General Hospital a tract of about 28 acres known as the Throne Lands. These were situated about five miles from the centre of Belfast, between the road to Antrim and the lough shore, and well away from the smoky atmosphere of the town. They were ideal for convalescents and long-stay patients, and steps were soon taken to establish a convalescent hospital, first for children, and after 1877, for adults.

The original gift of land by John Martin was made in memory of his son, a life governor who died of a violent fever; donors for the building included Edward Benn (£1,000), John Charters (£1,000), Lady Johnston (£500) and William Dunville (£300). Once opened in 1874, the Throne Hospital remained closely associated with the Belfast Royal Hospital and its successor the Royal Victoria Hospital, and its annual report was published along with theirs until 1948.

When the Throne Hospital opened, access to it was difficult but by 1884, when a meeting of the British Medical Association (BMA) was held in Belfast, the steam tram service on the Antrim Road had just been started. Children remained the principal group of patients at the Throne Hospital for many years, the majority of them suffering bone and joint tuberculosis. At this time and well into the twentieth century, tuberculosis anywhere in the body was treated by rest and fresh air, and in many cases this therapy lasted for a year or more. The hospital had an energetic Ladies' Committee which supplied additional food, clothes and toys for the children; one little boy called Tommy Vane who was there for three years (1886–89) is recorded as having received a suit of clothes on one occasion and a box of bricks on another.

In 1885 there was no specific provision in Belfast for treatment of pulmonary tuberculosis, or consumption as it was usually known. In that year Forster Green donated £5,000 to the Throne Hospital for the establishment of a consumptive hospital (or unit) there. This was only used for the treatment of advanced cases of the disease and, since there was no really effective treatment, there was a high mortality. The unit provided valuable nursing care for this terrible scourge, however, and served to isolate these patients until an even more generous donation from Forster Green established the Forster Green Hospital in 1896 on the outskirts of south Belfast. The consumptive unit of the Throne Hospital was in the charge successively of Dr (later Professor) James Lindsay, Dr Strafford Smith and Dr William Calwell.

NURSING IN THE NIGHTINGALE ERA

Training of the nurses for most of the nineteenth century was nonexistent, and indeed it was only in the 1870s that doctors at the General Hospital began to see that organised nursing measures such as cleanliness, antisepsis and isolation of infected patients were valuable. Perhaps it was an episode of smallpox spreading via patients and nurses from the smallpox wards to the surgical patients that alerted the hospital doctors to a serious problem. At that time nurses' training schools were being set up in England; the first had been established at St Thomas's by Florence Nightingale herself in 1860, and another began in Liverpool in 1862. The planned training at Belfast General Hospital was sparse, but at least there was a three-year course with some lectures in the first year and an organised apprenticeship

No 45
9. March

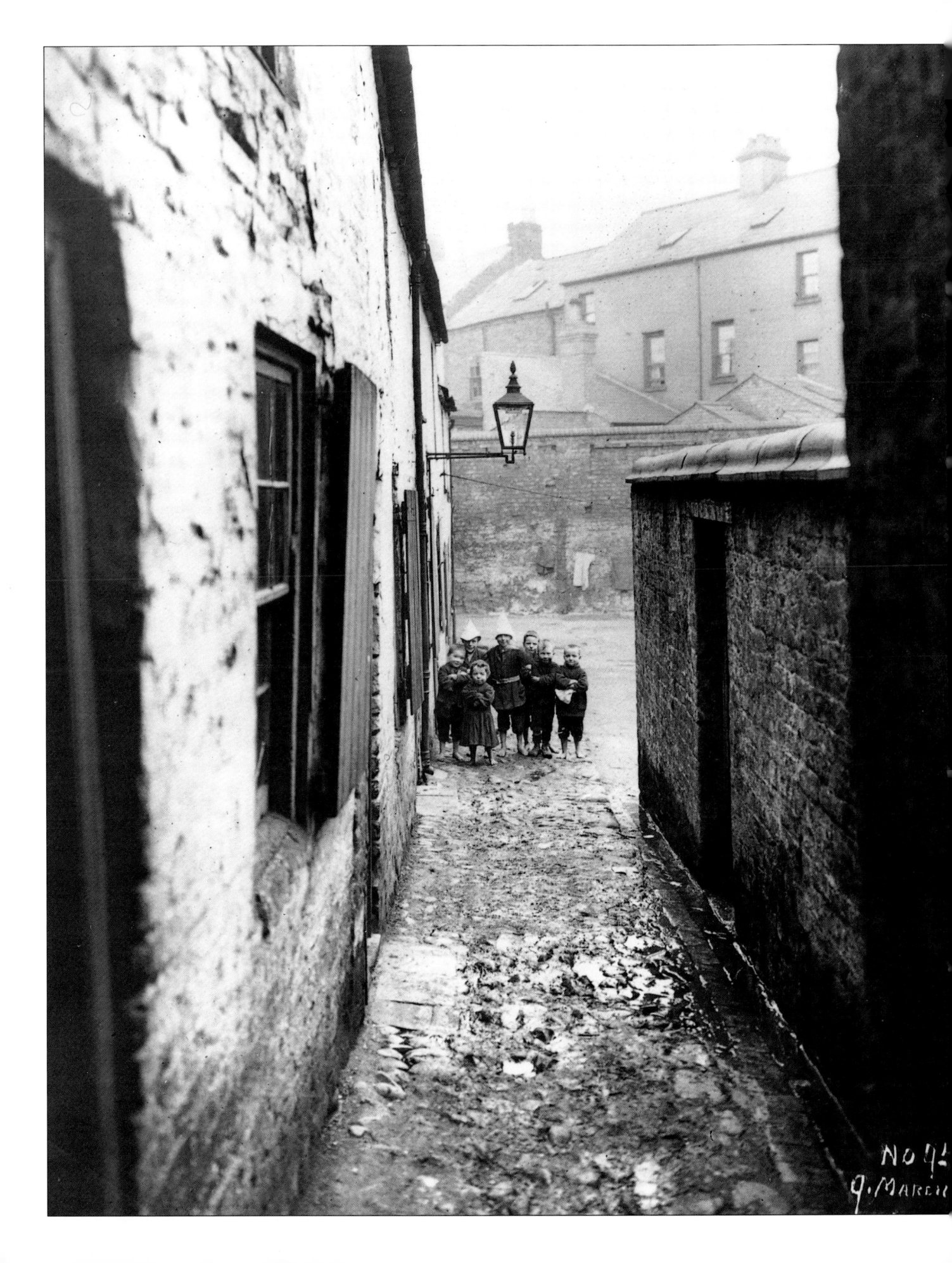

in the wards throughout. A nurses' home was opened at 2 Frederick Street (opposite the hospital) in 1872. The nurses in the home were under the care of a lady superintendent (rather than the hospital housekeeper), but the doctors still insisted on ultimate control. Some nurses were still kept in the hospital itself, sleeping in the damp basement, in case they were needed in an emergency.

From the nurses' point of view the most useful change that came with the opening of the nurses' home was being relieved of the heavier cleaning chores by extra ward maids. Ward maids had to be paid, however, whereas, in their first year at least, probationer nurses cost the hospital nothing. Necessary economies left these nurses still scrubbing floors daily into the 1890s.

Finance for the training system came partly from fundraising but mainly from fees charged for private nursing which some of the probationer nurses had to do in their second and third years. On completion of training, each nurse was given a testimonial, but from 1890 a more rigorous system with examinations and certificates was introduced. With the high demand for private nurses in Belfast, the home planned to take in more nurses than the hospital needed, so that the surplus would be available for paid private nursing. The money that the nurses earned would then be used to finance the home and help towards the cost of the hospital nurses. The house at 2 Frederick Street soon proved inadequate, so the adjoining house was rented, and in 1875 a purpose-built, four-storey nurses' home was opened at 32 Frederick Street.

Administrative arrangements were far from satisfactory; the lady superintendent and Ladies' Committee ran the home in frequent conflict with the hospital. The main source of conflict was financial for it was quite impossible for the nurses' home to be self-financing while nurses were provided free to the hospital. During the 1880s and 1890s the hospital was persuaded to pay annually for each nurse according to her year of training. Then there were personality clashes over who had the ultimate authority over the nurses. In 1874 the Board of Management issued a new rule (or a reversion to the 1832 rule) that the resident House Surgeon would have the power, with the concurrence of a member of the board, a senior doctor or the Housekeeper, to fine or dismiss any nurse for neglect or improper conduct. The lady superintendent resigned following this erosion of her authority; indeed there were eight lady superintendents over the fifteen years 1872–87. As the row continued, in 1875 there appeared an anonymous letter about the home in the *Belfast News-Letter* and Miss Otway, honorary secretary of the Ladies' Committee of the nurses' home, wrote to say, 'It strikes me that all this has arisen from the hospital Board forgetting they have given up having any nurses of their own.' However after this exchange her own committee forced her to resign. Other points of conflict included the home taking a nurse away from the hospital to

Opposite:
A group of Belfast children living in slum conditions at the turn of the century; photograph by A.R. Hogg
ULSTER MUSEUM

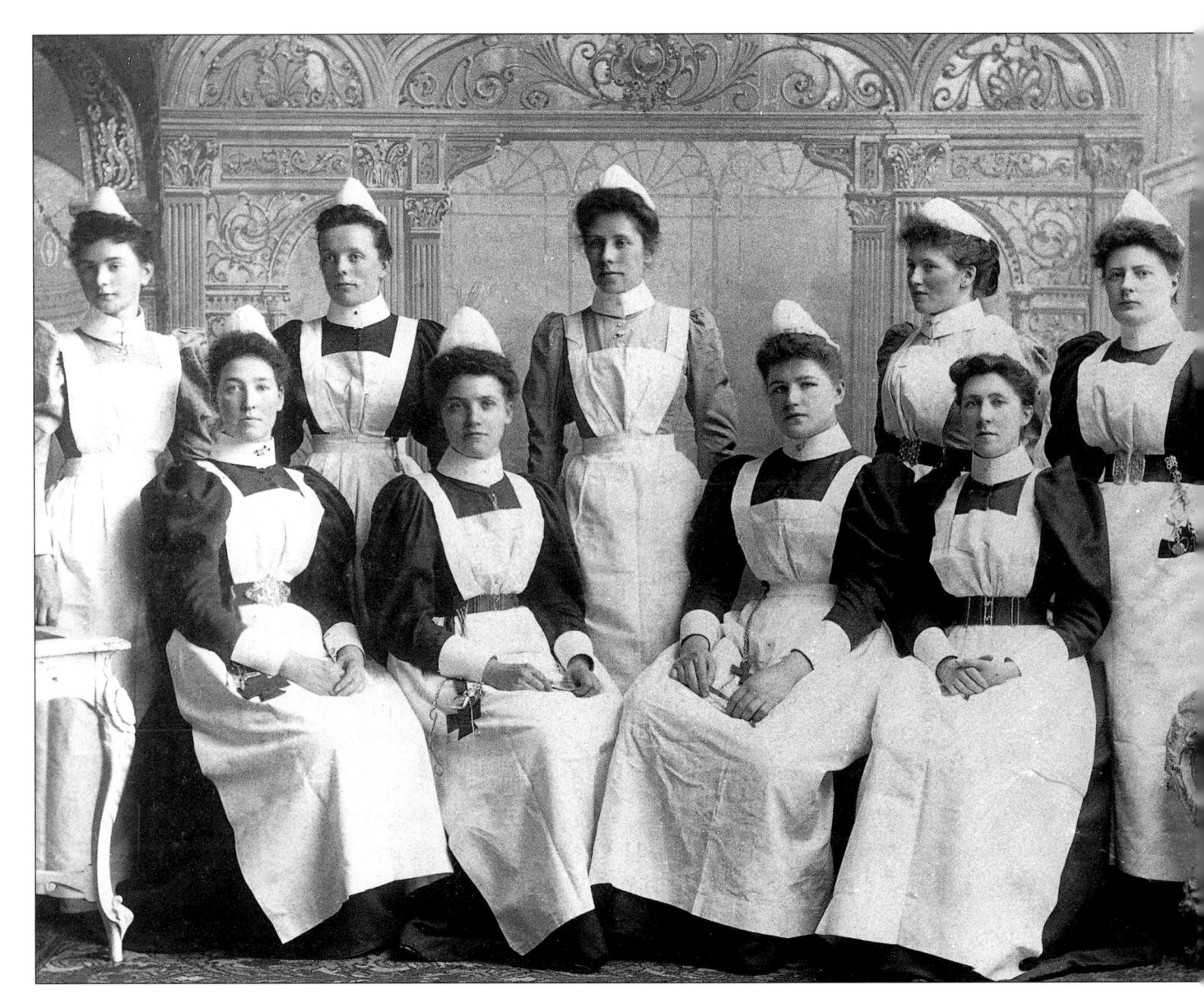

A group of recently qualified nurses in 1895: Marianne Harden, *front left*, said that her abiding memory of this period was of endless floor scrubbing.
ROYAL VICTORIA HOSPITAL

nurse privately, and such trivial matters as the state of the hospital mattresses. The most successful of the lady superintendents was Miss Lydia Newman, who had trained at St Bartholomew's Hospital, London, and who remained at the Belfast Royal and later the Royal Victoria Hospital from 1886 to 1928. Because of its financial basis, the nurses' home continued to function as a private nursing agency when the hospital moved in 1903; it was eventually destroyed in the German air raids of 1941.

Nursing uniform in the mid-nineteenth century included bonnets and buttoned jackets, which were the height of fashion at that time. By 1895, however, when we have the first group photographs of the hospital's nurses, the uniform was essentially that familiar to us throughout the twentieth century. It included a small cap – not by any means covering the hair as has often been suggested – and an apron of the classical style. Both apron and the blue dress underneath extended, of course, below the ankles; just as nowadays, they were worn with a tight belt with (usually) a silver buckle. The fact that the nurses in that 1895 photograph are not smiling as they would be now is probably a result of the problems of long-exposure photography, rather than of any severity in the ethos or discipline.

In the five decades before this first group photograph was taken, the hospital had undergone many changes. Since 1847, when it had become a general rather than a fever hospital, the hospital had grown enormously, and the royal charter was a worthy recognition of this. Its medical and nursing staff had more than doubled and it was a momentous half-century particularly in terms of surgical advances. In earlier times it had been a small provincial hospital coping with epidemic after epidemic as best it could. Now it was undertaking regular planned admissions, though pressure on it as the town's main accident hospital was already heavy. Finally, it was a centre of medical teaching, with distinguished chairs and a steady flow of students studying for their MB degrees (even if they still had to go to Dublin to be awarded them). Nevertheless the expansion and success were to bring intolerable pressures before the end of the century.

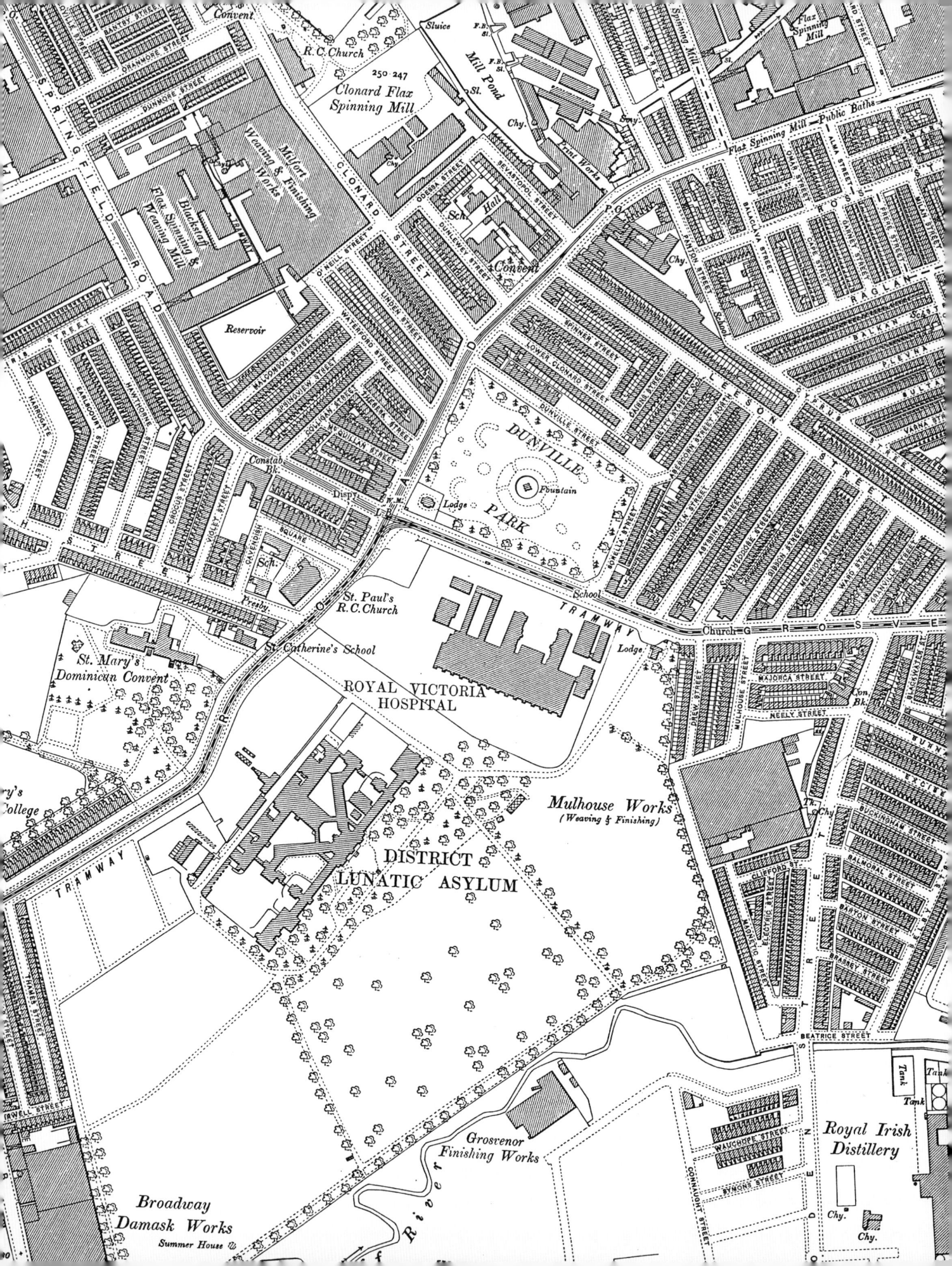

ROYAL VICTORIA HOSPITAL

DISTRICT LUNATIC ASYLUM

Mulhouse Works (Weaving & Finishing)

Dunville Park

Clonard Flax Spinning Mill

St. Paul's R.C. Church

St. Catherine's School

St. Mary's Dominican Convent

Grosvenor Finishing Works

Broadway Damask Works

Royal Irish Distillery

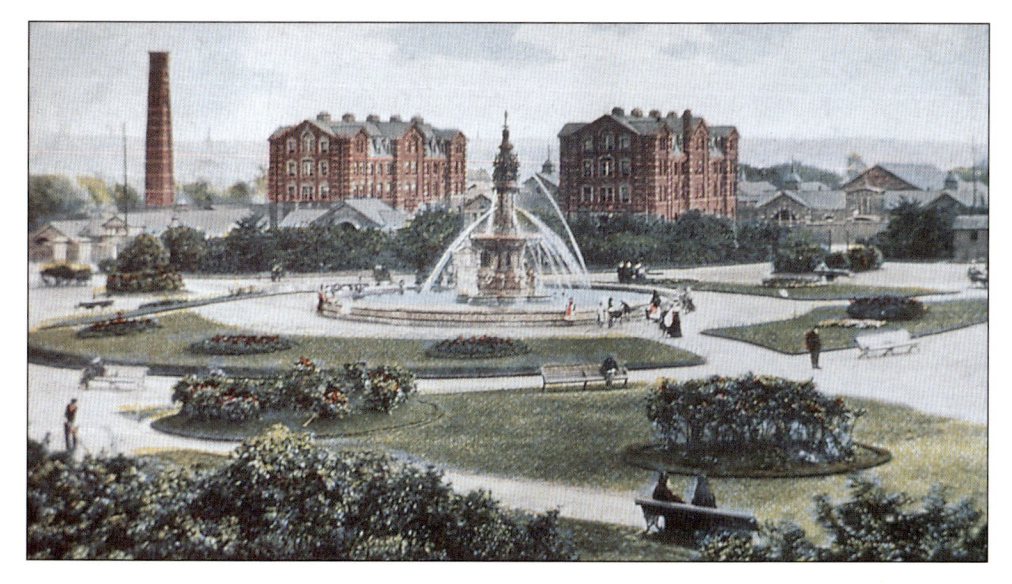

View of Dunville Park, *c.* 1905, given to the city by Robert Dunville in 1889, with its formal lawns, flowerbeds and terracotta fountain: behind are the East and West wings of the Royal Victoria Hospital, the tall chimney to the left and the extern building to the right
ROYAL VICTORIA HOSPITAL

3
THE ROYAL VICTORIA HOSPITAL BUILDING AND ADMINISTRATION
1903–1948

Opposite:
Map of 1907 showing the Royal Victoria Hospital in a corner of the large asylum grounds: to the north is Dunville Park; the main entrance to the asylum, with its gate lodge on Grosvenor Street (now Grosvenor Road), is the start of the present hospital road.
ORDNANCE SURVEY OF NORTHERN IRELAND

THERE WAS INCREASING DISSATISFACTION IN THE 1890s with the site of the Belfast Royal Hospital in Frederick Street which had become more and more cramped, but extension was almost impossible. The Charters and Mulholland wings had been completed as far back as 1866, but the population of the city had risen from 175,000 in 1871 to double that figure in 1901. By the turn of the century Belfast was one of the great commercial cities of the British Empire. It was the centre of the Ulster linen industry, the home of the great

65

shipyards Harland and Wolff and Workman Clark, and of a large ropeworks and a major harbour. Everywhere there were visible signs of prosperity; a new City Hall would be completed in 1906 and Queen's College would be upgraded to Queen's University in 1908.

The prosperity did not benefit everyone equally, however. Much of the population was now concentrated to the west of the centre, round the linen mills, and as a result there was heavy air pollution both from domestic fires and factory chimneys. Doctors had already begun to move away from College Square to the more salubrious University Square and College Gardens, and the more prosperous classes were spreading out along the Malone ridge. Housing for the poor was slow to improve and although rear access was mandatory for all houses built after 1878, at the turn of the century there were still twenty thousand houses without back access, and all their refuse, including the contents of the dry privy, had to be carried out through the living room into the street.

Meanwhile the demands on the hospital were increasing in spite of the elaborate vetting scheme. Those who were subscribers through contributions at their workplace, or were recommended by annual subscribers, were accepted as patients after examination by a doctor. Others were questioned closely about their financial resources because, as a notice in the extern said, 'This Hospital is for the Poor. Advice and Treatment are intended only for those who are unable to pay for medical attendance. The Visiting staff give their services free.' Paying patients were taken into the hospital and made a significant contribution to the funds, but their proportion had fallen over the previous half-century and was down to about 10 per cent by 1900. The alternative, of course, was treatment at home or in a nursing home, and these remained the options for those who could afford them until the advent of the National Health Service. However, in the new century, particularly after the advent of National Insurance in 1911, the less prosperous middle-class patients who had probably made donations to the Royal Victoria Hospital were beginning to feel that they should have access to it, free or at low cost. In the case of more complicated surgery this was also much safer than management outside hospital.

At the end of the nineteenth century the number of beds in the hospital had been constant for some years at about 186; of these 55 were in the fever wards and reserved for contagious cases. The case for rebuilding was made in considerable detail by Professor Whitla at the annual meeting of subscribers on 16 November 1896. Essentially he argued that patients were constantly being refused admission and despite recent upgrading of the theatres, the old buildings were inadequate. Belfast had 470 hospital beds in its various institutions whereas Dublin, Edinburgh and Glasgow had about twice as many per head of population. His case was supported by the great educationalist and philanthropist Vere Foster and other committee members, and a rebuilding fund was launched three weeks later.

FUNDING AND PLANNING

The Lord Mayor, William James Pirrie, was asked to convene a special meeting in December to discuss fund raising for the rebuilding and was subsequently elected chairman of the executive committee set up. The meeting took place in the old town hall in Victoria Street and immediately large sums for a rebuilding fund were forthcoming. The Lord Mayor gave £5,000 and the Lady Mayoress gave £2,000; Pirrie's own business, Harland and Wolff, gave £5,000, and there were many donations of lesser sums, so that by the end of the first day over £20,000 had been subscribed. The target aimed for was £100,000, enough to erect a hospital of 300 beds on a new site with plenty of room for expansion. By January 1897 the list of subscriptions totalled £40,000 and included £5,000 from the York Street Flax Spinning Company and £1,300 from the medical and surgical staff of the Belfast Royal Hospital. Thanks to widespread efforts throughout the north of Ireland the target of £100,000 was reached by July 1897; all subsequent donations were credited to an endowment fund.

Ground-floor plan of the Royal Victoria Hospital, showing Grosvenor Street (now Grosvenor Road) in the foreground, from which the main entrance leads directly between the East and West wings to the front door. Beyond this are the 'connecting corridor' and the original seventeen wards; to the left of the entrance are the boiler house, ventilation and laundry blocks, and to the right are the extern building, mortuary ('pathological') and ophthalmic and isolation wards.

ROYAL VICTORIA HOSPITAL

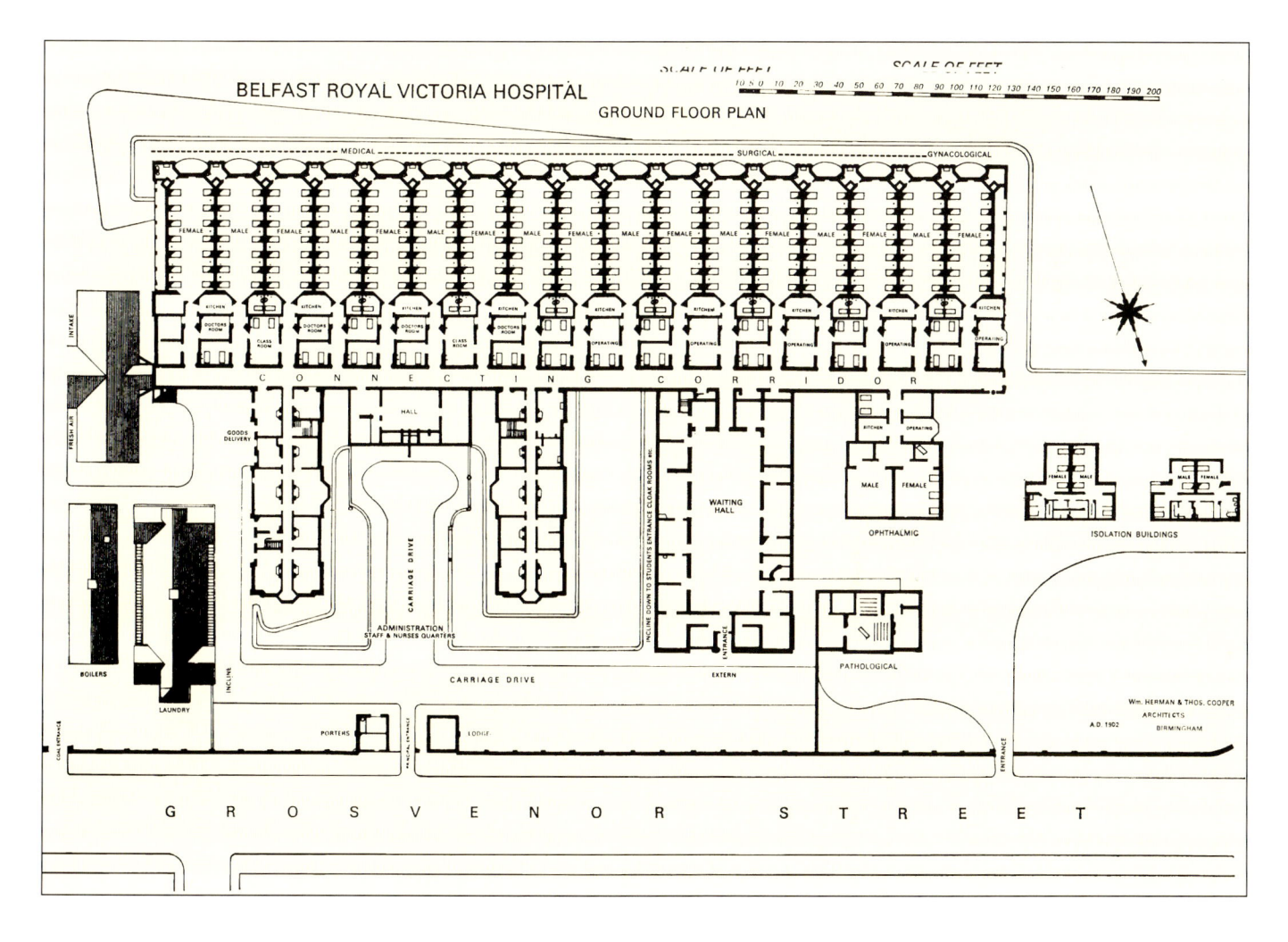

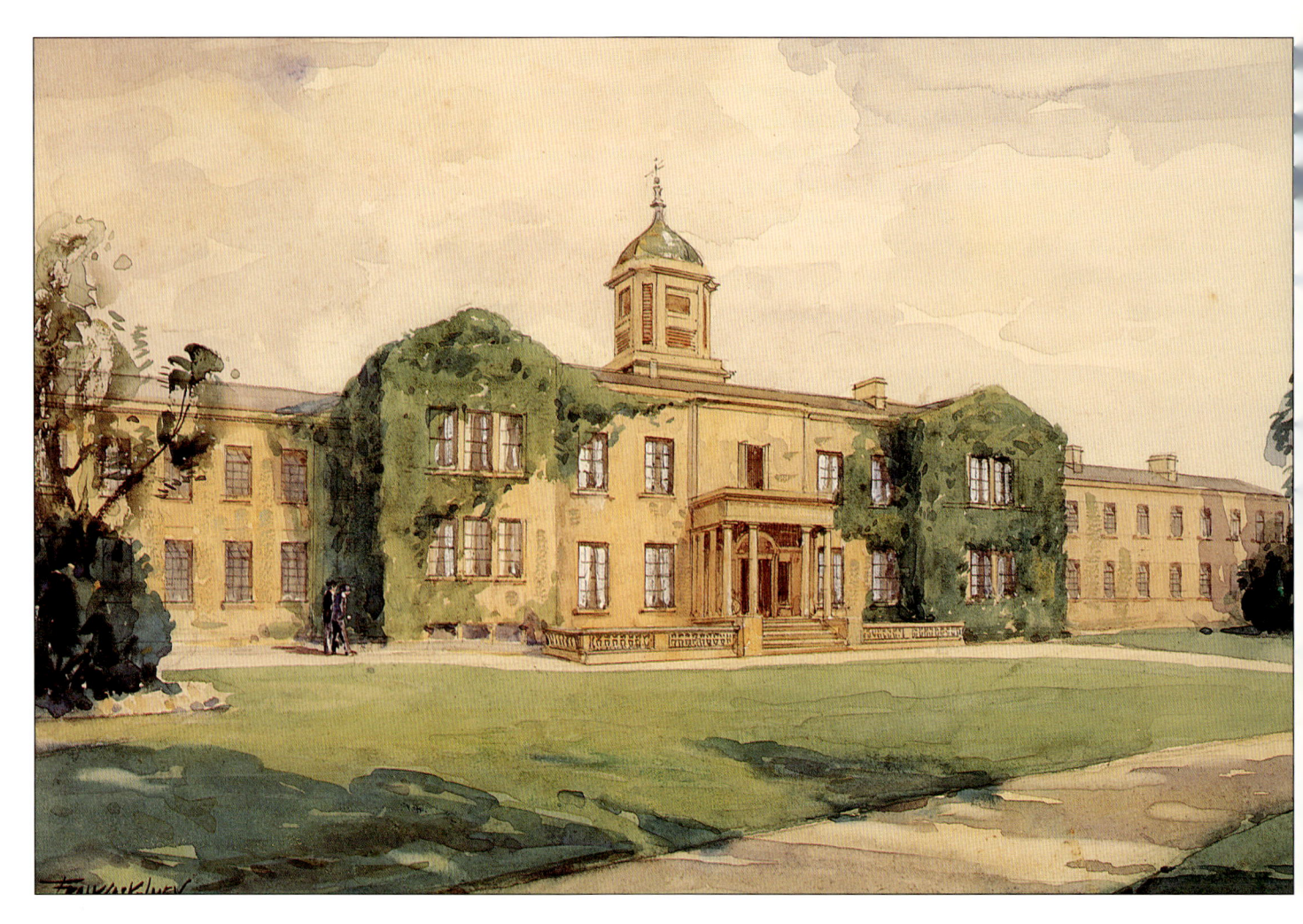

The Belfast Lunatic Asylum, from a watercolour by Frank McKelvey: the asylum was in the middle of the grounds at present occupied by the Royal Group of Hospitals, approximately where the Royal Maternity Hospital now stands. Although Purdysburn Hospital was opened for patients in 1906, the old asylum continued to be used throughout World War One and remained standing in a dilapidated state until *c.* 1930.
ULSTER MUSEUM,
COPYRIGHT ROBERT McKELVEY, ESQ.

While funds were being raised, special committees looked into other matters, the most urgent being the finding of a site for the new hospital. The places considered were at Peter's Hill, the Belfast Flour Mill site on the Falls Road, the Victoria Barracks, the Poor House, Ormeau Park, and the Lunatic Asylum grounds to the west of the city centre, but only the last of these was satisfactory when financial and other restrictions were considered. The aim had been to acquire 10 acres, but the site committee was prepared to accept the 4 acres at the corner between the Falls Road and Grosvenor Street (now Grosvenor Road), on the understanding that if and when the asylum vacated the site the hospital could acquire the remainder. Negotiations with the asylum and Belfast Corporation, which effectively controlled the site, lasted throughout 1897 but by December a construction committee, also chaired by W.J. Pirrie, was approved and the detailed planning and building stage could begin. The minutes include a reference to a Mr O'Neill's public house at the corner of the Falls Road and Grosvenor Road, which had to be bought for demolition in 1899.

In the meantime a nursing committee met in December 1897 and resolved to change the system of management of the nurses when the hospital moved. In Frederick Street the nurses lived in the self-financing nurses' home, controlled by an independent management committee and a lady superintendent. For the new hospital it was proposed that the nurses should live in a block that was part of the hospital (later known as the West Wing) and that the superintendent of the nurses should be appointed by and responsible to the hospital. The new block would provide separate bedrooms for up to eighty nurses as well as the necessary domestic servants. The cost of the new arrangements would be £2,500–£3,000 annually.

The executive committee and the new construction committee met monthly from December 1897, both chaired by the Lord Mayor. The first requirement was to take soundings from the medical staff on the type of hospital that was required. After this an architect could be appointed and detailed plans drawn up. Almost half the members of the construction committee were medical staff (Professor Cuming, Dr Lindsay, Dr Mitchell, Professor Whitla, Professor Byers and Dr Nelson). The executive committee, on the other hand, was entirely composed of lay members, with the exception of Professor Whitla. The lay people over the years of building consisted of prominent figures in business and the Churches such as the Right Honourable Thomas Sinclair, Sir Daniel Dixon, Sir William Crawford, James Cunningham, Otto Jaffe, Henry Musgrave, the Moderator of the Presbyterian Church and Dean Seaver, together with two from the Working Men's Committee and a number of ladies.

The medical staff felt that the new building should provide the following facilities, giving 296 beds in total:

1 a large extern waiting room with small rooms surrounding it
2 an administrative block to include resident doctors' accommodation and rooms for the superintendent
3 a nurses' block with accommodation for 100 nurses
4 a block for teaching, with a lecture theatre and an operating theatre
5 a block for mortuary, postmortem examinations and pathology
6 an isolation block for 24 medical (fever) cases and 8 surgical cases
7 8 large wards and 8 small wards and a 4-bed delirium tremens ward.

The engine room with the steam-engines which drove the fans for the Plenum ventilation system via shafts and belting
ROYAL VICTORIA HOSPITAL

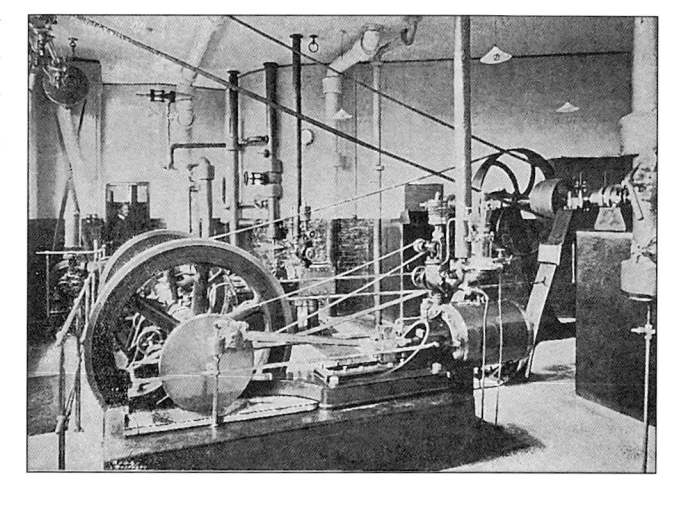

The layout of the hospital would be totally dependent on the type of ventilation adopted and by January 1898 opinion was already divided. A new hospital had opened in Birmingham in 1896 with a novel method of artificial ventilation known as the Plenum System. Its function was to provide all the patient accommodation with air that was fresh, clean and warmed. It meant that there would be no possibility of opening windows and no coal fires. The architect of the Birmingham General Hospital, William Henman FRIBA, believed that the best way to use the Plenum System was to have the wards side by side in a continuous block with roof lighting throughout. He had extolled the virtues of such a system in an article in the *Builder* of 1896, and on the strength of this he was invited to Belfast. Members of the subcommittee responsible for appointing an architect had already visited hospitals in England, including Birmingham, and by December 1898 the company of William Henman and Thomas Cooper was appointed.

The fact that it had taken most of 1898 to come to this decision is an indication that there was a considerable degree of dispute among the medical staff and reluctance on the part of some to abandon the old maxim of 'the open window'. Professor Cuming on the appointment committee was highly respected, however, and carried along with him Dr Lindsay, Professor Byers and Professor Whitla so that gradually the doubters were won over.

The other major change to the medical staff's plans was that they reduced greatly the concept of an isolation block. The old fever hospital had not given up all such patients when the Union Infirmary and the new Union Fever Hospital were opened in the 1840s, and the old isolation block remained at the back of Frederick Street. The medical patients had mainly typhoid, diphtheria and scarlatina, while there continued to be surgical patients with cellulitis and erysipelas. The medical staff therefore felt that isolation beds were needed in order to maintain the status of a complete teaching hospital and to cope with fevers and severe sepsis whether from within the hospital or admitted from outside. However, the medical staff paid only lip service to isolation and could still suggest that 'patients suffering from typhoid fever could be nursed in the ordinary wards'. The first medical staff scheme asked for 24 fever beds and 8 surgical beds but these numbers were reduced to a maximum of 8 fever and 8 surgical beds in the final plans. The argument for a smaller isolation unit was helped by plans for the opening of a new fever hospital at Purdysburn, to the south of Belfast, though in fact this did not come into operation until 1906. At the same time pressure for general beds was reduced by the opening of the greatly enlarged Mater Infirmorum Hospital in 1899–1900, with 150 beds. The Mater hospital had been opened in 1883 by the Sisters of Mercy and from that time had been in the attractive Bedeque House on the Crumlin Road. It had recently proved quite inadequate and was demolished to make way for the larger building.

THE REVISED CHARTER

It was felt that a new hospital justified a new charter, and the most obvious feature of the revised charter of 1899 was the change of the hospital's name from the Belfast Royal Hospital to the Royal Victoria Hospital. Under the new charter, the sums required for becoming a life governor were essentially unaltered but the conditions were broadened to allow previous donations to be taken into account when deciding eligibility.

Eligibility for the title 'annual subscriber' was broadened to include those who paid one guinea a year; these contributors were entitled to recommend for treatment one intern and two extern patients per year. The number of patients a subscriber could recommend increased steadily with the size of subscription paid, up to £40 per year. Likewise church ministers and managers of businesses received entitlement to recommend patients in proportion to the sums collected in their organisations. These privileges were valuable in a time of much greater general poverty than now, and no significant provision of health care, but they did cause trouble in extern departments between those recommended by subscribers and those who arrived without a 'line'. The life governors and annual subscribers amounted to over eight hundred individuals in 1900 and were all represented on the General Committee by about sixty members. This number was again further reduced in the more workable Board of Management, which had around thirty members. New regulations suggested that one-fifth of the General Committee should if possible be ladies, and on the Board of Management there should be a total of six.

THE PIRRIE FAMILY

The work of Dr John Miller Pirrie, Attending and Consulting Physician to the hospital, has been already described (see pages 46–47). Dr Pirrie died in 1873; some two decades later, his nephew William James Pirrie, though not a doctor, was to play perhaps an even more important role in the development of the hospital.

After education at the Royal Belfast Academical Institution, William Pirrie entered the newly established company of Harland and Wolff in 1862 as an apprentice. Twelve years later, when still only twenty-seven, he became a partner; he eventually became chairman, and remained the ruler and driving force of the company until his death. William Pirrie became Lord Mayor of Belfast early in 1896 and this led to his involvement with the various committees for the new hospital, though he had already been a life governor since 1892. He used his role with Harland and Wolff on several occasions to benefit the hospital, notably at the launch of the *Oceanic* in January 1899, when money raised from the sale of tickets to a specially constructed stand was donated to the rebuilding fund. Again in 1910, when the first of the giant liners, the *Olympic*, was launched, tickets were sold to spectators and £456 was raised for the hospital; there was also a public viewing for the ship's refitting in 1920 in aid of the hospital. William Pirrie tried to keep out of politics but, whilst certainly a Unionist, he had distinct sympathies with the concept of Home Rule, and this estranged him from hard-line Unionist opinion. There was an unpleasant incident at the opening of the new hospital in 1903 when the King remarked to Mr Pirrie, 'And so, Mr Pirrie,

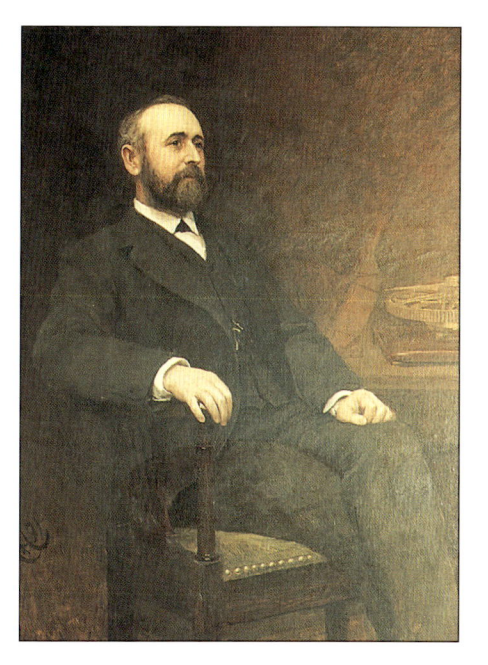

William Pirrie, Chairman of Harland and Wolff, Lord Mayor of Belfast, and Chairman of the Executive Committee and Construction Committee for the new hospital
ROYAL VICTORIA HOSPITAL

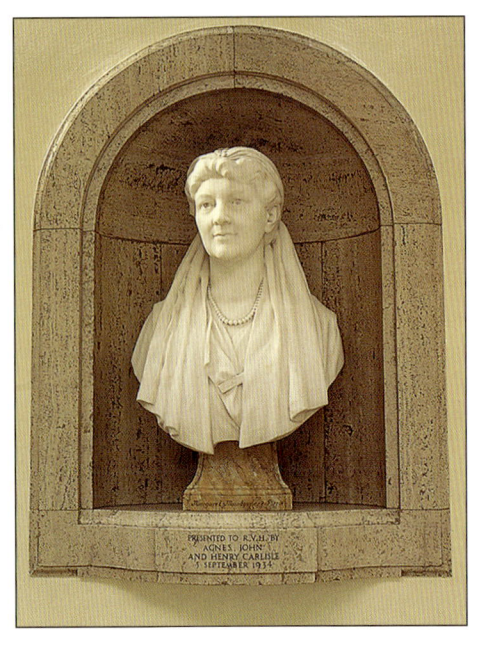

this significant building is your great work.' Pirrie bowed modestly in acknowledgement, but a third gentleman brusquely interposed, 'Yes, his wife collected the money.'

William Pirrie continued to chair the construction committee until its winding-up in 1904 and made a final donation of £11,000 to enable the hospital buildings to be opened free of debt. He was created Baron Pirrie in 1906 and died on 7 June 1924; he is buried in the City Cemetery. He and his wife Margaret had no children, and this must partly explain their generosity in time and money to a cause they valued.

Lady Pirrie was not content with simply donating money, however; she chaired the Ladies' Committee and the Nursing Committee and was, indeed, probably even more involved in the new hospital than her husband, not only raising £10,000 for naming Ward 5 but also collecting over £100,000 for naming beds. In the course of her life she did more for the hospital than any other single benefactor, and she was president of the hospital from 1914 until her death in 1935.

Bust of Margaret Montgomery Pirrie, Lady Mayoress, and the major fundraiser for the new hospital; by A. Bertram Pegram
ROYAL VICTORIA HOSPITAL

DESIGN AND BUILDING OF THE HOSPITAL

During the early months of 1899 planning of the hospital took shape. It was based on the original staff request (see page 69) and 300 beds were to be divided as follows:

8 medical and 8 surgical wards (16 beds each)	256 beds
1 gynaecological ward	18 beds
1 ophthalmic ward (across the corridor)	6 beds
1 isolation ward for medical (fever) cases	8 beds
1 isolation ward for infected surgical cases	8 beds
1 ward for patients with delirium tremens	4 beds
	300 beds

Each ward unit was to consist of a long open ward of fourteen beds and a two-bed side ward as well as a number of shared doctors' offices and classrooms, a kitchen and, for the general surgical wards, a total of four operating theatres. The gynaecological and ophthalmic units were similarly independent, with their own theatres. The extern waiting hall and its accompanying examination rooms were across the corridor from Ward 12; the isolation buildings were to the west of this. The resident doctors, nurses and domestics, as well as the administration, were to be accommodated in the East and West wings and the low building adjacent to the corridor; the connecting block on the north side did not come until later. The wings initially included a suite of rooms for the Medical Superintendent. The

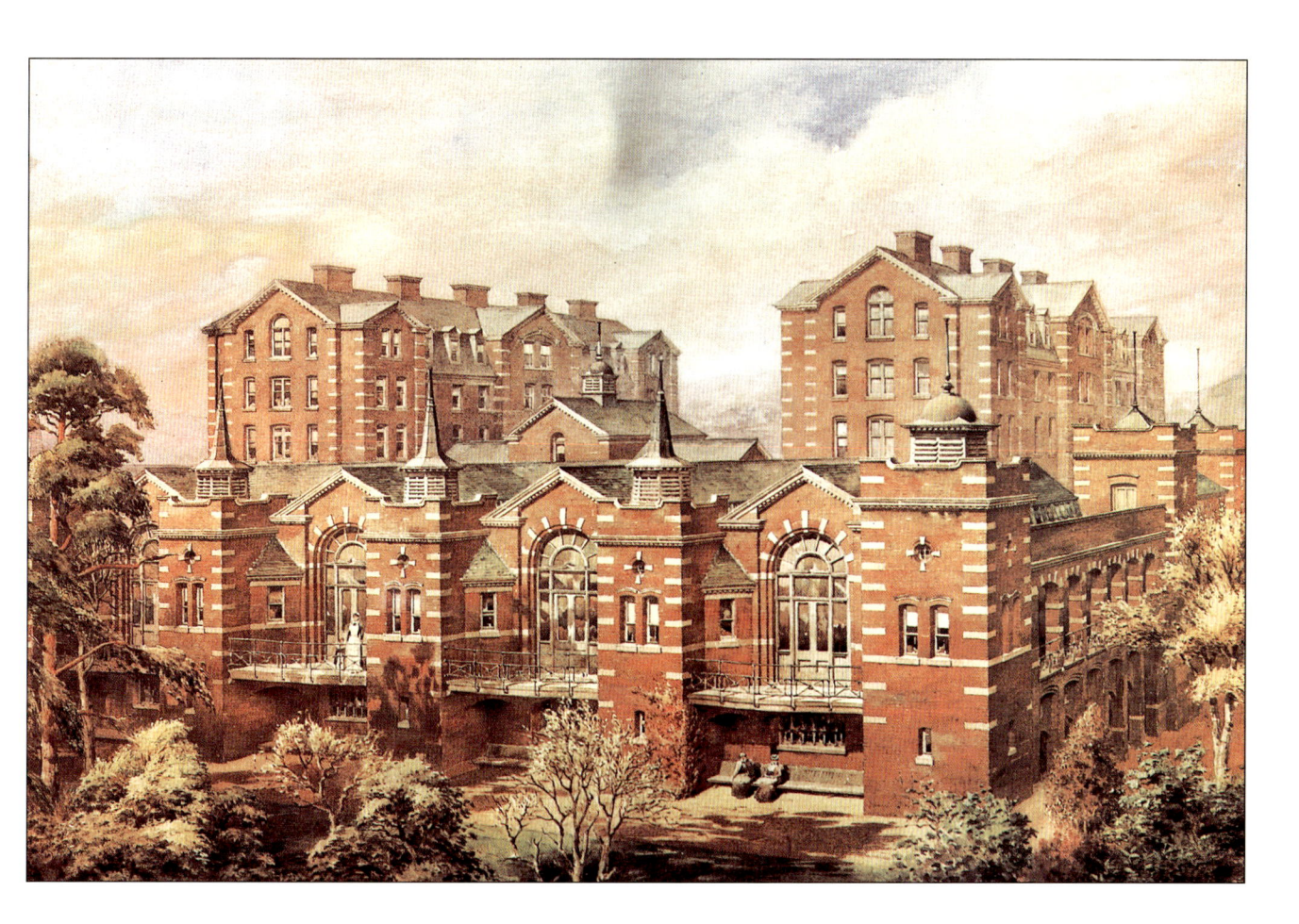

The hospital viewed from the south, as originally designed, with projecting bays and individual balconies; drawing by the architect, William Henman, 1901
ROYAL VICTORIA HOSPITAL

mortuary, postmortem room and pathology department had a separate entrance (this still exists), which also served the isolation buildings. The main entrance from Grosvenor Street, with its porters' lodge, faced the space between the East and West wings.

The inlets for the Plenum ventilation system were to be at the east end of the main corridor but at a lower level. The main ventilation duct therefore would run under the main corridor with side ducts to the wards and outpatient block. The boiler house and laundry were also to be at this end of the site; the laundry was only finally removed in 1995. The kitchens and workshops were to be in the basement of the East and West wings, and the students' cloakrooms were to be in the basement of the outpatients' block, with a stairway up to the central corridor.

Discussions about details of the plans continued with the architects throughout 1899, and the building was ready to go out to tender at the end of the year. By this stage, however, estimates of the total cost had risen to £140,000. Efforts were now made to bring this figure down below £100,000, while still allowing for 300 beds and accommodation for 76 nurses. It was therefore not until September 1900 that the tender of McLaughlin and Harvey was accepted. The hospital now had 4 acres of ground with the option of a further 6 acres as soon as required, though some ground was given at the corner of the site for the widening of the Falls Road.

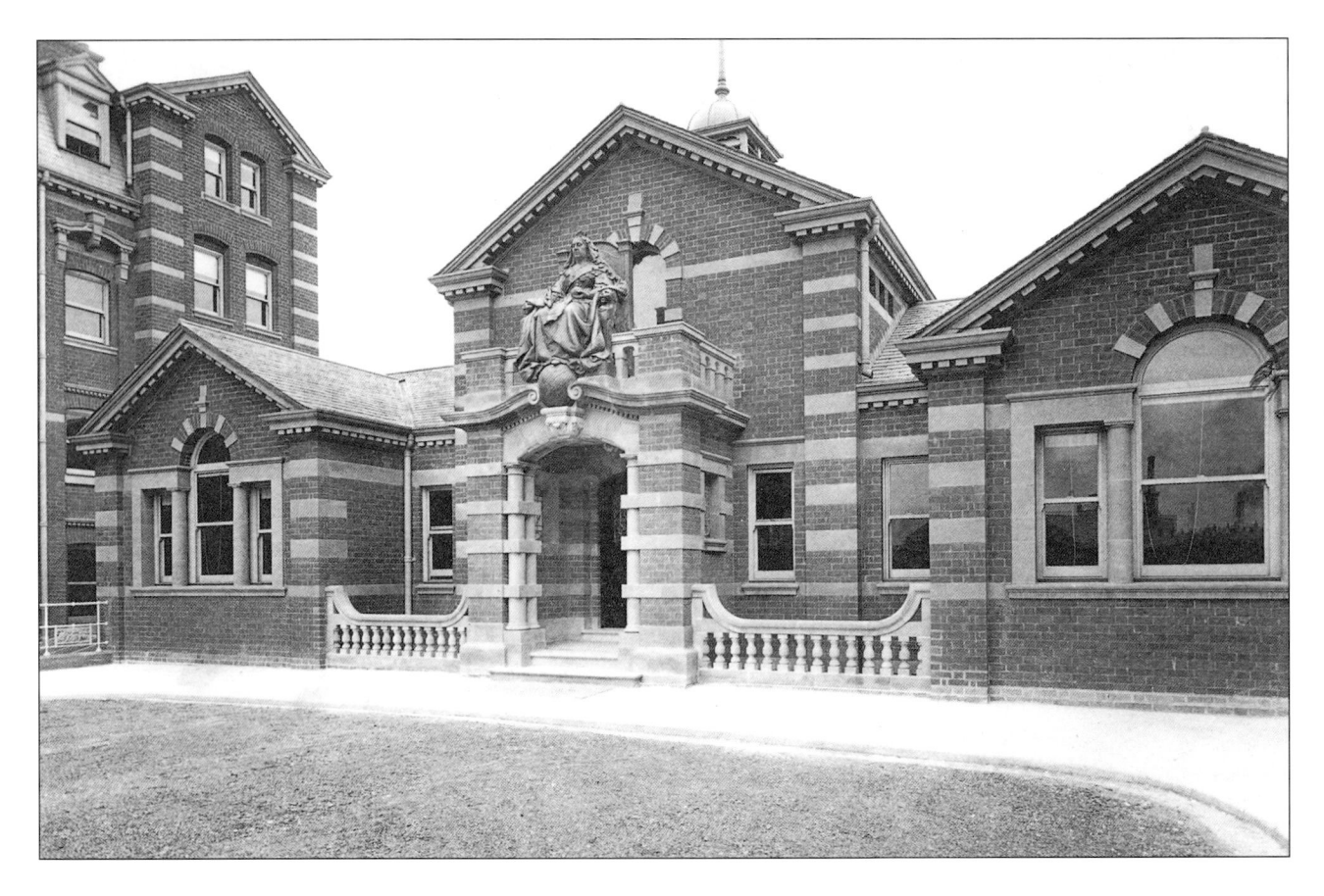

The porch and front entrance to the hospital with the bronze statue of Queen Victoria above the door and before the shelter of steel girders and glass was put up by the Working Men's Committee in 1962; photograph by R.J. Welch
ROYAL VICTORIA HOSPITAL

A wooden fence was to be erected separating the hospital from the asylum, and a wall was to be built along part of the Grosvenor and Falls roads.

The foundation stone for the new hospital was laid early in 1901 and work proceeded so rapidly that the medical staff were able to hold their monthly meeting in the new hospital on 18 October 1901. During all this period the construction committee continued to meet regularly, chaired by the indefatigable William Pirrie. Details that came before the construction committee (and frequently the Medical Staff Committee) included questions relating to the boundary wall, the sewers (again and again), the supply of electricity, boilers, the supply of water, the type of floors (terrazzo was chosen for corridors), cooking appliances, the type of beds and bed linen.

THE OPENING OF THE WARDS

Parts of the new building were ready for occupation before the end of 1901, but the official opening did not take place until 27 July 1903 when King Edward VII and Queen Alexandra arrived and with much ceremony received the Loyal Address from Sir John Walton Browne. At the same time the larger-than-life statue of Queen Victoria by J. Wenlock Robins was unveiled in its place above the main entrance door of the hospital outside the 'black and white hall'. The transfer of patients took place on 17 September 1903, under the direction of the Medical Superintendent and the Matron. A sufficient number of ambulances and buses had been acquired in advance and 'not a single patient complained of the process of transfer nor did any of them get the slightest back-set by it'.

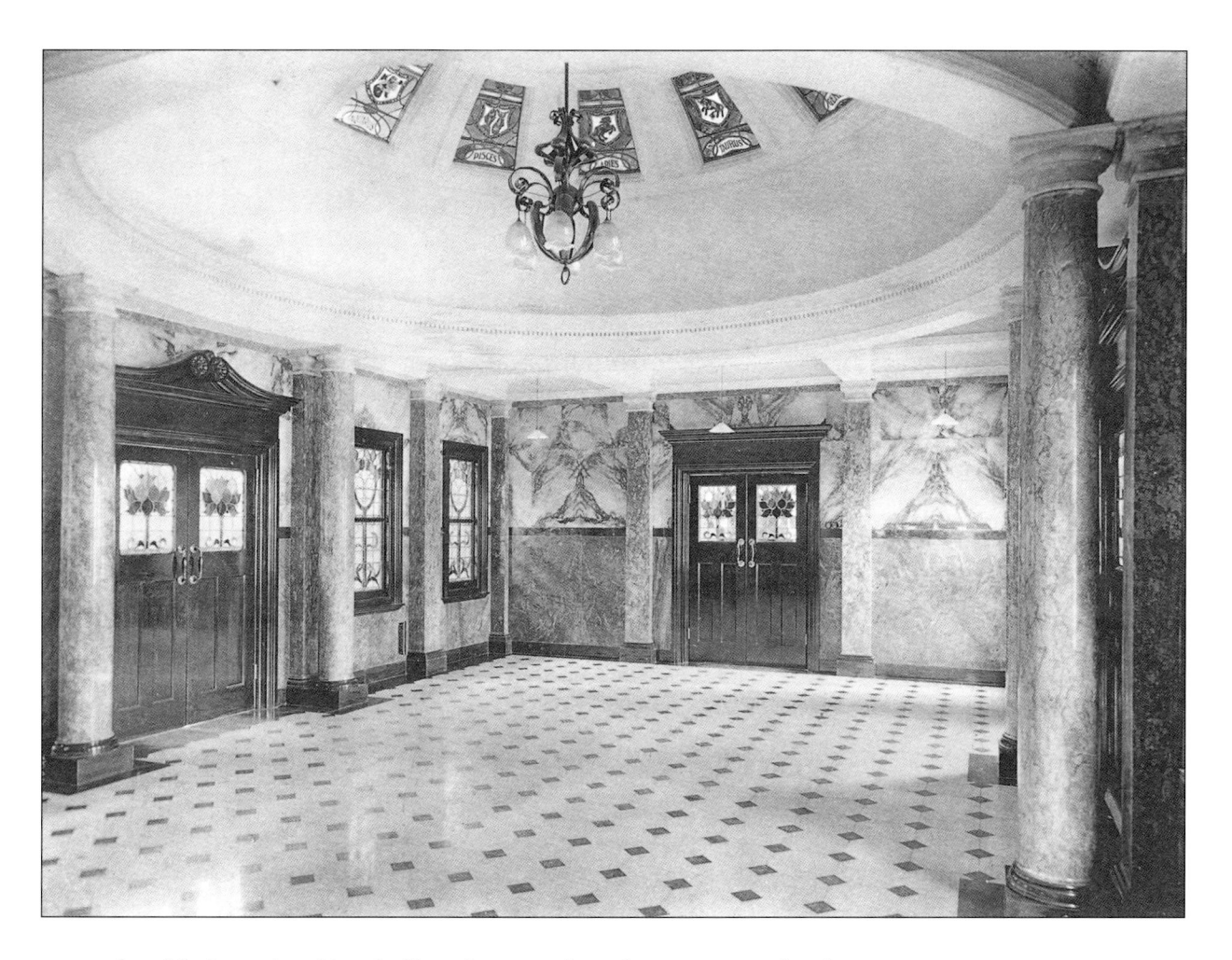

It was decided that the old hospital should be sold and as many as possible of its historical memorabilia were transferred for preservation and to give character to the new building. Probably the most conspicuous object transferred was the Good Samaritan window, originally donated to the Belfast Royal Hospital in Frederick Street by Dr William Whitla in 1886 (see page 44). It shows the Samaritan helping the man who had 'fallen among thieves' nearly two thousand years ago – an image as common now as it was then, while the Priest and the Levite walk past thinking 'It's not my problem.' The four coats of arms in the window highlight the early history of the hospital and of Queen's University: they are of the Belfast Royal Hospital (comprising the royal arms and those of the city of Belfast), the Queen's University of Ireland, Queen's College Belfast, and the Royal University of Ireland. This window was placed high in the extern waiting hall, but in 1947 it was moved to its present location in the main corridor. Immediately below the window in the corridor is the

The entrance hall (known as the 'black and white hall'); the doors to the left lead to the connecting corridor and the doors in the background lead to the board room. Some signs of the zodiac can be seen in the glass dome; photograph by R.J. Welch
ROYAL VICTORIA HOSPITAL

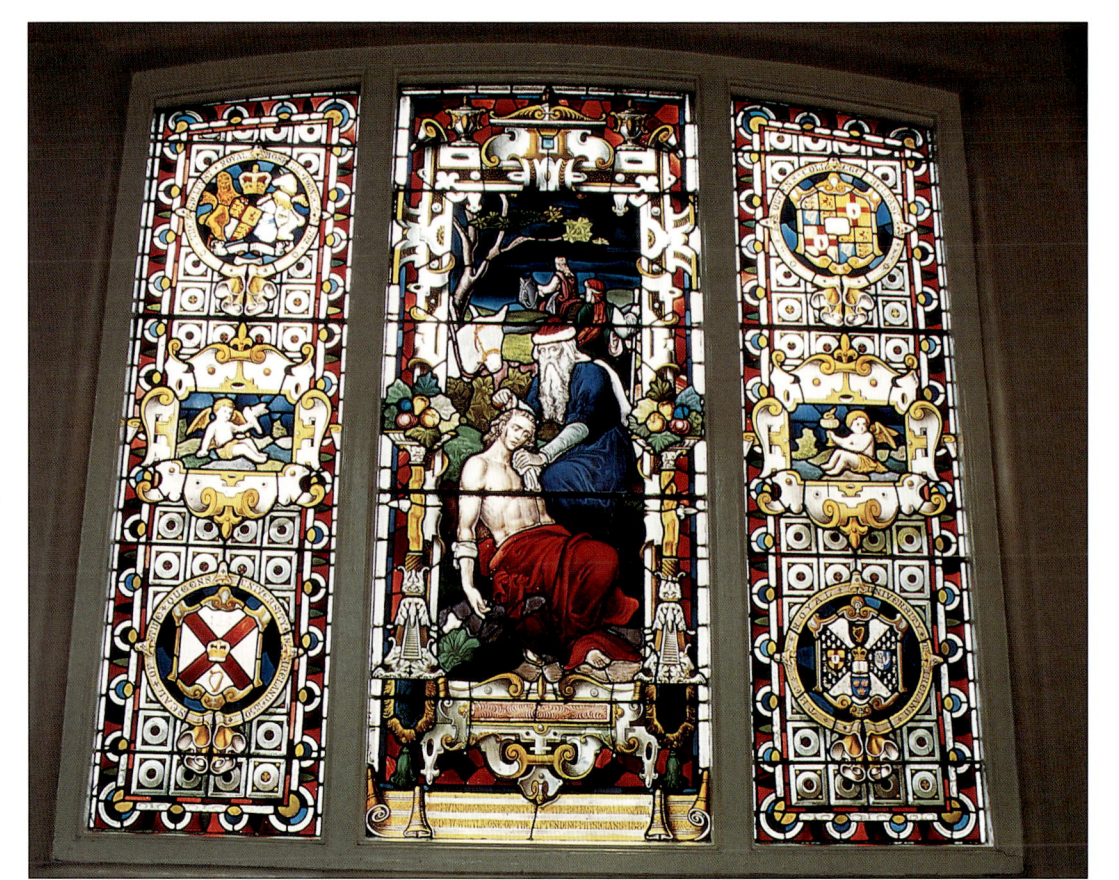

Right:
The Good Samaritan window donated by Sir William Whitla to the Royal Belfast Hospital in 1886: it was transferred to the extern waiting hall of the new Royal Victoria Hospital in 1903.
ROYAL VICTORIA HOSPITAL

Below:
The extern waiting hall, 1903, showing the Good Samaritan window installed above the door; photograph by R.J. Welch
ROYAL VICTORIA HOSPITAL

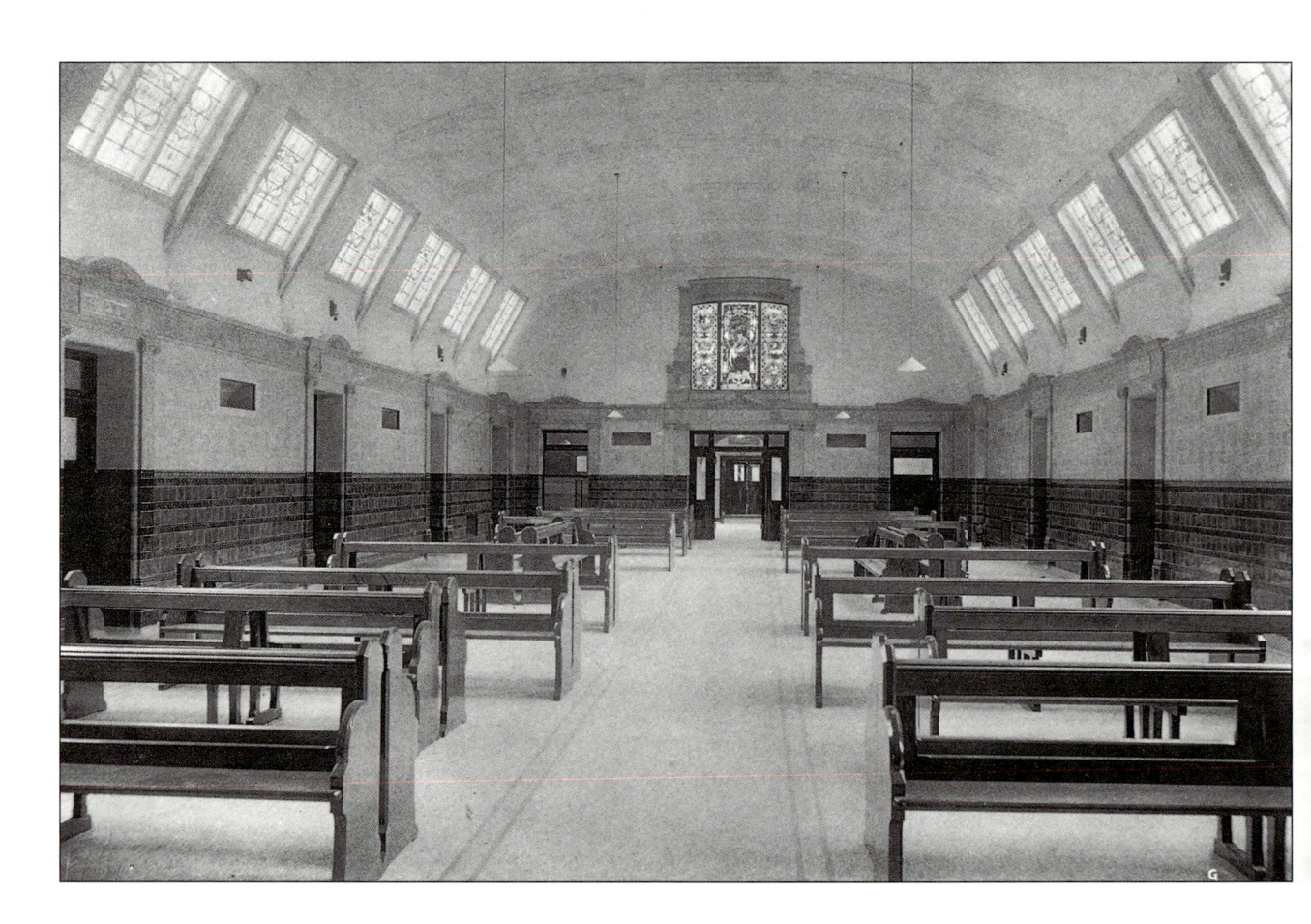

tablet commemorating James Girdwood which was originally erected in the boardroom of the Belfast General Hospital (see pages 30–31).

Also transferred were memorial tablets to Dr Alfred Anderson, who died in 1847 of typhus, and to Dr Walter B. Croker, who died in 1890; both were mounted in the basement below the new wards. Memorial tablets to Dr A.G. Malcolm, Mr David Moore and Dr Anderson were transferred but are now lost. The old date stone (1817) from the General Hospital was removed from the building but it also went astray, and portraits of Mr W.B.T. Lyons (briefly president of the Royal Hospital in 1883) and the solicitor Mr A. Macrory (who was honorary secretary 1860–78) which were in that hospital are now also lost.

ADMINISTRATIVE AND MEDICAL STAFFING

The new hospital of 1903 perhaps justifies a review of the administrative arrangements. In overall control was the Board of Management with the 6th Marquess of Londonderry as president (1890–1914), but the person who made the decisions was the chairman, William Crawford JP (later Sir) (1901–08 and 1914–18). There was an honorary treasurer and honorary secretary, but the day-to-day running of the hospital was in the hands of the Medical Superintendent who, as we have seen, had a flat in the administrative wing. These administrative arrangements were to continue, with few changes, until the introduction of the National Health Service in 1948.

Colonel Andrew Deane MD had taken over as Medical Superintendent of the Frederick Street hospital in July 1901 and continued in the post until 1920. Minutes indicate that he played a considerable part in the final planning of the new building, which included visits to look at

View of the hospital from Grosvenor Street (now Grosvenor Road), complete with tram lines, *c.* 1905: it shows the East and West wings and the entrance courtyard between them, before the North (Musgrave) Wing was built. To the left are the gate lodge and boiler-house chimney; photograph by R.J. Welch
ROYAL VICTORIA HOSPITAL

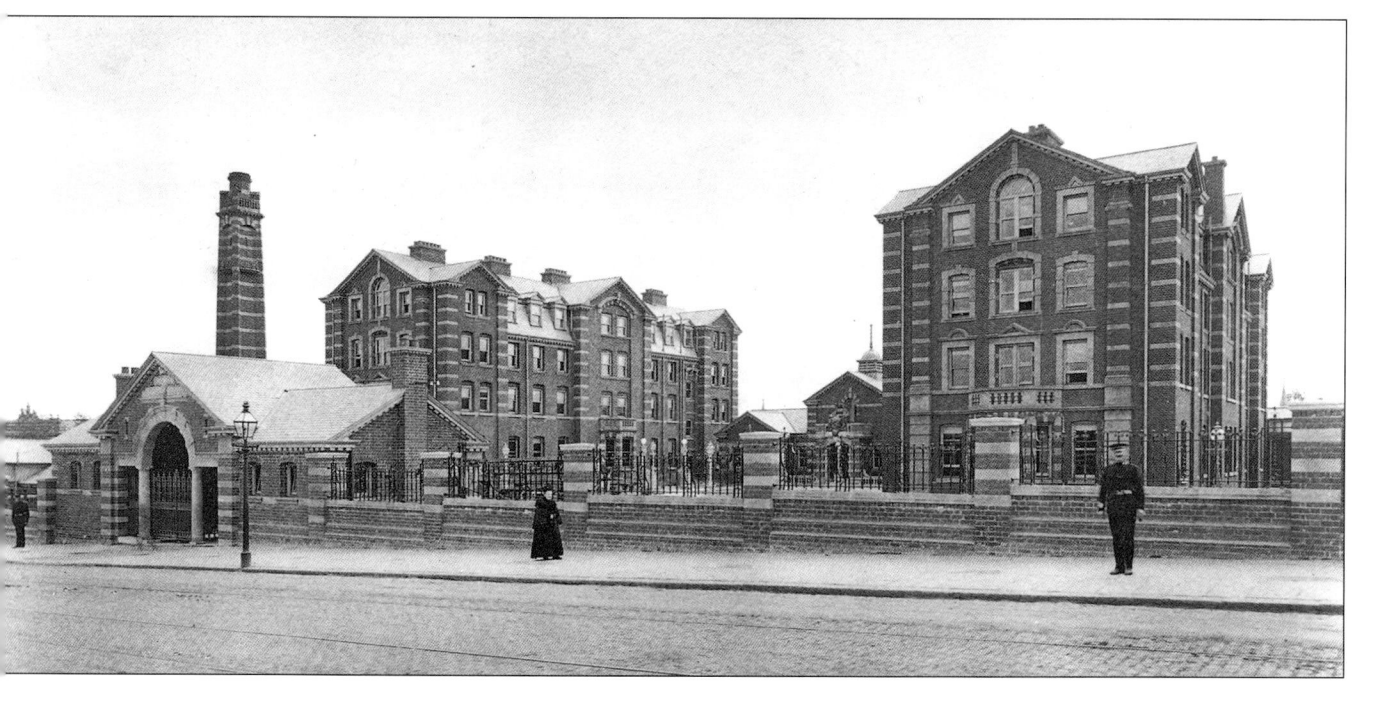

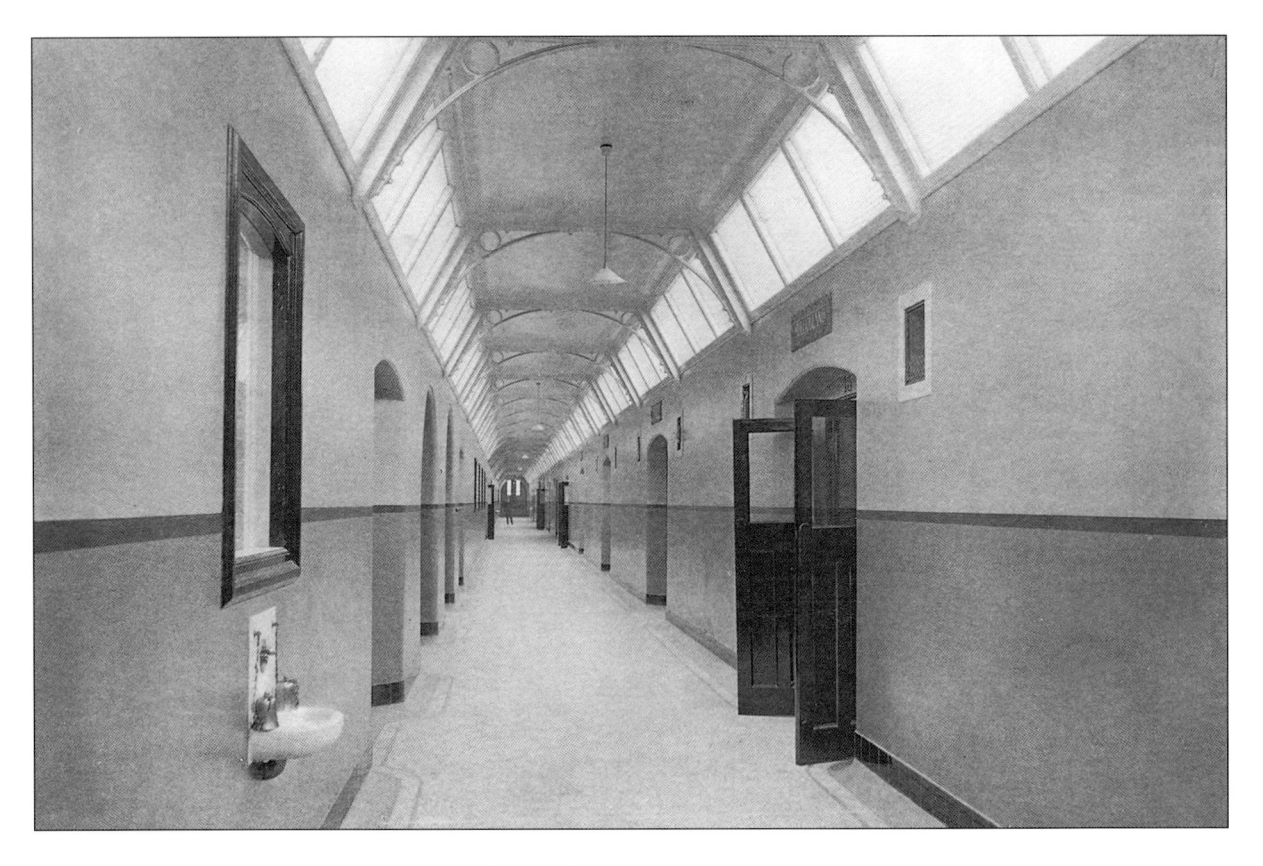

The main 'connecting' corridor of the hospital, 1903, before the fire doors and plethora of notices arrived; photograph by R.J. Welch
ROYAL VICTORIA HOSPITAL

arrangements in hospitals in Great Britain.

On 1 January 1921 Colonel John Forrest took up the post and when he resigned in 1931 he was succeeded by Colonel J.W. Langstaff. He remained until 1944, to be followed (after a short gap) in 1946 by Brigadier Thomas Davidson, the first medical graduate of Queen's to hold the position.

The other major change was in the post of Matron. There had been a succession of matrons (see Appendix 6) in the late nineteenth century with little real influence on the hospital. The last of these, Mrs Waters, retired at the end of 1901 and it was decided to appoint the Matron at the Throne Hospital, Mary Frances Bostock, to the post in the new Royal Victoria Hospital. Thus both Miss Bostock and Colonel Deane were in post well before the transfer of patients to the new hospital.

By 1903 there was one resident House Physician, two House Surgeons, one extern House Surgeon and a Pharmaceutical Chemist, also one Medical and one Surgical Registrar. There were two Assistant Physicians, two Assistant Surgeons, one Assistant Gynaecologist and one Assistant Pathologist; the Assistant staff had essentially the same privileges as Attending staff but only a small number of beds. The Assistant staff also included three honorary Anaesthetists. Attending staff now numbered four Physicians, four Surgeons, a Gynaecologist, an eye, ear, nose and throat Surgeon, a Dermatologist and a Pathologist.

The nursing staff consisted of the Matron (who was also Lady Superintendent of the nurses and Housekeeper of the hospital), the assistant superintendent, the night superintendent, 8 sisters, 4 staff nurses,

11 night nurses, and 47 probationers. There were 33 maidservants of all types and 12 men, one of whom was a male nurse.

The Attending staff were responsible for wards in the new hospital as follows:

Wards 1 and 2 (medical)	Sir William Whitla
Wards 3 and 4 (medical)	Dr W. Calwell and Dr H.L. McKisack
Wards 5 and 6 (medical)	Professor J.A. Lindsay
Wards 7 and 8 (medical)	(unfilled)
Wards 9 and 10 (surgical)	Mr T.S. Kirk
Wards 11 and 12 (surgical)	Mr John Walton Browne
Wards 13 and 14 (surgical)	Professor Thomas Sinclair
Wards 15 and 16 (surgical)	Mr A.B. Mitchell (wards not opened)
Ward 17 (gynaecological)	Professor John Byers
Ophthalmic ward	Dr J. Nelson

THE NAMING OF THE WARDS

Early in 1903 the Relations Committee met to decide on the naming of the wards in the new hospital. It was planned that all should be given names to commemorate generous benefactors of the Belfast General Hospital or donors of £10,000 (see table below).

DEDICATIONS OF THE CORRIDOR WARDS
OF THE ROYAL VICTORIA HOSPITAL, WITH DATES

1. Shaftesbury, 1903
2. Riddel, 1904
3. Ruby Gallaher, 1930
4. Sir Milne Barbour Bart., 1944
5. The Viscountess Pirrie, 1903
6. Cuming, 1903
7. Belfast Co-operative Society Limited, 1944
8. Our Day, 1920
9. The Honorary Medical Staff, 1953
10. Sinclair, 1903
11. Charters, 1903
12. Pirrie, 1903
13. Mulholland, 1903
14. Ismay, 1903
15. James and Eliza Jane Moore, 1944
16. Harland, 1904
17. Clarence, 1903
18. RVH Working Men's Committee, 1992
19. Thomas Gordon Herald, 1944
20. Shaw, Holywood, 1944

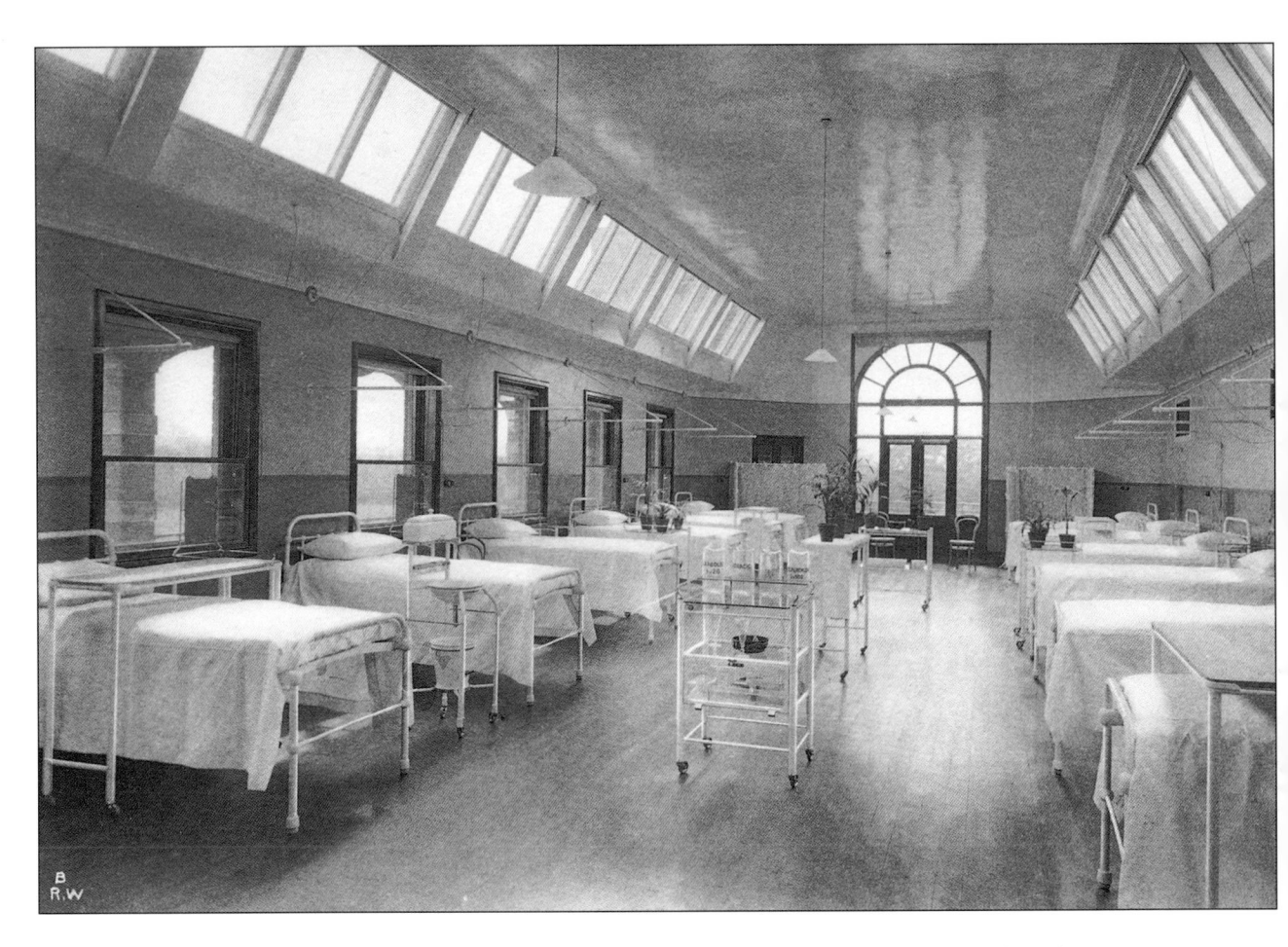

Ward 1 (Shaftesbury Ward) with its door leading onto the balcony: when the wards were extended in the 1930s, more utilitarian doors were put in place. To the left are the windows to the side balcony, which were blocked when the metabolic unit was added; photograph by R.J. Welch.
ROYAL VICTORIA HOSPITAL

Ward 1 was named after the Shaftesbury family, the name commemorating Anthony, 8th Earl of Shaftesbury (1831–86) who in 1857 married Harriet, daughter and heiress of the 3rd Marquess of Donegall. They and their son, the 9th Earl of Shaftesbury (1869–1961), had continued the family interest in the Belfast Royal Hospital and in 1869 the 8th Earl and his wife sealed this with a gift of the ground in Frederick Street on which the hospital was built. When the Royal Victoria Hospital moved, Harriet, Countess of Shaftesbury, and her son extended this gift and a tablet in the ward records gratitude for their 'allowing the site of the old Belfast Royal Hospital in Frederick Street to be sold free of rent for the benefit of the endowment fund of this Hospital'. The 9th Earl of Shaftesbury became Lord Mayor of Belfast in 1907 and first Chancellor of the newly created Queen's University of Belfast in 1908. He gave Belfast Castle and grounds to the city in 1934.

Ward 5 was named after Margaret Montgomery Pirrie (Viscountess Pirrie from 1906) who in donations and fundraising had done so much for the new hospital. Her bust (sculpted by A. Bertram Pegram and donated in 1934) is displayed facing the front entrance in the corridor (the Marquess of Dufferin and Ava described her as 'the most charming and most popular Lady Mayoress who ever sceptred a city or disciplined a husband'). William Pirrie's work and generosity is commemorated in the naming of Ward 12;

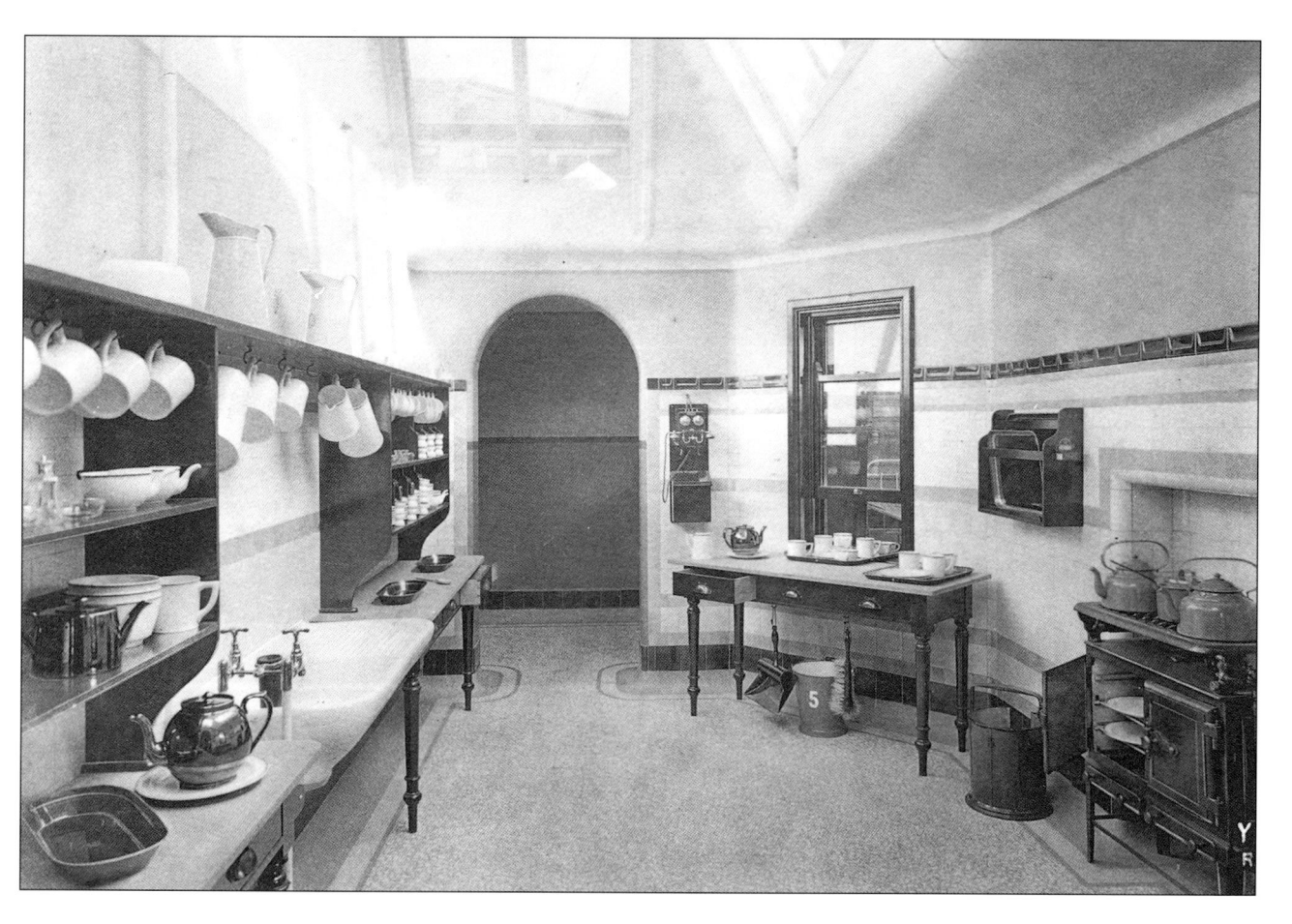

A ward kitchen, complete with gas cooker and kitchen utensils; photograph by R.J. Welch
ROYAL VICTORIA HOSPITAL

his portrait hangs in the King Edward Building.

Ward 6 was named after Professor James Cuming to mark his great involvement in the planning of the new hospital as well as his previous contributions to medical studies. During fundraising for the new hospital, Mrs Pirrie had undertaken to raise £10,000 to name a ward in his honour and this was completed by March 1903. The ward, when opened, contained a tablet recording this dedication and a bust of Professor Cuming, but they were lost somehow during refurbishment of the ward in the 1970s (as indeed was the Pirrie tablet in Ward 5).

Ward 10 was named after the Sinclair family. The tablet commemorating the Sinclair Memorial Ward (see page 28) was moved to Ward 10 from the old hospital.

The name Charters was allocated to the new Ward 11, commemorating John Charters's gift of 1865 which enabled a wing of the Belfast General Hospital to be built; his bust and commemorative tablets were transferred accordingly. The name Mulholland was given to Ward 13 to commemorate St Clair Kelburn Mulholland's donation of 1863; the gift had been made in memory of his only son who died in Sorrento, Italy, on 4 April 1861, a fact that is recorded on three separate tablets which were transferred in 1903.

The name Ismay, associated with Ward 14, is not as well known in

Belfast as those mentioned previously, as the family did not live in Ireland. But they had important local business connections, and Thomas Henry Ismay really did contribute to Belfast by his support of shipbuilding as well as by his company's donation to the Royal Victoria Hospital's building fund. He was born on 7 January 1837 in Maryport, Cumberland, the eldest son of Joseph Ismay, a shipbuilder. Thomas Ismay left school at sixteen and was apprenticed to the Liverpool firm of Imrie and Tomlinson, Shipowners. He subsequently started business independently and in 1867, at the age of thirty-one, he founded the White Star Line of Australian clippers. He went on to form the Oceanic Steam Navigation Company (1869) with William Imrie. From this time he decided to introduce iron vessels to replace wooden ships, and it was this change that connected him with Belfast. The American route was clearly the important one for both passengers and cargo, and in 1869 Ismay's company ordered from Harland and Wolff no less than six large transatlantic steamers to sail between Liverpool and New York.

T.H. Ismay was given the Freedom of Belfast in 1898 in recognition of his contribution to the city's prosperity, and in return he gave £1,000 to the hospital building fund. After his death on 23 November 1899 the White Star Line gave £10,000 to dedicate a ward as a memorial to him. The commemoration tablet in the ward includes this dedication:

> In memory of the late Thomas Henry Ismay, founder of the White Star Line, this ward bears his honoured name. A sum of £10,000 was generously voted by the shareholders in the Oceanic Steam Navigation Company Limited at their Annual Meeting held 1 May 1901, towards the funds of this hospital, as a permanent memorial to one who was closely identified with the prosperity of Belfast and its charities.

Below these words are approximately one hundred names of shareholders.

The last of the wards to be named by the time the Royal Victoria Hospital was opened was Ward 17. When King Edward VII and Queen Alexandra opened the hospital on 27 July 1903, they asked for a ward to be named after their eldest son, the late Prince Albert Victor, Duke of Clarence. He had been born in 1864 and in due course went into the army; he developed pneumonia in 1892, and died at the early age of twenty-eight.

THE NAMING OF THE REMAINING WARDS

It is convenient to mention the dedications of the remaining wards here, even though the process of their naming took place over the following ninety years.

Ward 2 is named after the Riddel family of Beechmount, in Belfast, and specifically with the donation of Eliza and Isabella Riddel in memory of

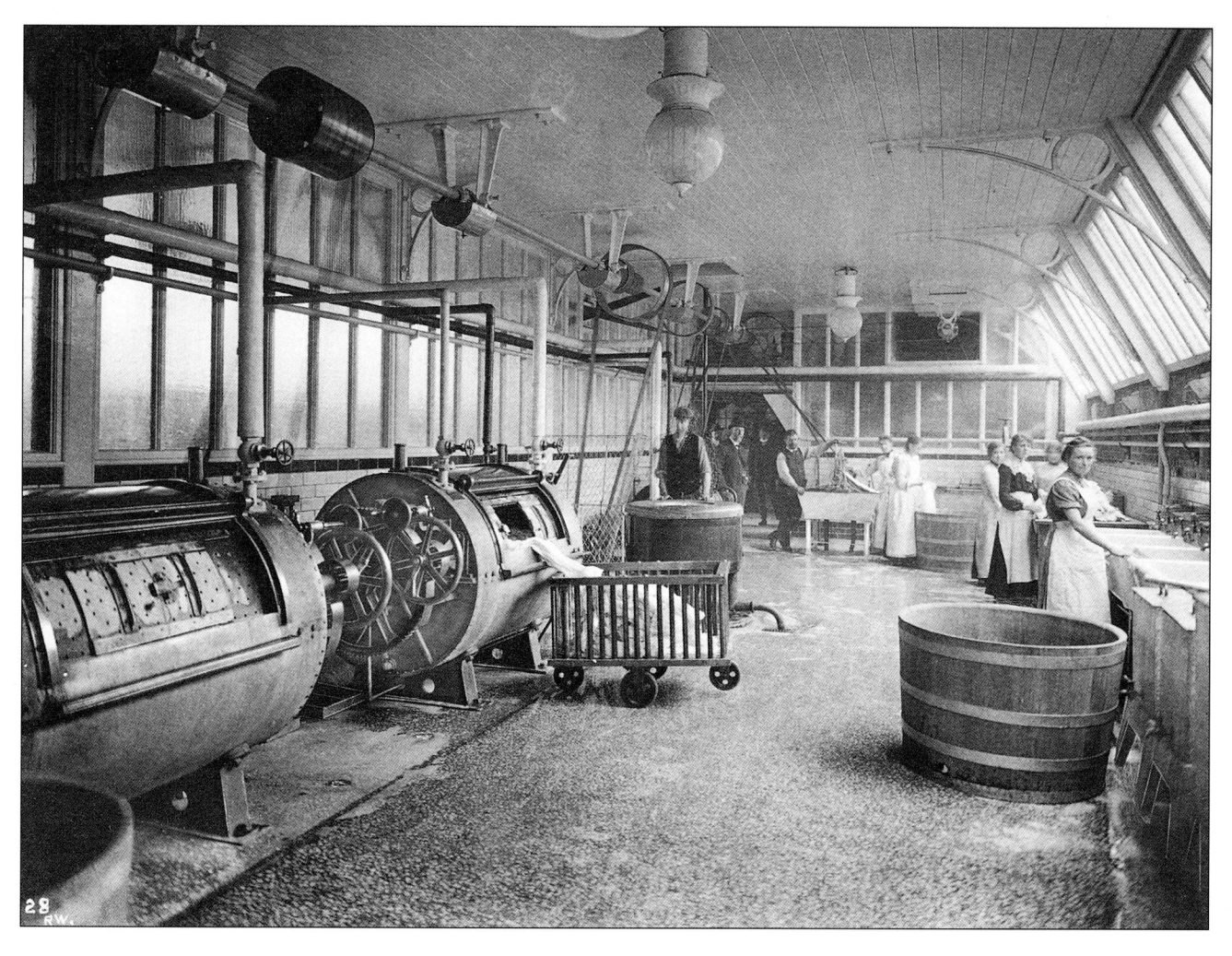

The laundry, 1903: at that time, and until c. 1960, all hospital laundry was dealt with on the site; photograph by R.J. Welch
ROYAL VICTORIA HOSPITAL

their father John, who was a successful hardware merchant. They not only donated £10,000 in 1904 but bore the cost of building the house for the Medical Superintendent, endowed a demonstratorship in pathology (1904), and in 1912 gave £45,000 to build and endow Riddel Hall as a hall of residence for women students of the university.

Ward 3 commemorates Ruby Gallaher, daughter of Thomas Gallaher of Whitehouse, the tobacco manufacturer, who had moved to Belfast from Londonderry in 1870. He died in 1927 and his wife Robina died in 1930, leaving £10,000 to name the ward in memory of their daughter, who had died some years earlier.

Ward 4 was named in 1944 after Sir Milne Barbour Bart., head of what was at one time the largest linen thread company in the world. It had grown, over three generations of the family, in the Lisburn–Hilden area and had swallowed up smaller firms along the Lagan and Upper Bann. John Milne Barbour was chairman of the Linen Thread Company, a Minister of Finance in the Northern Ireland Government, and president of the Royal Victoria Hospital from 1939 until 1948.

The Belfast Co-operative Society, under its chairman James McCombe, decided to endow Ward 7 to commemorate its centenary in 1944.

McCombe was certainly the prime mover in this (and in other projects such as the pasteurisation of milk in Belfast) and was able to raise the £10,000 from members of the society and from employees.

The significance of the title 'Our Day' over Ward 8 may be obscure to many of us now, but it harks back to the middle of World War One when the British Red Cross Society and the Order of St John made a massive fundraising effort. Between 1916 and 1918 Ulster raised a total of £146,000 for the Our Day effort, which was much needed as until well after the war the hospital had many soldiers as patients. In 1920 the joint committee for the two organisations decided to give the sum of £10,000 to the hospital to name a ward in recognition of Belfast's contribution to the welfare of the armed forces.

Ward 9 was named in 1953 in recognition of the work of the honorary medical staff who had given their services free until 1948.

Ward 15 commemorates the Moore family, Eliza Jane and her brother James. George C. Moore, their brother, was a solicitor from Limavady, County Londonderry, who had graduated with honours from Queen's University Belfast and practised as a solicitor in Belfast for twenty years. He seems to have been a particularly successful investor, and when he moved to Forest Hill in London to engage in other business interests he was said to have an annual income of over £1 million. In 1920 he undertook to donate £20,000 over a number of years, but the donation was not completed until 1944 when the balance was received by the will of Miss Anna L.C. Moore, the residuary legatee.

Ward 16 commemorates Sir Edward James Harland, founder of the shipbuilding firm Harland and Wolff. He died in 1895 and his widow Rosa donated £10,000 to name a ward in his memory in 1904.

Ward 18 was the last of the corridor wards to be named. It commemorates the contributions of the Working Men's Committee from its foundation in 1888. During more than a century the committee collected over £1 million for the hospital and in 1992 a plaque was unveiled by Sir Ian Fraser, then the senior Consulting Surgeon, to acknowledge the committee's dedicated work.

Ward 19 is named after Thomas Gordon Herald who died in 1918. His father, Samuel Herald of Windsor Avenue, Belfast, was managing director of the Irish Preserve and Confectionery Company, and when he died in 1922 he left £20,000 to name a ward in memory of his son. However Samuel's widow Sarah had a life interest in the capital, and the bequest did not come to the hospital until after her death, in 1944.

Ward 20 was also dedicated in 1944, following the bequest of Mrs Hetty Hamilton Shaw, widow of William Shaw of the company Shaw and Jamison, wholesale druggists. The company had a five-storey warehouse in Townhall Street, Belfast, and had a very successful business in all kinds of groceries as well as chemical and patent medicines.

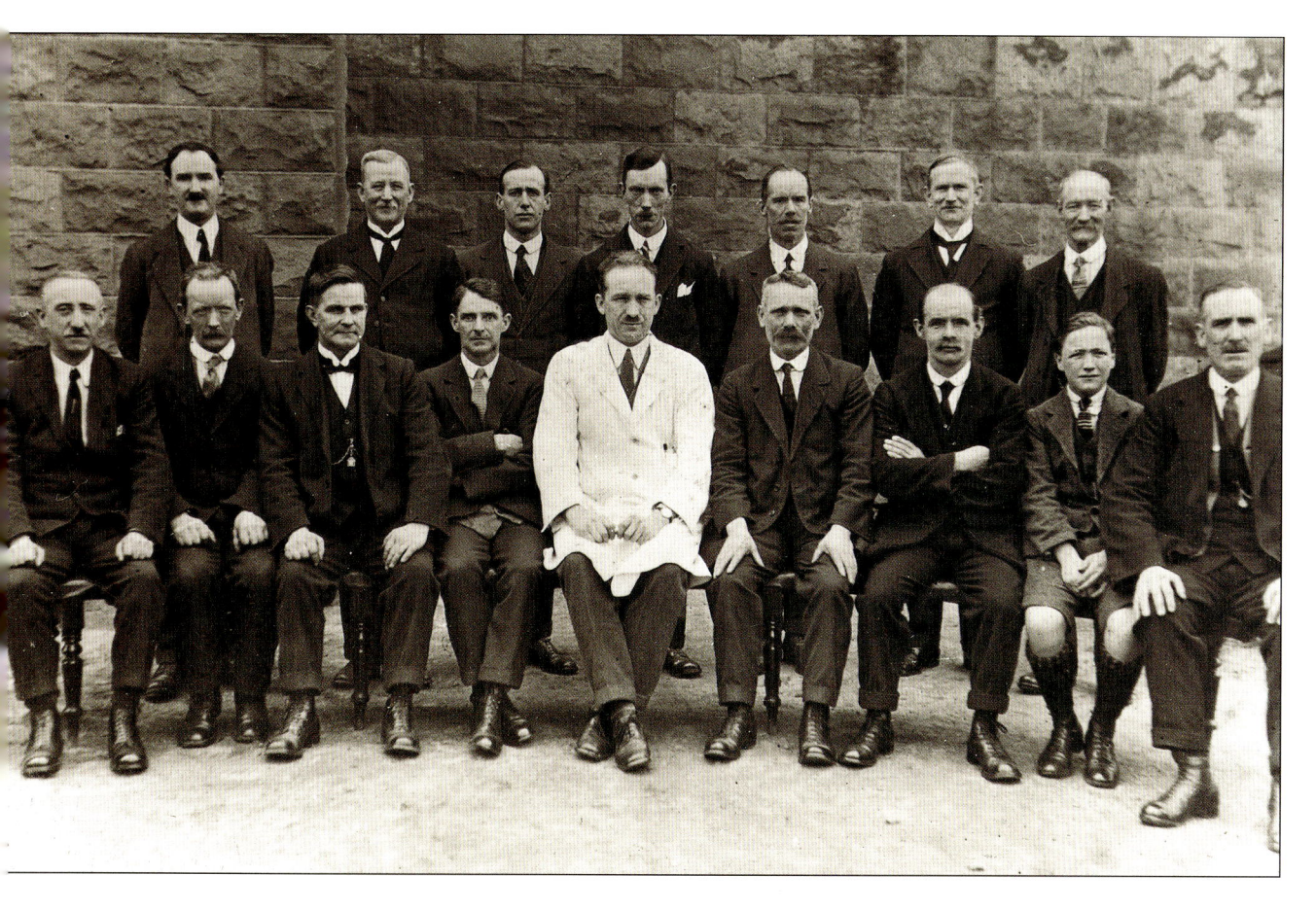

THE WORKING MEN'S COMMITTEE

Regular financial support was provided for the new hospital not only by wealthy sponsors but also by the Working Men's Committee. This developed from a Hospital Saturday collection in 1888 to bring in the subscriptions of the working man to help to run the hospital. However, its greatest financial significance was in the period from 1916 until the advent of the National Health Service (1948). Before 1888, as well as straightforward donations, it had been possible to raise money for charitable causes by the employer making a deduction from his workers' wages. However in 1887 this practice, which could have allowed employers to filch money from their workers, was forbidden by the Truck Amendment Act, and the following year the Working Men's Committee was set up to collect money from men at their workplace in a formal way. Over the committee's first decades there was a steady increase in the number of workers involved, the number of companies agreeing to participate, and the sums raised. Fundraising always relied on both channels – place of work and street collections – and indeed included collections all over east Ulster as well as Belfast. The first working chairman was John Ginty who remained a major force in the committee for many of the early years.

In return for their contributions to the cost of running the hospital, the working men demanded increasing representation on the Board of Management. This was resisted by the board and a running battle went on

The ambulance class of the Working Men's Committee, 1925, with the Extern Surgeon, Dr T.J. Gibson, centre front
ROYAL VICTORIA HOSPITAL

in private and in public correspondence. For instance, in 1931 the Board of Management minutes record that the Medical Superintendent had received letters from the secretary of the Working Men's Committee, 'at least one being couched in discourteous terms and containing a threat of drastic action at the next meeting' of their committee. The issue was resolved by both groups agreeing to get together and talk it over. The Working Men's Committee gradually gained more influence – mainly through the life governorship system. In 1940, for example, when the committee wanted its representation to be raised to two, it was suggested that their honorary secretary, Mr Lavery, should be made a life governor, which would give them a voice in addition to that of their elected representative, and this was arranged.

The Working Men's Committee members also felt that they should have a say in improving patient comfort. The members were always around the hospital at visiting times, the retired members coming during working hours, and were quick to pass on complaints and grievances to the Medical Superintendent and medical staff. They also passed on praise, and they played a valuable part in improving amenities and organising entertainment such as live concerts in the 1890s and cinematograph entertainments in the early 1900s. These were particularly valuable for the long-stay and convalescent patients of the Throne Hospital.

The 1920s and 1930s were the most important decades in the history of this committee. In spite of the Depression, men in work had more disposable income, and the improved standard of living was seen particularly among the more poorly paid. They saw the importance to themselves of good health care, not least in maintaining their ability to work, and their contribution as a proportion of the hospital's income rose to a peak of 50 per cent in 1930 (approximately £26,000).

Although the importance of the Working Men's Committee and street

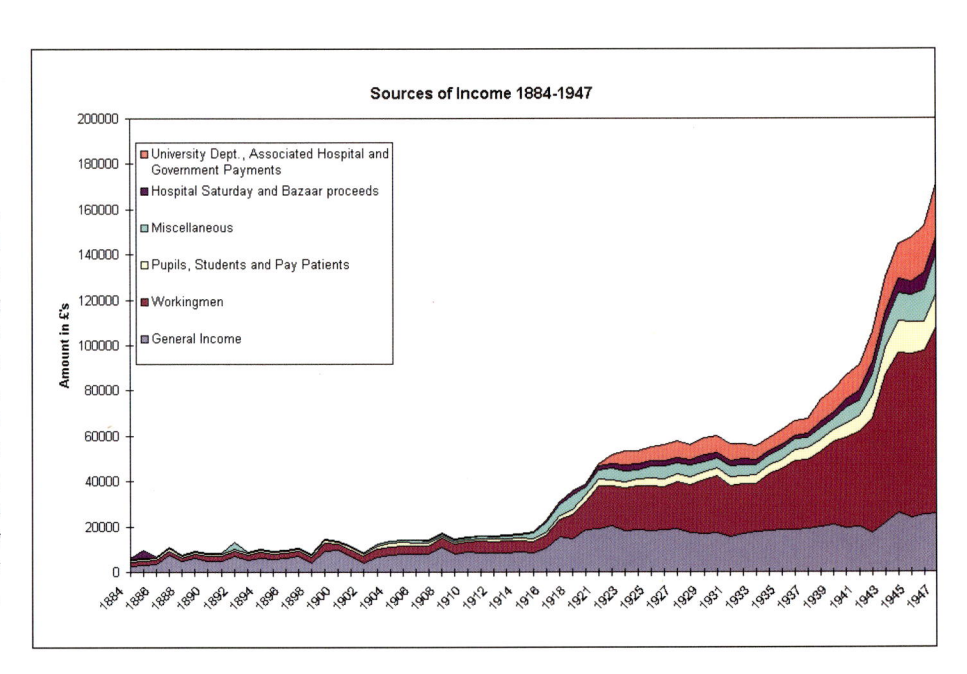

Sources of income of the Belfast Royal and Royal Victoria hospitals: in 1930 the contribution of the Working Men's Committee reached a peak of 50 per cent of the hospital income as a whole, and was between 40 and 50 per cent in most of the years between 1920 and 1945; reproduced from Clarkson and Litvac, *The Working Men's Committee*, 1996, by permission of the authors.

collections generally declined in 1948 with the introduction of the National Health Service, it remains an important contributor to the present day. This was recognised in the centenary history by Professor Leslie Clarkson and Marianne Litvac (published in 1996), and by the memorial plaque erected in Ward 18 in 1992.

THE HOSPITAL AND THE WORLD OUTSIDE, 1903–1939

The events of the twentieth century that influenced the UK also had their effects on the hospital. The effects of World War One brought an influx of wounded which filled the unoccupied wards at times, as well as the old asylum building. In 1919 when the last of them left the hospital, 1,209 soldiers and sailors had been treated, with only 9 deaths – but of course it was only possible to bring back the less seriously injured from the fighting. Many of the staff who were of an age to serve in the armed forces did so, leaving the hospital to be manned by the older or less fit staff, and women doctors appeared in the wards for the first time.

After the war came the partition of Ireland with the creation of a separate parliament for Northern Ireland and a separate police force. This did not really affect the running of voluntary hospitals, though in the investiture following the opening of the new Parliament in Belfast in June 1921, Mr William J. Pirrie was created a viscount and Dr John Walton Browne a knight. On the other hand, the troubles of 1920 and 1922 had a considerable impact for, as in later periods of rioting and murder, the hospital received most of the casualties of Belfast. At one time in 1921 there were so many male gunshot admissions and other casualties of civil violence that the female Ward 7 was appropriated for men. However, at last things settled down to an uneasy truce and there was relatively little civil violence during the remaining inter-war years.

In the 1920s and 1930s, in spite of unemployment, there was a 12 per cent increase in the labour force in the UK mainly due to expansion of tertiary services and the building trade. For those out of work, insurance benefits were higher in relation to incomes in Northern Ireland than in Britain, so those qualifying for benefit had some improvement in the quality of life. However, there was also extreme poverty, highlighted by a violent demonstration in 1932, significantly involving Shankill Road Protestants and Falls Road Catholics at the same time. In the course of this several people were killed and thousands of pounds' worth of damage was done.

MAJOR CHANGES TO THE HOSPITAL BUILDINGS BEFORE
    WORLD WAR TWO

We can trace the changes to the hospital in maps of the site (see pages 64,

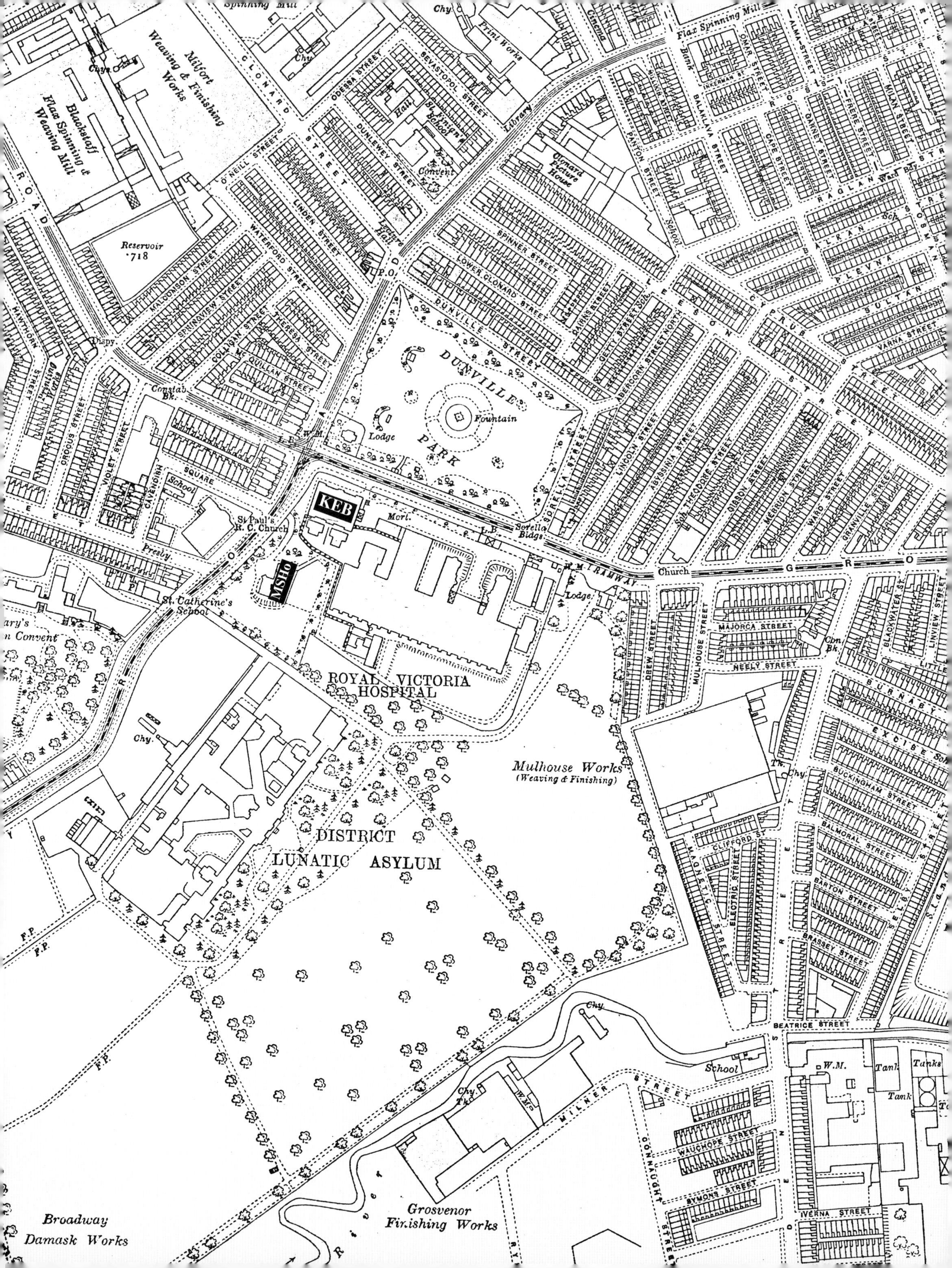
Milfort Weaving & Finishing Works
Blackstaff Flax Spinning & Weaving Mill
Reservoir ·718
CLONARD STREET
O'NEILL STREET
ODESSA STREET
SEVASTOPOL STREET
DUNLEWEY STREET
Hall
St. Finian's School
Convent
Print Works
Cinema
Flax Spinning Mill
Library
Clonard Picture House
LINDEN STREET
WATERFORD STREET
MALCOMSON STREET
SPRINGVIEW STREET
COLLIGAN STREET
THERESA STREET
McQUILLAN STREET
SPINNER STREET
LOWER CLONARD STREET
DUNVILLE STREET
DUNVILLE PARK
Fountain
Lodge
CAIRNS STREET
GETTY STREET
ABERCORN STREET NORTH
LINCOLN STREET
ABYSSINIA STREET
THEODORE STREET
GIBBON STREET
MERRION STREET
WARD STREET
GRANVILLE STREET
SORELLA STREET
Sorella Bldgs.
OMAR STREET
INKERMAN ST.
BALAKLAVA STREET
CAPE STREET
GARNEY STREET
FRERE STREET
MILAN STREET
PANTON STREET
RAGLAN STREET
PLEVNA STREET
SULTAN STREET
VARNA STREET
ALMA STREET
School
Dispy.
Constab. Bk.
HAWTHORN STREET
GROCUS STREET
VIOLET STREET
CAVENDISH SQUARE
School
KEB
MSHo
St. Paul's R.C. Church
Presby.
Mort.
St. Catherine's School
Convent
ROYAL VICTORIA HOSPITAL
W.M. TRAMWAY
Church
Lodge
Chy.
DISTRICT LUNATIC ASYLUM
Mulhouse Works (Weaving & Finishing)
DREW STREET
MULHOUSE STREET
MAJORCA STREET
NEELY STREET
BLACKWATER ST.
LINVIEW STREET
BURNABY STREET
EXCISE STREET
BUCKINGHAM STREET
BALMORAL STREET
BARTON STREET
BRASSEY STREET
CLIFFORD ST.
ELECTRIC STREET
MAGNETIC STREET
BEATRICE STREET
School
W.M.
Tanks
Tank
MILNER STREET
WAUCHOPE STREET
SYMONS STREET
IVERNA STREET
CONNAUGHT STREET
Grosvenor Finishing Works
Broadway Damask Works
F.P.
River

88 and 91), which provide evidence of steady growth in the numbers of patients treated, and of staff employed, and in the scope of facilities on the site. The first addition was a house for the medical superintendent built through the generosity of the Misses Riddel and opened in 1905. It was situated where the outpatient block now stands, with an entrance from the Falls Road, and was demolished in 1964 to make room for that block. From 1946, it had provided accommodation for nurses and administrative offices, whilst the medical superintendent now lived off the site in a hospital house in Malone Park.

The King Edward Building was a much more important addition to the hospital; it was used to hold all the hospital facilities not adequately provided in the 1903 building. After the death of King Edward VII in July 1910, the Board of Management immediately decided to erect a distinguished building of three storeys above a basement, with a conspicuous clock, in his memory. The architects were the Belfast firm of Young and McKenzie, and McLaughlin and Harvey again took on the building contract (at a cost of £20,000). The lower floors were to serve Dr Thomas Houston's Department of Vaccine Therapy and Haematology, the former being a line of treatment much in favour at the time. The Electrical (x-ray) Department under Dr John Rankin was also in this area. The two upper floors of the building were to house additional nurses and ward maids. The building was to be in the space to the west of the extern department, and was not properly started until 1913. Unfortunately the outbreak of war delayed the completion of the building until May 1915; even then the laboratories were not in use until the war was over and Dr Houston returned to the hospital. The bronze bust of King Edward VII by Bruce Joy in the fine central hall was presented by Sir William Crawford. The hall was now available for social gatherings and the annual meeting of the hospital.

Although the King Edward Building opened to accommodate radiology, laboratories and nurses' bedrooms, its functions changed frequently over the years. When two honorary Dental Surgeons were appointed, a room was found for them in a spare pathology laboratory, although their patients had to wait in the corridor. In 1925 the eye, ear, nose and throat outpatient clinics were moved to the building. In 1926, when the nurses had moved out, the top floor of the building was converted for use as a Dental Department and functioned as such for thirty years.

Opposite:
Map of 1923 showing the King Edward Building and the Medical Superintendent's house; the asylum is still in position.
ORDNANCE SURVEY OF NORTHERN IRELAND

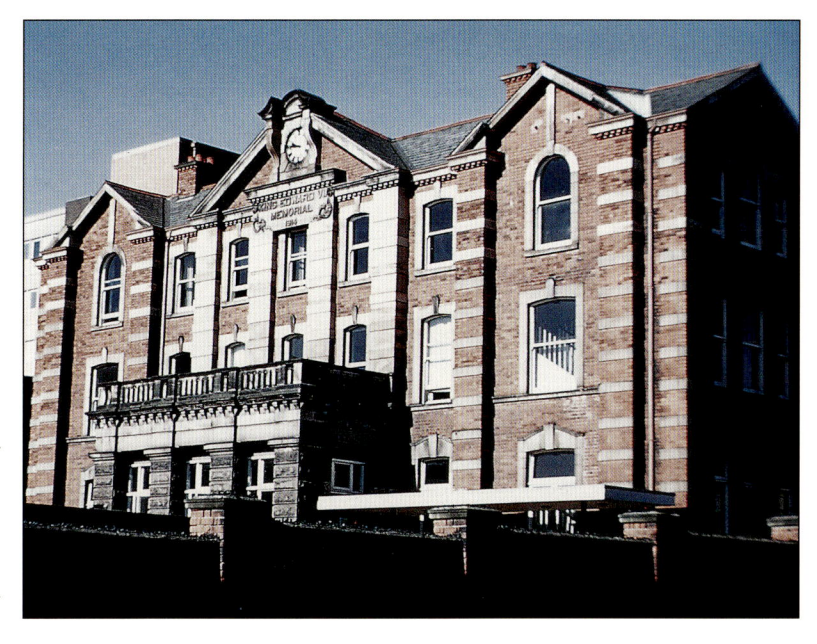

The King Edward Building, completed in 1915, as it appeared before the extension of the cardiac surgical intensive care and X-ray facilities, which now block the view of the façade.
ROYAL VICTORIA HOSPITAL

Opposite:
Map of 1937 showing the new buildings to the east and south of the original hospital: the Institute of Pathology, the boiler house and chimney, the Royal Maternity Hospital, the Musgrave Clinic, the nurses' home and the Belfast Children's Hospital; as yet there are no hospital buildings to the east and south of the hospital road.
ORDNANCE SURVEY OF NORTHERN IRELAND

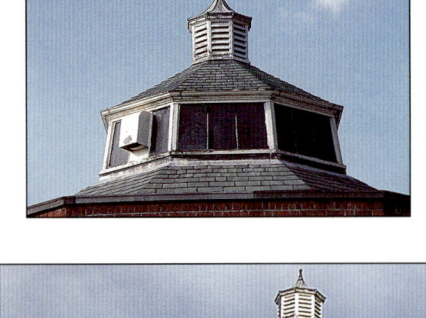

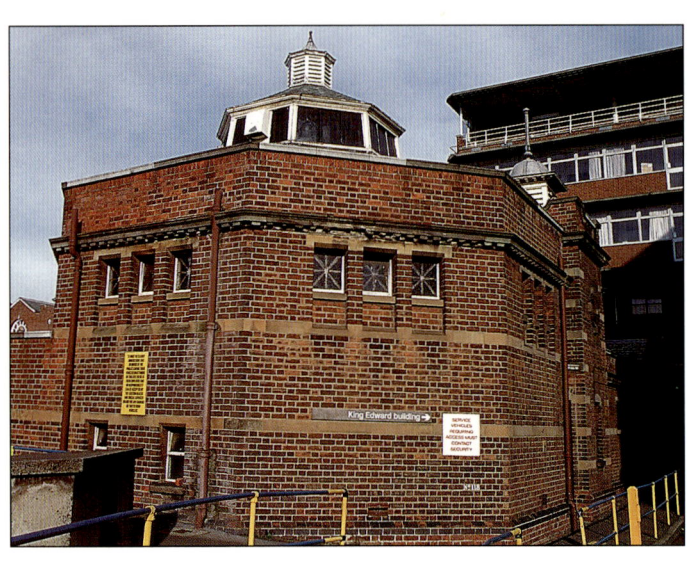

Above:
The old mortuary, built in 1924 and demolished in 1995: it was designed to tone in architecturally with the hospital, and at demolition the particularly attractive cupola, *top*, was preserved.
ROYAL VICTORIA HOSPITAL

Another minor department in the building was patient case records, which were bound up into black books and stored in one room. This department seems to have opened in 1918 under Miss M.V. Lutton, who also looked after medical student placements and received their hospital fees. She was still looking after medical records and students thirty-five years later and only retired when the new outpatient building opened.

The move of the nurses from the King Edward Building was made possible by the opening in 1925 of a North Wing (named the Musgrave Wing, following Henry Musgrave's donation), which joined the East and West wings to complete a quadrangle. As well as accommodating additional nurses, it provided a billiard room for the doctors and a 'boudoir' for the 'lady doctors' who had by now arrived on the site.

It would seem that because of shortage of money and nurses, wards 7/8 and 15/16 were not in regular use for civilians until after World War One, and the hospital's effective capacity initially was thus about 200 rather than 300 beds. Once peace returned, however, hospital activities (including the care of chronic injuries to soldiers) increased to fill all the existing wards. Then, at the annual meeting of 1923, it was announced that the hospital had received a bequest of over £50,000 from Mr Henry Musgrave of Musgrave and Co., engineers and ironfounders, whose father Sir James Musgrave had funded the university chair of Pathology. This enabled a further three wards to be added (18, 19 and 20), doubling the number of gynaecological beds and adding a complete new surgical unit and operating theatre. These were opened in 1925. From the outset, they were longer than the original wards and provided a stimulus for the changes to take place in 1936–37.

At about the same time (1924), a new mortuary with a large steep observation rotunda was built to the south of Ward 1, designed by Young and McKenzie in harmony with the original building. In 1926 the Young family gave a window in memory of R.M. Young who was a noted architect and local historian; the window was eventually transferred to the new replacement mortuary in 1994. The 1924 mortuary was demolished in 1995.

The last building to be added to the original Royal Victoria Hospital site was the Institute of Pathology in 1933. It had been planned from 1928 by Queen's University Belfast, and from the beginning it was very much a joint enterprise between the hospital and the university. The site was bounded approximately by the old avenue to the asylum (now the main road through the hospital), and the institute was built in the narrow space between the laundry and this road. The opening of this building meant that

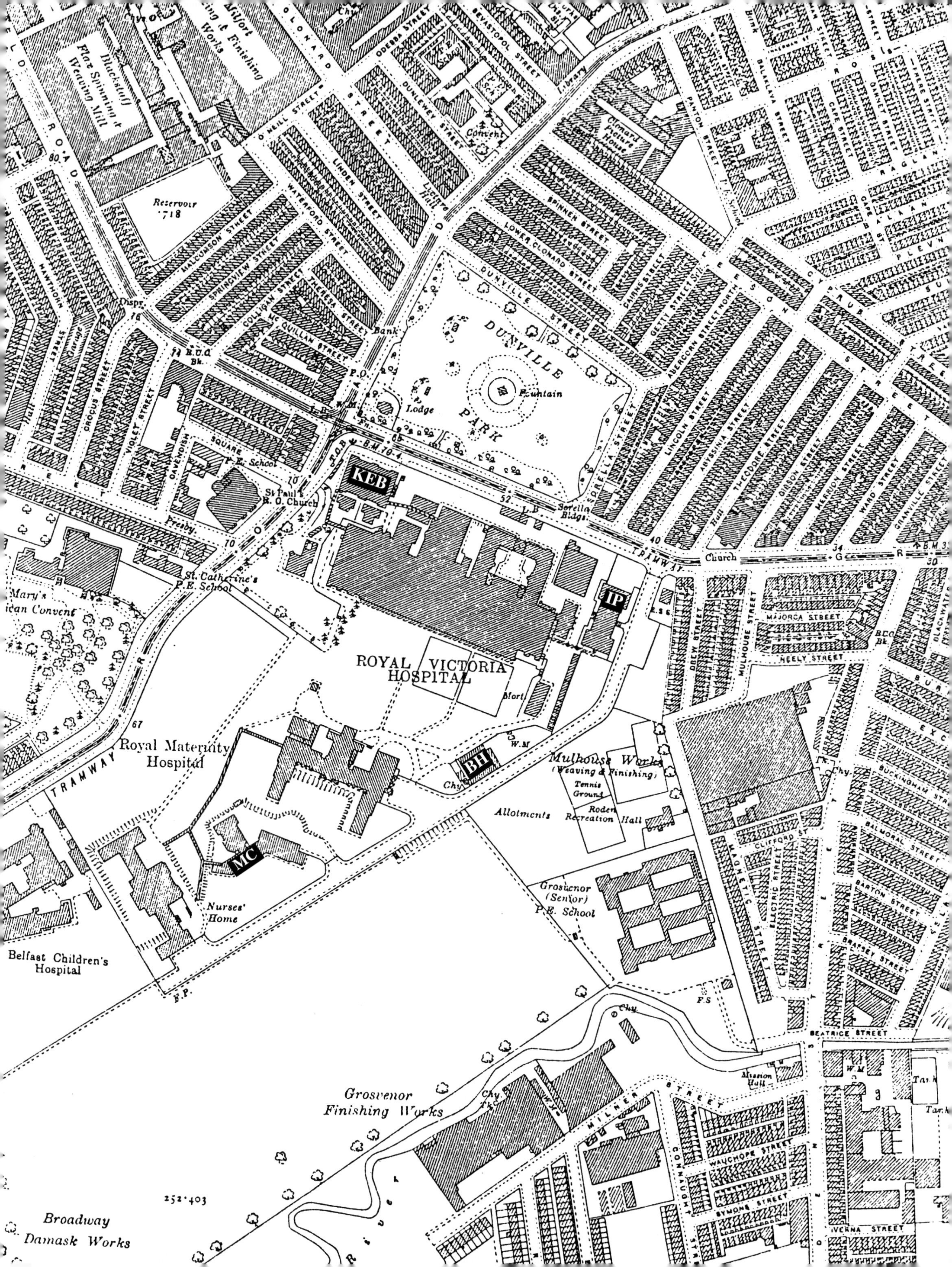

Blackstaff Flax Spinning & Weaving Mill
Milfort
Works
Reservoir
DUNVILLE PARK
Fountain
Lodge
KEB
IP
BH
MC
ROYAL VICTORIA HOSPITAL
Royal Maternity Hospital
Nurses' Home
Belfast Children's Hospital
St. Catherine's P.E. School
St Paul's R.C. Church
Mulhouse Works (Weaving & Finishing)
Tennis Ground
Roden Recreation Hall
Allotments
Grosvenor (Senior) P.E. School
Grosvenor Finishing Works
Broadway Damask Works
Mission Hall
TRAMWAY
SPRINGVIEW STREET
MALCOMSON STREET
WATERFORD STREET
LINDEN STREET
DUNLEWEY STREET
ODESSA STREET
SEVASTOPOL STREET
O'NEILL STREET
COLLIGAN STREET
THERESA STREET
McQUILLAN STREET
DUNVILLE STREET
LOWER CLONARD STREET
SPINNER STREET
SORELLA STREET
LINCOLN STREET
ABYSSINIA STREET
THEODORE STREET
GIBSON STREET
MERRION STREET
WARD STREET
GRANVILLE STREET
CAVENDISH SQUARE
VIOLET STREET
CROCUS STREET
MAJORCA STREET
NEELY STREET
MULHOUSE STREET
DREW STREET
BEATRICE STREET
MILNER STREET
CONNAUGHT STREET
WAUCHOPE STREET
SYMONS STREET
IVERNA STREET
MAGNETIC STREET
ELECTRIC STREET
CLIFFORD ST
BUCKINGHAM ST
BALMORAL STREET
BARTON STREET
BRAGSEY STREET

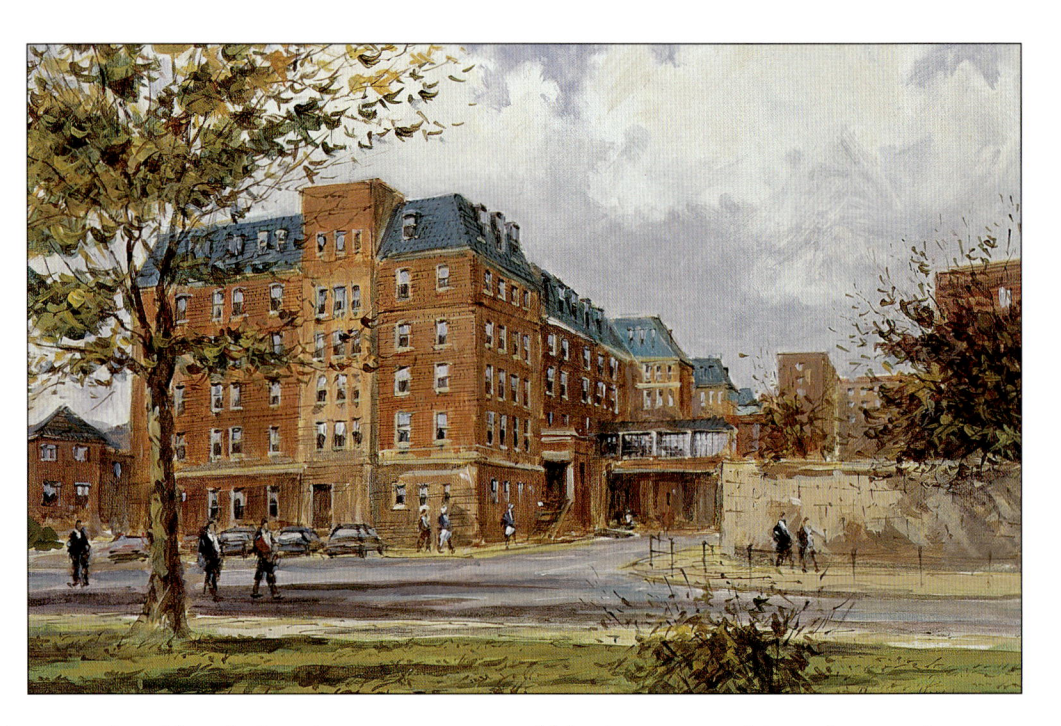

The first freestanding nurses' home at the Royal Victoria Hospital, opened in 1937 and named Musson House in 1951 after the recently retired Matron, Anne Musson. In the background is Bostock House, to the left is a new part of the Children's Hospital and to the right is part of the Musgrave and Clark Clinic; painting by Colin Gibson and reproduced by permission of the artist

the old pathology/mortuary area could be incorporated into the growing extern area and the laboratory space in the King Edward Building could also be vacated.

The Purdysburn estate was purchased in 1895 for a new asylum and Purdysburn House was opened for patients in 1906. Then, as villas were built nearby, the old asylum building in Belfast was used less and less and the remaining six acres were transferred to the Royal Victoria Hospital in 1921. The last patients were shell-shock victims from the army. The old building remained in position until 1930, by which time it was becoming difficult to maintain its safety and the decision was made to demolish it. As had been promised, the whole site northwest of the old avenue to the asylum was now made available for additional hospital buildings, and on it the new Belfast Hospital for Sick Children was opened in 1931 (it gained the title 'Royal' in 1948), and the Royal Maternity Hospital in 1933. These were separate institutions, of course, but their proximity to the Royal Victoria Hospital was of great clinical benefit. All these additions necessitated the building of a new boiler house with its tall chimney, completed in 1931 near the Royal Maternity site and beside the hospital road.

A new nurses' home was opened to the south of the hospital in 1937 with 208 rooms for nurses and 75 for domestics. It was designed to bring some comfort to the life of the nurses, having no less than eleven sitting rooms, three day rooms, a sitting room where nurses could entertain their friends with its own kitchen, a hairdressing salon, and a wing for the training of student nurses. In 1951 this block was named Musson House after Anne Musson, the Matron from 1922 to 1946.

The additional wards opened in 1925 had given the hospital a temporary respite from problems of accommodation, but outpatient attendances kept increasing and by 1930 pressure on beds was again severe. In that year, therefore, a new appeal was launched: for £100,000 to build an extension to each of the original seventeen wards. With the accession of King George VI this became known as the Coronation Extension Fund. It was decided that half of the money should be raised by the Working Men's Committee ('Million Shilling Fund') and half by the honorary officers, Board of Management and the life governors. In the event neither group was able to reach its target and by the end of 1938 only £55,000 had been raised. World War Two finally blocked all hope of completion.

But despite the financial problems, extensions to the wards proceeded, with the addition of projections out into the lawn behind the hospital and a rather unattractive iron balcony running its whole length. Essentially the idea was to increase the capacity of each ward from seven beds along each side to ten beds; the total per ward (including the centre bed and side wards) would increase from nineteen to twenty-five. The extensions to wards 5 to 17 were opened in 1937 and those to wards 1 to 4 in the following year, adding about 100 beds in all and bringing the hospital's theoretical total up to 538.

At best this extension was a makeshift, though, and the wards were always too large to be manageable. The patients at the far end were remote from the administrative hub of the ward at the corridor end. The wards were noisy and, in spite of the addition of new toilet and sluice arrangements, facilities were overstretched. In addition, the sewers and Plenum ventilation system were having to take an excessive load, creating problems that would become apparent over the next sixty years.

The last major addition to the hospital before the 1939 war was the Musgrave Clinic. Funded by Henry Musgrave for 50 private beds and enlarged after World War Two by Sir George Clark's donation (see page 144), this was not simply an amenity for the wealthy but contained beds specifically reserved for those of middle income. It was hoped that this would provide income for the hospital and take some pressure off the beds for the truly needy patients.

In 1939 a new building was completed beyond Ward 20, away from the corridor and housing wards 21 and 22; Messrs McLaughlin and Harvey were once again the builders. It was designed to accommodate up to 36 septic and isolation patients in small wards. This was intended to free space beside the main wards and outpatient hall for an x-ray department, though in fact the latter was not built until well after World War Two ended.

The changes described in this chapter show how enormously the hospital developed once it moved to the Grosvenor Road site. It was frequently on the brink of financial crisis, but thanks to energetic fundraising it stayed afloat. However, all this describes only the structures of the hospital. The work done and the staff involved are described in the next chapter.

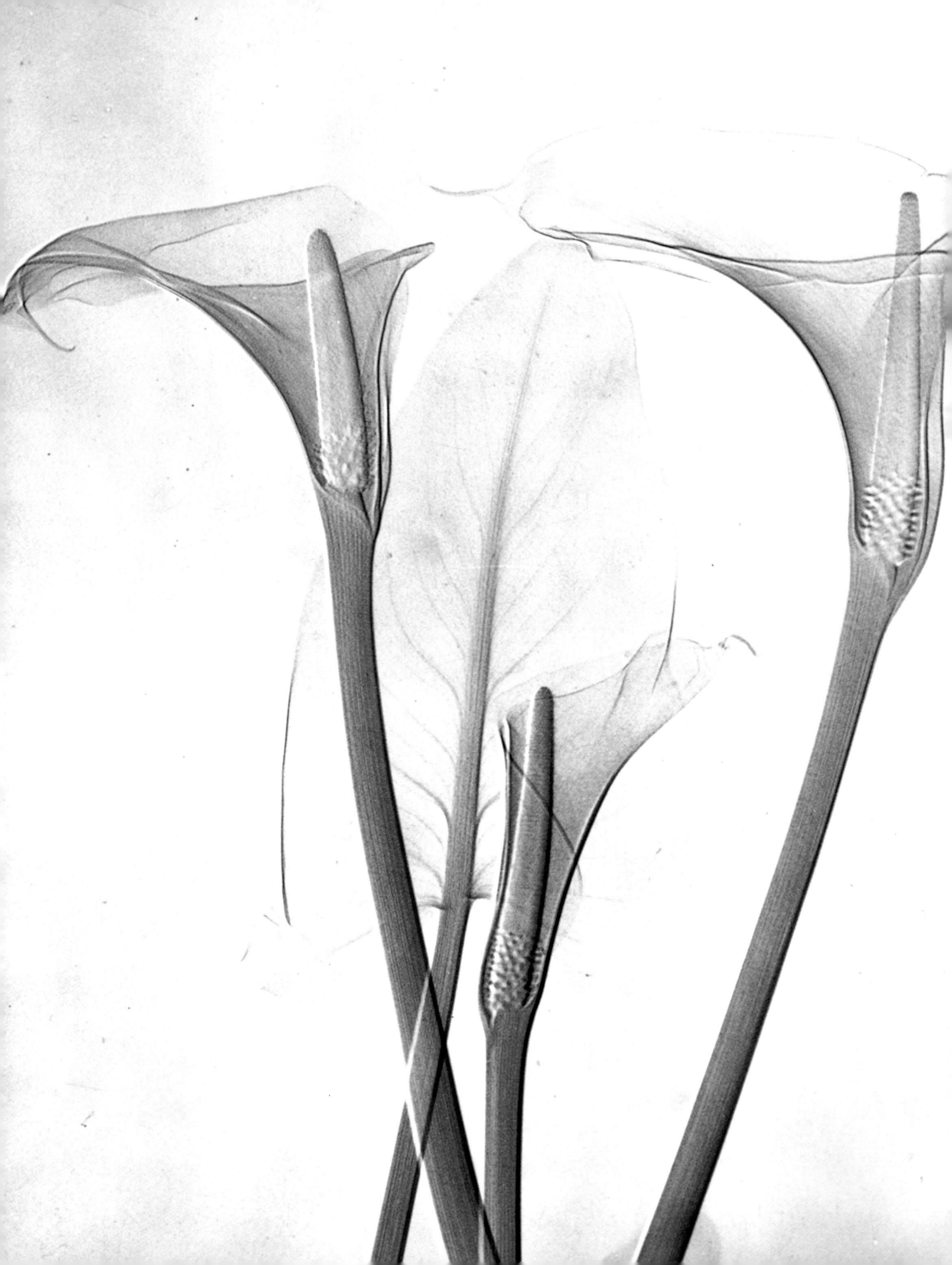

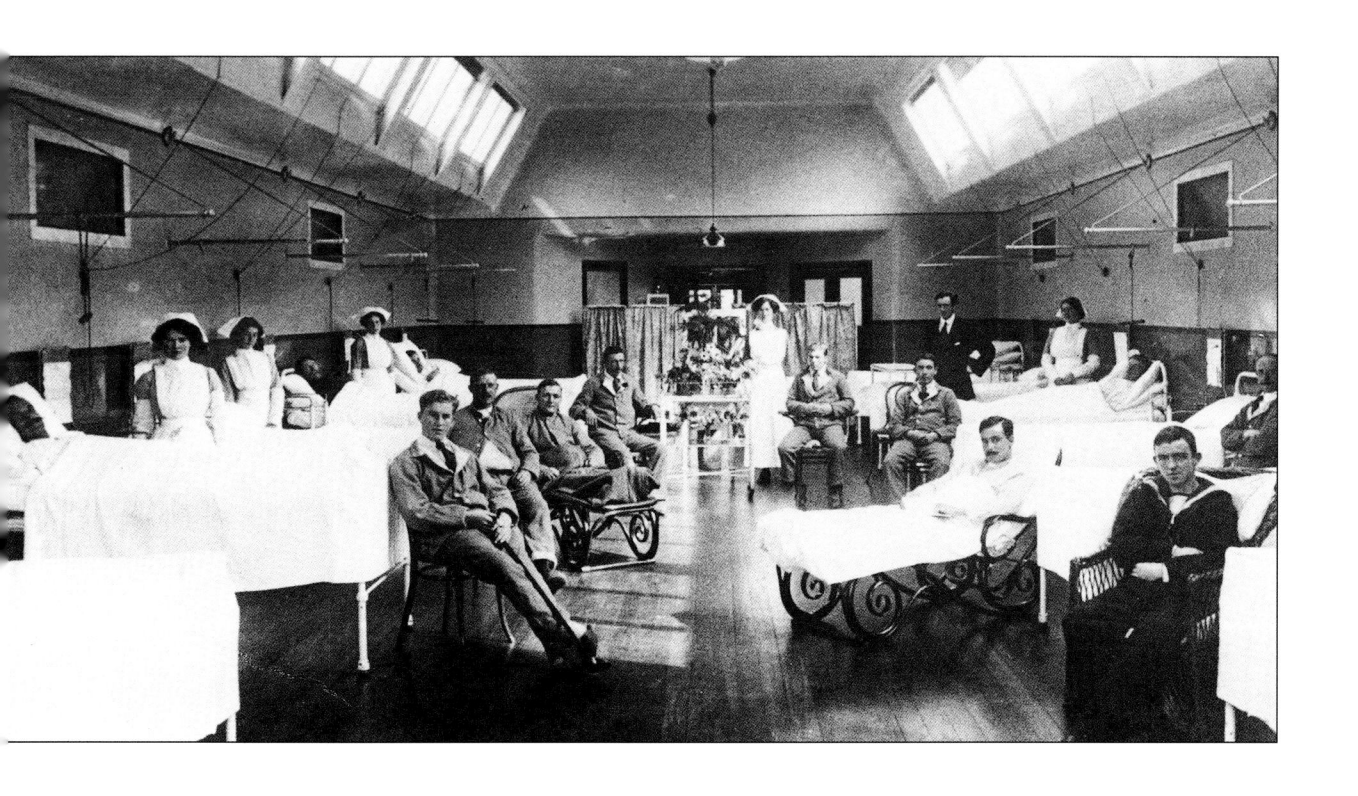

4
MEDICINE AND SURGERY IN THE ROYAL VICTORIA HOSPITAL
1903–1948

By THE BEGINNING OF THE TWENTIETH CENTURY, the Royal Victoria Hospital was caring for significantly fewer nonsurgical patients than previously: this was a result of the continuing decline in infectious fevers as well as the fact that such patients were mainly managed elsewhere. In 1903, for instance, the hospital's doctors admitted 888 new medical (including gynaecology) patients compared to 1,410 surgical patients, and there was a similar difference in the number of extern patients seen.

Above:
Ward 5 of the hospital, with wounded soldiers and sailors, August 1915; photograph by A.R. Hogg
ROYAL VICTORIA HOSPITAL

Opposite:
X-ray of an arum lily, one of many non-medical x-rays taken during the 1930s by Ralph Leman, pioneer radiographer at the Royal Victoria Hospital
ROYAL VICTORIA HOSPITAL

Medical complaints fell into all the groups with which we are familiar today – Bright's disease (kidney failure), bronchitis and pneumonia, chronic endocarditis, paralysis resulting from cerebral vascular accidents, gastric ulcer and 'gastritis', anaemia, rheumatism, fevers, and poisoning particularly by alcohol – but there were still few specific remedies available. However, if fevers were diminishing, venereal disease certainly was not, and the end of World War One brought an influx of cases into Belfast as soldiers returned home.

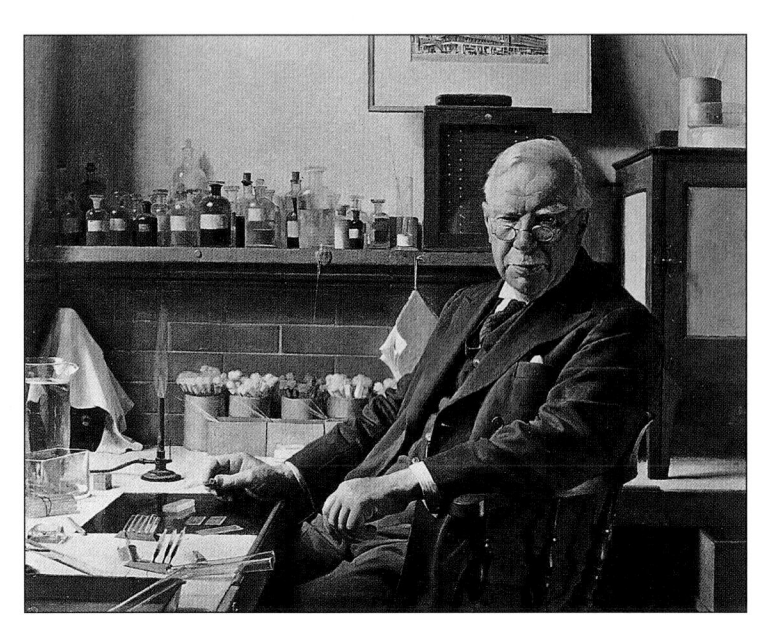

A significant feature of the medical treatment of many disorders at the turn of the century was the preparation of serum and vaccines against particular infections. One of the pioneers was Dr (later Sir) Almroth Wright, a Belfast man and a graduate of Trinity College Dublin (MB 1883), who worked for most of his life at St Mary's Hospital, London. His theory (much derided in George Bernard Shaw's *The Doctor's Dilemma*) was that infection could be overcome by stimulation of the body's natural resistance in the form of the phagocytes (white blood cells). The treatment involved taking a sample of the patient's blood or pus from an abscess, preparing a serum with supposed antibodies against the infecting organism, and injecting it into the patient again. The practice was totally superseded with the arrival of sulphonamides and specific antibiotics about the time of World War Two; it is hard nowadays, in the light of the massive growth since then in the numbers of effective treatments, to comprehend just what a large part vaccine therapy played in the treatment of all infections – from boils to tuberculosis – in the first forty years of the twentieth century.

Belfastman Sir Almroth Wright, who established the bacteriological and vaccine laboratory in St Mary's Hospital, Paddington, and influenced much of Sir Thomas Houston's work in the Royal Victoria Hospital
ROYAL VICTORIA HOSPITAL

The cardiology practised after 1903 in the new hospital was little changed from that of the nineteenth century, being still largely confined to administration of digitalis, and the first advance into the scientific era was the introduction of the electrocardiograph (ECG) to record the electrical activity of the heart. This had first been applied to humans in the 1880s, but the invention of the Einthoven string galvanometer in 1903 made it a practicable possibility. The first model reached the Royal Victoria Hospital in 1913 and the hospital's annual report for that year gives a detailed description of the working of the galvanometer under the general statement 'Medical Science has of late advanced with giant strides and new instruments of precision are being constantly devised for the better elucidation of disease.' The electrocardiograph was the first purchased in Ireland and credit must go to Dr John Elder MacIlwaine, newly appointed as an Assistant Physician, for his enthusiasm and to Mr James Mackie of the Albert Foundry for providing the money to buy it.

One of the great medical advances of the twentieth century was the discovery of insulin by Banting and Best. Before the introduction of insulin, life for diabetics was indeed miserable, for they had to try to regulate their blood sugar solely on the basis of food intake. If they took too much, the high blood sugar would push them into diabetic coma, a danger indicated by sugar in the urine. If they did not take enough, they would have no energy and would feel faint. In the end the patient usually developed disease of the arteries and nerves and died in middle life. Insulin was first used in the treatment of diabetes in Toronto in 1922 and in the following year it became available in the British Isles. A biochemistry laboratory was set up in the Royal Victoria Hospital in 1922 so that, among other tests, the level of blood sugar could be measured to supplement the detection of sugar in the urine (any sugar in urine is abnormal). This provided a basis for calculating the dosage of insulin needed, and this put diabetes management on a more scientific footing.

Not long after this it became possible to overcome another biochemical deficiency: by the administration of liver extract to patients with pernicious anaemia. The first reports of this treatment came from doctors Minot and Murphy of Boston in 1926 and in the following year its value was being investigated by Sir Thomas Houston in the Royal Victoria Hospital. By the early 1930s patients were being regularly treated in the hospital and the complicated connection between gastric juice, a vitamin of the B group (later called B12), anaemia, and degeneration of the spinal cord was becoming understood. With both diabetes and pernicious anaemia the Royal Victoria Hospital was in the forefront of medical research and early treatment. Subsequent years were to show that the liver treatment was indeed of genuine and life-saving value, though isolation of Vitamin B12 did not come until later.

THE VISITING PHYSICIANS

The four Attending Physicians in post in 1903 were Sir William Whitla, Professor J.A. Lindsay, Dr W. Calwell and Dr H.L. McKisack (see Chapter 2). The Assistant Physicians (see page 26) were Dr William Baird McQuitty and Dr John Morrow; this situation remained unchanged until 1910 when Dr McQuitty died of a cerebral haemorrhage at the age of forty-seven. He had been educated at Queen's College Belfast, winning a succession of prizes and studentships, and graduating with an MD in 1887. After further experience he was appointed honorary Surgeon to the Ulster Hospital for Women and Children, Templemore Avenue, in 1890, and he transferred to the medical side in 1893. He remained in that hospital until

Dr William Baird McQuitty, Assistant Physician at the Royal Victoria Hospital from 1900 until his death in 1910
ROYAL VICTORIA HOSPITAL

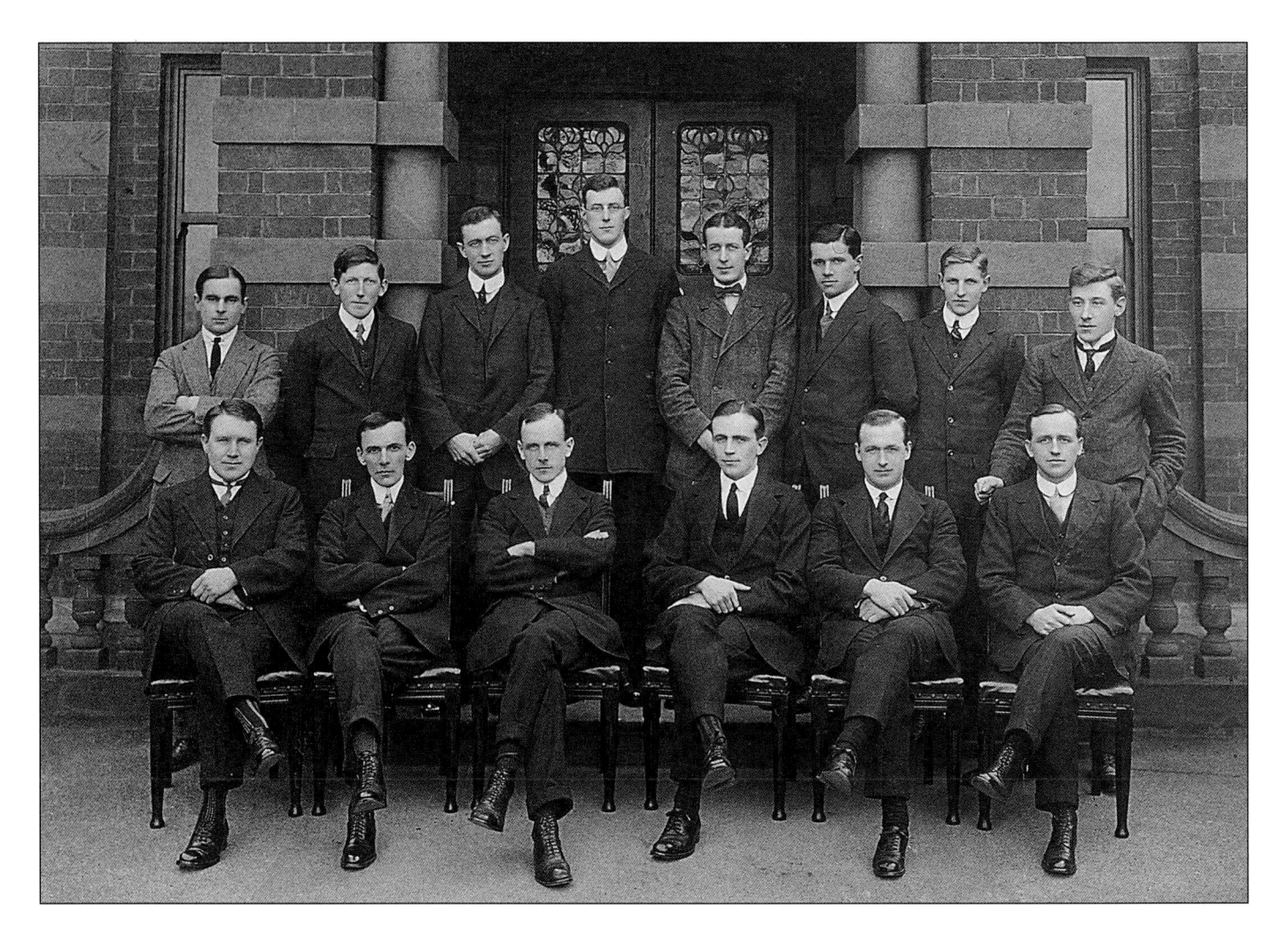

The Resident Medical Staff of the Royal Victoria Hospital, January 1913: standing *left to right:* G.D. Latimer, E.U. MacWilliam, R.S. Ross, W. McDermott, H.P. Hall, S. Geddis, S.E. Picken and W.M.H. McCullagh; seated *left to right:* J. Cathcart, S.I. Turkington, E. Morison, R. Marshall, S. Davison and F. Jefferson
ROYAL VICTORIA HOSPITAL

he was appointed Assistant Physician at the Royal Victoria Hospital in 1900, when he resigned his previous post. McQuitty's post at the RVH carried no rights to beds and he practised mainly in the extern department. In this field he achieved great popularity on account of his kindness and consideration to the poorer patients. He was clever enough to have doubts about most of the medical treatments of his day, but tactful enough to advise and help all who came to him. The story is told of the high-society lady who came to him, whose only treatable condition was dirtiness. His prescription was a supply of sugar-coated pills containing only bread, to be taken daily after a hot bath. When he died a vast crowd followed his coffin to the City Cemetery and (very unusually) a public subscription was begun which eventually endowed the McQuitty Scholarship at the Royal Victoria Hospital.

Dr John Smyth Morrow studied medicine at Queen's College Belfast, and graduated MB in 1890 and MD in 1895. He became an Assistant Physician in 1903, and served in the RAMC during World War One (being awarded the OBE). On Sir William Whitla's retirement in 1918, Morrow was elected Attending Physician. He was a medical officer to Harland and Wolff and was always the general physician, avoiding any temptation to specialise. He was unusually earthy and irascible in manner, and many stories are told of his uproarious ward rounds. On one occasion he addressed the patient with 'Good morning, Moses', and turning to the class went on, 'Gentlemen, Moses means beloved of the Lord, but unfortunately Moses harbours the spirochaete.' Dr Morrow retired as a Consulting Physician in 1930.

Dr John Elder MacIlwaine replaced Dr McQuitty as Assistant Physician in 1910 and immediately took a special interest in cardiology and the use of the new electrocardiograph. He had an engineering B.Sc. of Glasgow University and qualified MB from Queen's College Belfast in 1901. After service in the RAMC during World War One, he returned to the hospital and was appointed Attending Physician on the retirement in 1921 of Professor J.A. Lindsay. In the same year he was also appointed Professor of Materia Medica and Therapeutics, the modified title of the chair vacated by Sir William Whitla in 1919. Dr MacIlwaine resigned from the chair in 1928 but his eyesight deteriorated rapidly and (presumably fearing a malignant cause) he shot himself on 6 August 1930.

The next physicians appointed to the Visiting staff were Professor W.W.D. Thomson and Dr Foster Coates, who replaced Dr Calwell and Dr McKisack on their retirement in 1924. Professor William Willis Dalziel Thomson was the son of the dispensary doctor of Annahilt, County Down. He studied medicine at Queen's College Belfast, graduating with an MB in 1910 with first place and first-class honours, following this achievement by gaining an MD with gold medal in 1916. After travel for further study, and war service, Dr Thomson returned to Belfast as Assistant Physician at the Royal Victoria Hospital in 1918. When Professor Lindsay retired from the chair of Medicine in 1921, Dr Thomson succeeded him. He was the last of the old-style professors who made their mark not by research but by bedside teaching, and indeed he was the last of the part-time professors of medicine. These professors were part-time Attending Physicians or Surgeons of the hospital (unpaid), part-time teachers in hospital and university (paid a small emolument), and part-time engaged in private practice. Inevitably they had no time (and little inclination) for research. Professor Thomson had a wise but friendly and relaxed approach to all students, patients and medical colleagues, and his opinion was sought as often by general practitioners in the country villages as by colleagues in University Square. He was knighted in 1950 and died in the same year. After his death his colleagues on the staff presented a bronze medal to be awarded annually in his memory. His only son, Captain Humphrey Barron Thomson RAMC, was killed in 1942 on active service in the Far East, and is commemorated by the Thomson Room in the medical library.

Dr Foster Coates was the son of Dr Stanley Coates of University Square,

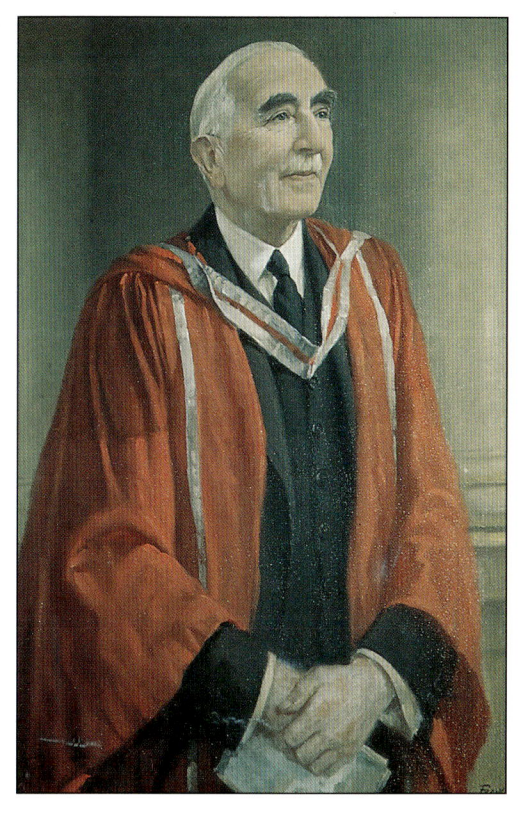

Professor W.W.D. Thomson (later Sir), Professor of Medicine at Queen's University Belfast, 1921–50, and Visiting Physician at the Royal Victoria Hospital; portrait by Frank McKelvey
QUEEN'S UNIVERSITY BELFAST

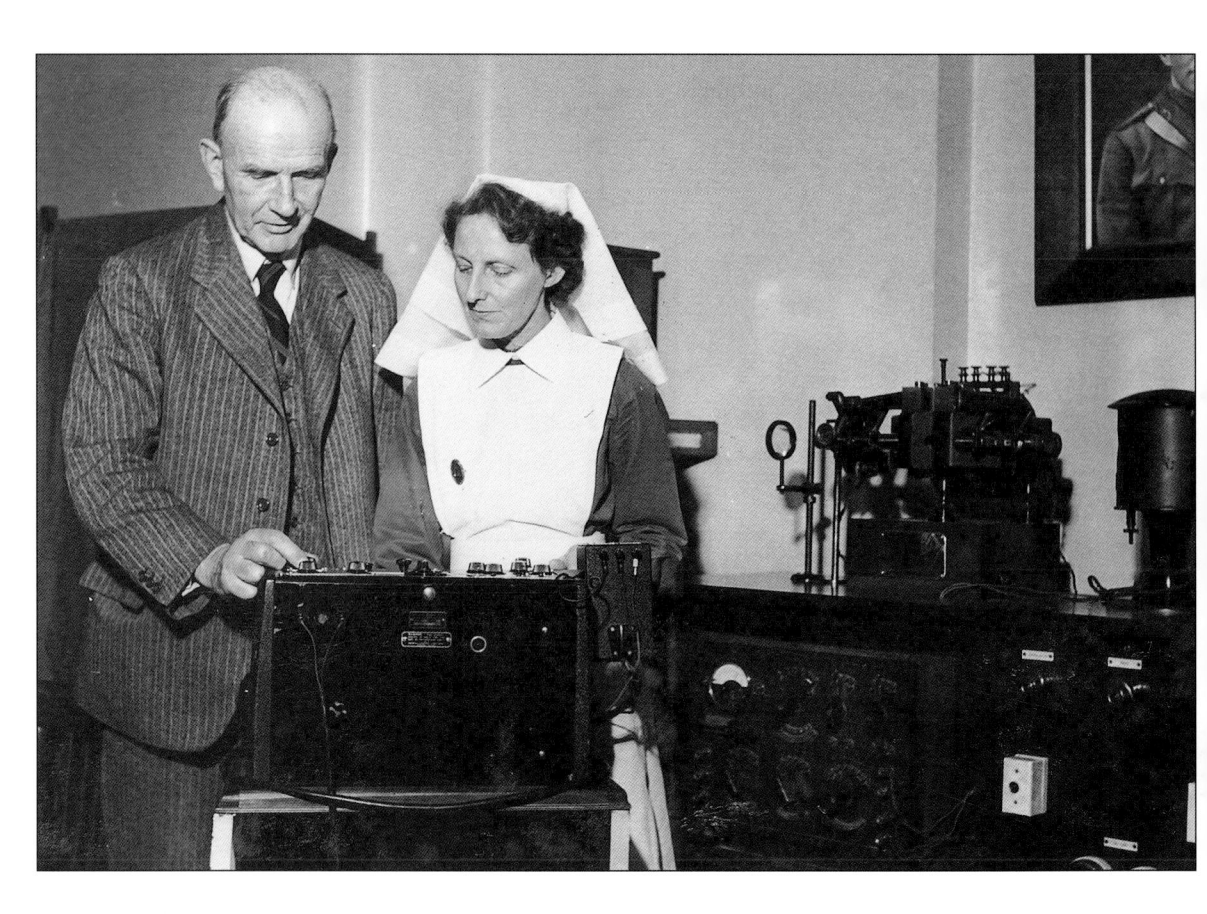

Dr Boyd Campbell, Visiting Physician to the Royal Victoria Hospital, 1921–54, and Sister Thelma McMath, with an electrocardiograph machine of the period
ROYAL VICTORIA HOSPITAL

Belfast, and studied at Queen's College Belfast, graduating MB in 1905, and MD in 1907; he was the first doctor to obtain the Diploma of Public Health from the new Queen's University in 1908. He served with the RAMC during World War One and on his return in 1918 he was appointed Assistant Physician at the Royal Victoria Hospital. He was Attending Physician to wards 3 and 4 from 1924 with a special interest in neurology and was one of the first people to note the prevalence of multiple sclerosis in Northern Ireland. He was also a specialist in chest medicine, being also on the staff of the Forster Green Hospital, but he is remembered best as a sound and unassuming general physician 'not vain, nor flamboyant, nor a poseur, nor a simpleton' (J.S. Logan). He retired in 1945.

Dr Samuel Burnside Boyd Campbell was born in India, graduated MB with first-class honours from Edinburgh in 1912 and served in the British army during World War One, being awarded the Military Cross. After the war he settled in Belfast where in 1921 he was appointed Assistant Physician at the Royal Victoria Hospital and graduated with an MD. He worked with Dr MacIlwaine, taking over his interest in electrocardiography, and succeeded him as Attending Physician in 1929 (wards 7 and 8); he was given charge of the ECG department in 1930. He retained a strong interest in cardiology all his life but was also on the staff of the UVF Hospital. Outside hospital he was best known as a lifelong enthusiast of rugby. He retired in 1954; by this time his son, Dr Wilfred Campbell, was a paediatrician on the staff of the Royal Belfast Hospital for Sick Children.

Dr Robert (Bertie) Marshall was appointed Attending Physician to wards 5 and 6 in 1930 on the retirement of Dr Morrow. He had graduated MB with honours from Queen's University in 1912 and trained in cardiology in London before service with the RAMC in World War One. He joined the Royal Victoria Hospital in 1924 as Assistant Physician and from his appointment as Attending Physician he had a strong interest in cardiology. He had his own electrocardiograph, published much, and throughout his career always had a bitter rivalry with Dr Boyd Campbell, who was in charge of the adjoining wards and the ECG department. Dr Marshall was probably the more academically distinguished. A fluent raconteur, he often lapsed into Latin on appropriate (or inappropriate) occasions and he also wrote historical papers and a history of the Royal Victoria Hospital from 1903 to 1953. Nevertheless, within the hospital and beyond, Dr Boyd Campbell had at least as many friends and supporters. Both men retired in 1954. Dr Marshall's daughter Dorothy married Desmond Neill, the first full-time biochemist to the hospital.

There were no further major changes among the physicians of the hospital until after World War Two. Dr S.I. Turkington was assistant physician from 1924, Dr J.T. Lewis from 1929 and Dr R.S. Allison from 1930; they retained these titles until their return from war service.

Dr Samuel Ireland Turkington graduated at Queen's University in 1912 and throughout his career had a particular interest in chest disease, being also on the staff of the Forster Green Hospital. He spent most of his career in the Royal Victoria Hospital as Assistant Physician or Physician in Charge of Outpatients, and was highly regarded as a clinical teacher and as an exponent of old-fashioned physical examination. He was appointed

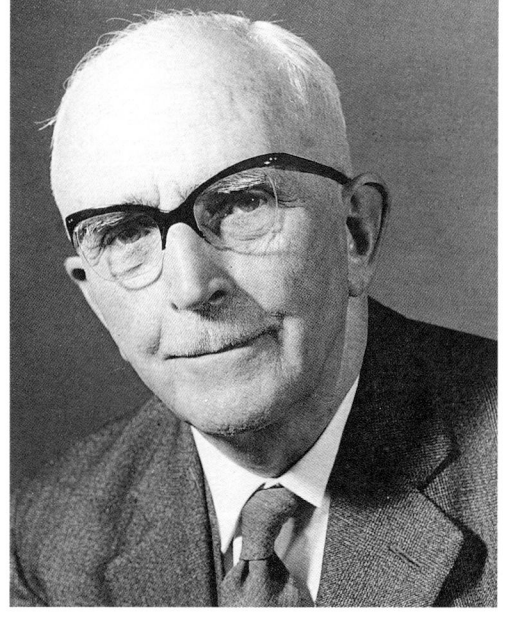

Dr Robert Marshall, Visiting Physician to the Royal Victoria Hospital, 1924–54
ROYAL VICTORIA HOSPITAL

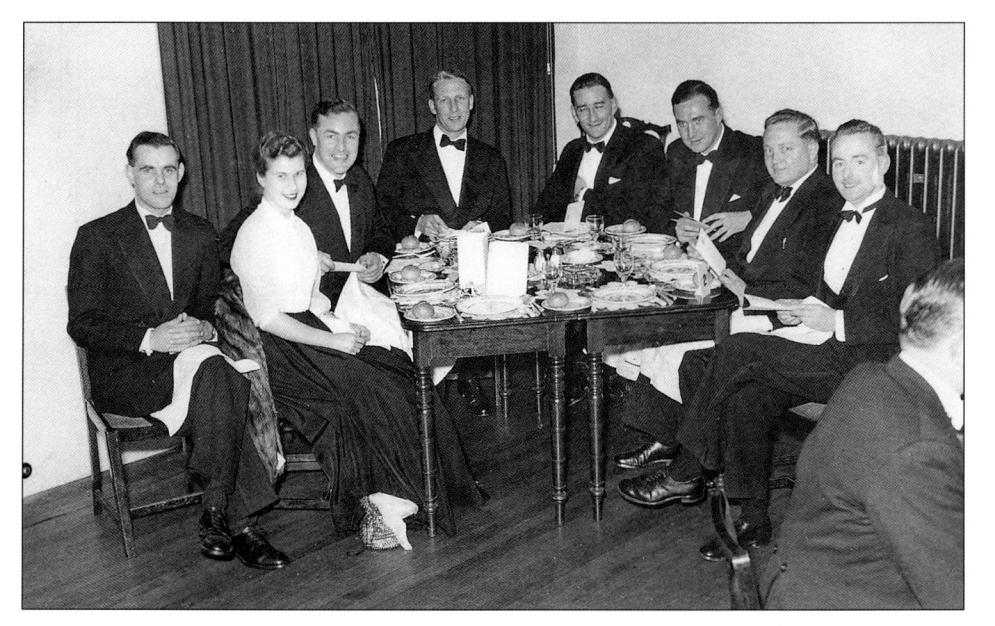

Dr Robert Marshall's farewell dinner, 1954; *left to right:* Dr Hugh Graham, Dr Beatrice Russell (later Mrs Graham), Mr Alex McAllister, Dr Neill Beck, Dr Bob Weir, Mr Willoughby Wilson, Mr Ken Roddie and Dr S. Bateman
ROYAL VICTORIA HOSPITAL

Attending Physician in 1945 and retired in 1950, a year before his death.

Dr Joseph Tegart (Ted) Lewis graduated MB at Queen's University in 1921 with first-class honours and MD in 1924 with gold medal. He joined the RAMC in World War Two, and was wounded in North Africa and then was a prisoner-of-war in Italy; later he was in charge of the unit sent in to provide medical care on the liberation of Belsen concentration camp. Dr Lewis described this experience in a lecture to the Ulster Medical Society in 1945 (it was only published, in an abbreviated form, in 1985). He was appointed an Attending Physician on the medical staff in 1946. The war took a heavy toll of his energies, but he worked on until his retirement in 1962.

Dr Richard Sydney Allison studied medicine at Queen's University, was a surgeon probationer in the Royal Navy during World War One, and qualified MB with honours in 1921 and MD in 1924. From 1922 he worked in various hospitals in London, then from 1925 to 1930 in Ruthin Castle, north Wales, always with a main interest in neurology and particularly in multiple sclerosis (or 'disseminated sclerosis' as it was then called). In 1930 he was appointed Assistant Physician to the Royal Victoria Hospital, in 1937 physician to the outpatients (with some beds) and in 1939 Visiting Physician to Claremont Street Hospital. Then came World War Two and he went back to the Royal Navy as a specialist physician. On returning to the Royal Victoria Hospital after the war, he gave up his general medical responsibilities and in 1947 was designated Physician in Charge of the Department of Neurology. He was a prolific lecturer and writer, and his work culminated in his book *The Senile Brain* (1962). After he retired in 1964 he was invited to become honorary Archivist of the Royal Victoria Hospital and produced his history of eye, ear, nose and throat surgery in Belfast, *The Very Faculties* (1969), his much larger history of the Royal Victoria Hospital from 1850 to 1903, *The Seeds of Time* (1972), and his *The Surgeon Probationers* (1979). His name is remembered in the hospital by the Allison Lecture and Prize.

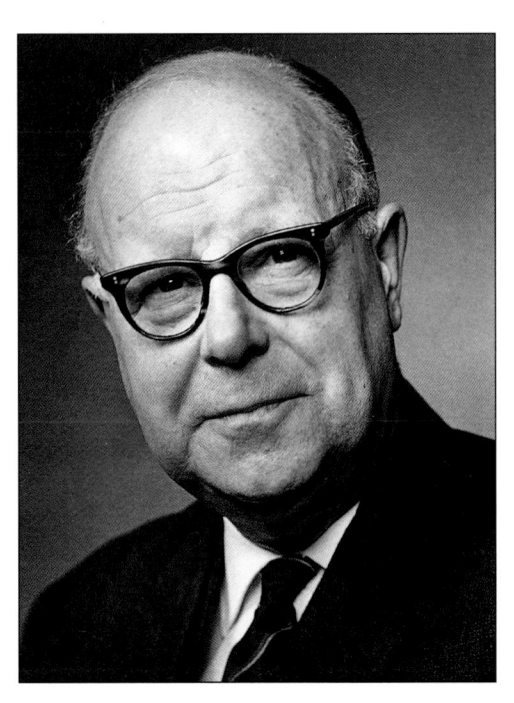

Dr Sydney Allison, Visiting Physician to the Royal Victoria Hospital, 1930–64, and founder of the Department of Neurology; he was the first honorary Archivist to the hospital.
ROYAL VICTORIA HOSPITAL

Dr Thomas Howard Crozier graduated with an MB at Queen's University in 1921 and with an MD in 1924. He was appointed physician to the Belfast Infirmary (later the Belfast City Hospital) in 1926 and held this post throughout his life. During World War Two he served with the RAMC; on returning to Belfast in 1945 he was appointed Assistant Physician in Charge of Outpatients to the Royal Victoria Hospital, to become a Consultant Physician in 1948. He was author of *Aids to Medical Treatment*, which ran to four editions, and co-editor with Dr R.S. Allison of the ninth edition of Whitla's *Dictionary of Medical Treatment*. He was an erudite physician and a sound teacher but he is particularly remembered for his at times bitter wit, as when during an examination of the eardrum of an elderly lady she asked him, 'Doctor, are ye lookin' at me brains.' To which he replied under his breath, 'Madam, this is an auriscope, not a microscope.'

Dr Crozier is only one of many authors associated with the RVH. A steady flow of publications had come from the hospital physicians from the mid-nineteenth century onwards. These included works of poetry (Drennan), of history (Malcolm, Marshall, Allison) and, most frequently, medical textbooks (Whitla, McKisack, Crozier). There were also, of course, many papers in medical journals, but before 1948 these were isolated, occasional productions, and it is only in the last fifty years that the output of papers has become an avalanche.

DERMATOLOGY

Dermatology was the only medical speciality that was recognised from the nineteenth century as distinct, and throughout the first half of the twentieth century it was the only one in the Royal Victoria Hospital that was organisationally separate. This was partly because of the frequency of skin diseases associated with dirt and poverty (for example, impetigo) and also because, then as now, any skin condition worried the patient out of all proportion to its true importance. Dr William Calwell had been Attending Physician in this field from 1900 (see pages 48 and 58), though he always combined dermatology with the role of general physician. He held a separate skin clinic – in the extern block and later in the King Edward Building – until he retired in 1924.

Dr Ivan McCaw, who succeeded Dr Calwell in a junior capacity, was the first 'pure' dermatologist to be appointed to the staff. He was the son of Dr John McCaw, a paediatrician on the staff of the old Children's Hospital in Queen Street. He was educated at Queen's University and in 1918, while serving in World War One, was severely wounded in the right arm. He returned to graduate in 1922 with honours, gained experience in skin diseases in Edinburgh, London and Belfast, and was appointed Assistant Physician in Charge of the Skin Department in 1933.

The inpatient treatment of skin diseases in Belfast took place in the Benn Hospital for Diseases of the Skin, and other noted dermatologists such as Dr Samuel Allworthy, Dr Elias Purdon and later Dr Jonathan Jefferson mainly worked there. This hospital was destroyed in an air raid in 1941 and after World War Two its financial assets were merged with those of the Royal Victoria Hospital, where a few dermatological beds were opened in Ward 22 from 1951. A dermatological ward opened in 1957, named the Purdon Skin Ward after Dr Henry Purdon (see pages 47–48).

During the war Dr Reginald Hall had a junior post in dermatology; he became Assistant Physician in the Department of Dermatology in the Royal Victoria Hospital in 1945. He had first been a barrister in Dublin, but graduated with an MB with honours in 1936 (QUB), and with an MD with gold medal in 1940. Subsequently he practised dermatology in the Royal Victoria, Belfast City and Ulster hospitals. He retired in 1971.

VENEREAL DISEASES

There was an upsurge in venereal diseases (mainly syphilis and gonorrhoea) after World War One, and the Board of Management decided to open a new clinic in the King Edward Building in 1919, under the clinical care of Dr John Rankin, with bacteriological support from Dr Thomas Houston. In the first year there were 578 new cases for treatment, mainly ex-servicemen, with a total attendance of 3,277. The laboratory carried out 50–60 Wassermann tests for syphilis weekly. This clinic became established on the first floor of the King Edward Building (approached from the outside door on the Grosvenor Road to ensure invisibility of patients and to keep them separate) and remained there until 1970, when it moved to the new outpatient building.

Treatment of syphilis at the beginning of the twentieth century included the time-honoured remedies of corrosive attack on the lesion followed by mercury administered by mouth, by rubbing into the skin and by hypodermic injection. The mercury was not given in heroic doses as in the Middle Ages, but it was still a very unpleasant, prolonged and unreliable form of treatment. In the 1930s the use of organic arsenicals had greatly improved outcomes but these drugs required to be given intravenously and with great care, and giving them was the main role of the clinics. Methods of treatment of gonorrhoea were more varied and even less reliable until the sulphonamides came into use in the 1930s and later penicillin.

Dr Rankin was joined in 1921 by Dr Hugo Hall, a son of Dr Robert Hall of Belfast and brother of Surgeon Commander Robin Hall, who graduated with an MB at Queen's University in 1916 and with an MD in 1929 and served in the Royal Navy during World War One. Dr Rankin and Dr Hall ran the Special Clinic, as it was called, with the help of male and female nurses until the outbreak of World War Two. At this time Hugo Hall returned to the navy, first to the naval base in Londonderry and later to the aircraft carrier HMS *Furious*. He returned to the RVH after the war, was given consultant status in 1949, and eventually retired in 1959. Dr Rankin retired in 1945; during the war he had been helped by Dr Sydney McCann as registrar, and the team was joined in 1947 by Dr Fred Bonugli.

SURGERY IN THE NEW HOSPITAL

When the Royal Victoria Hospital opened in 1903 it had three pairs of surgical wards: 9 and 10, 11 and 12, and 13 and 14; wards 15 and 16 opened as surgical wards only later.

An operating theatre was attached to each pair of wards, and the Visiting

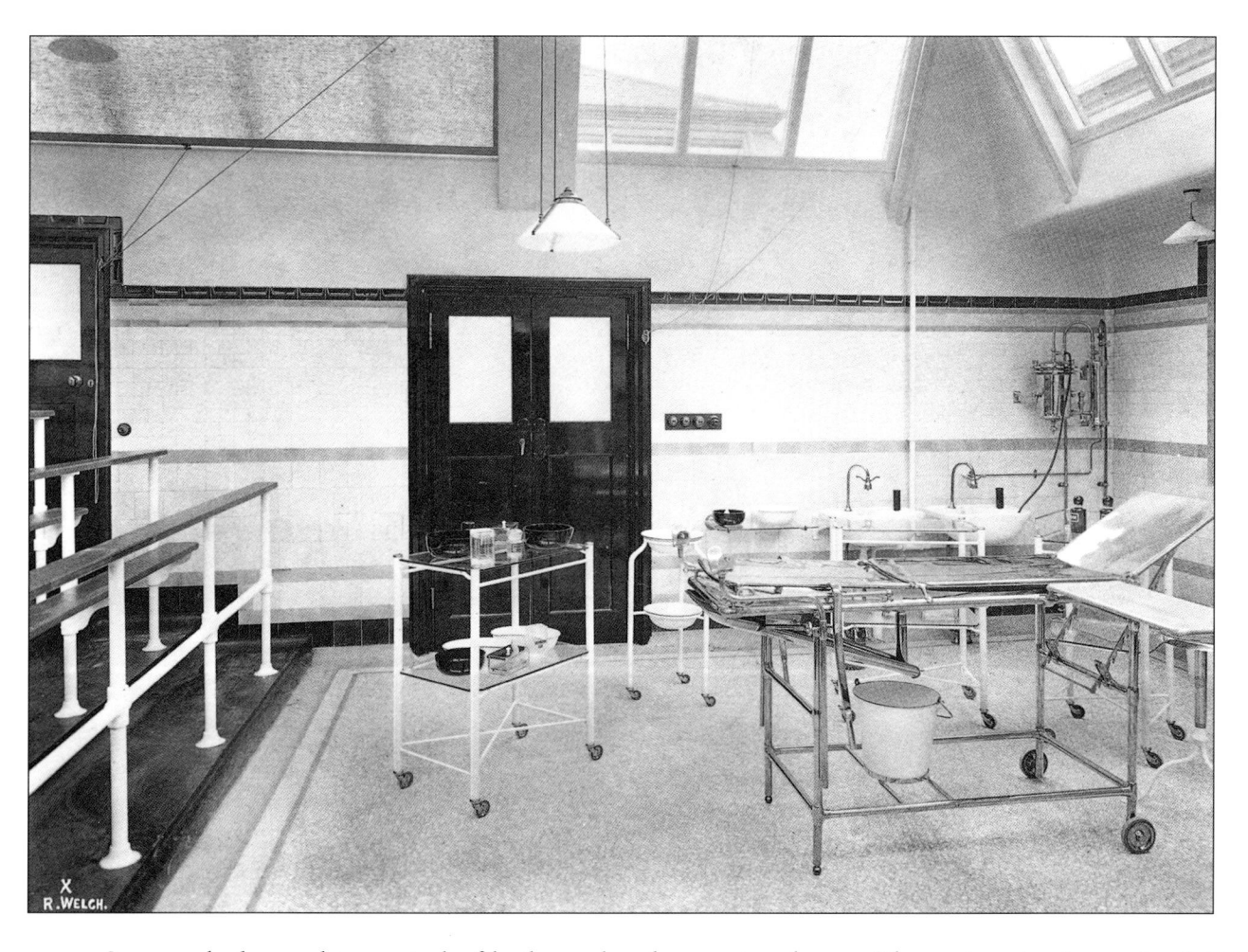

Surgeon had complete control of both ward and operating theatre. The theatres were tiled with white tiles and were provided with hot and cold running water so that scrubbing up, storage of instruments and the induction of anaesthesia could all be performed in them. The area of the theatres (26 x 16 square feet) might appear spacious, but it was reduced by one-third by the wooden benches provided to permit medical students to watch. Although the proximity of operating theatre to ward was very convenient, it readily permitted bacterial contamination, and moreover at that time the theatre staff still wore outside clothes during operations, with a gown on top to protect them from excessive soiling. The wooden benches were removed in the 1930s as one definite reservoir of infection, and although the surgeons were very much aware of the dangers of post-operative infection, it was not until the 1960s that rigorous ideas on theatre sterility became economic and practical possibilities. Another problem with the fact that each theatre opened off the ward corridor was that patients' relatives were often within easy hearing distance of noises inside and could see the patients as they were wheeled in and out of the theatre.

The Attending Surgeons at the hospital in 1903 were Mr J. Walton Browne MD, Professor Thomas Sinclair FRCSE, Dr A.B. Mitchell (later FRCSI) and Dr T. Sinclair Kirk MB. The Assistant Surgeons were Mr Robert

Operating theatre of wards 11 and 12, with wooden benches to the left for students to observe operations; these were later removed to give more space and to improve theatre sterility; photograph by R.J. Welch
ROYAL VICTORIA HOSPITAL

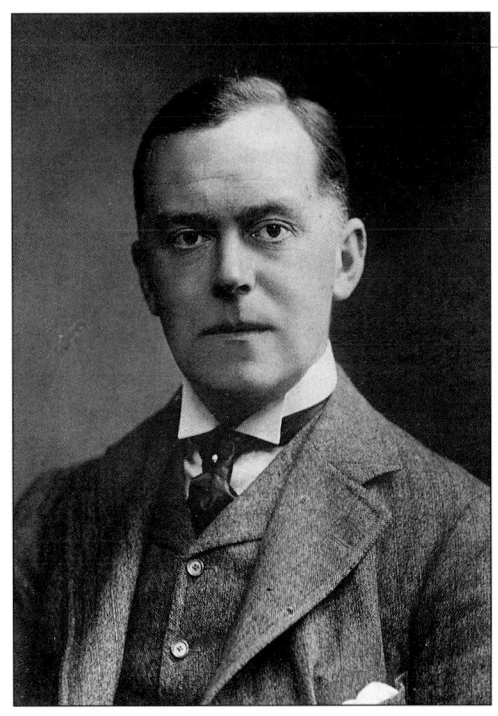

Dr T. Sinclair Kirk, known as 'Surgeon' Kirk, Visiting Surgeon to the Royal Victoria Hospital, 1897–1934
ROYAL VICTORIA HOSPITAL

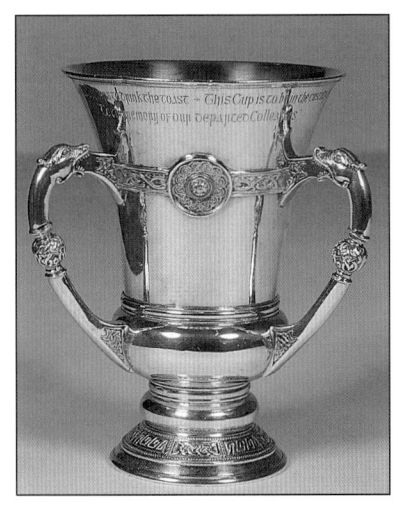

Surgeon Kirk's 'loving cup'; made of solid silver, it is still passed round at the annual staff dinner to drink a toast to departed colleagues. The cup was presented to Surgeon Kirk by the medical staff on his retirement in 1934 and returned to the staff on his death in 1940.
ROYAL VICTORIA HOSPITAL

Campbell FRCSE and Mr Andrew Fullerton MD, FRCSI. The first three of these surgeons have been described earlier; the fourth who transferred across from the old Royal Hospital was Dr T. Sinclair Kirk, known as 'Surgeon' Kirk or 'Pa' Kirk. He qualified in 1893 and, like many surgeons in the pre-NHS period, never obtained the FRCS. He was elected Assistant Surgeon to the hospital in 1897 and Attending Surgeon in 1902. He served in the RAMC during World War One, and was noted for a variety of unusual treatments (see page 109) which were still being used in living memory since he did not retire until 1934.

The Assistant Surgeon was, in modern terms, a junior consultant with a smaller number of beds in the ward (perhaps four) than his Attending Surgeon. Both, of course, were unpaid and relied on their private practice for a living. Private patients went for consultations to the surgeon's own home, but surgery was often performed in the private patient's house with instruments borrowed from the hospital and with the patient's general practitioner as anaesthetist (or the Assistant Surgeon if he was not assisting his senior with the operation).

During the whole of 1903, both before and after the move to the Grosvenor Road site, there were 859 surgical operations with 27 deaths (3.1 per cent, a figure that was up to the best national standards). These operations included 87 abdominal procedures, the commonest of which were appendectomy (21) and perforated (peptic) ulcer (14). There were 30 amputations, including 7 on the upper limb which probably resulted from accidents. Other common problems included adenitis (presumably tuberculous glands in the neck) (30), varicose veins (30), hernia (36), trephining of the skull (17), carcinoma of the breast (19), and a large number of fractures, bone infections and deformities. Notably, there were only 5 prostatectomies, one of which was fatal, compared with 16 external urethrotomies, 3 of which were fatal, and 7 suprapubic cystotomies. There were no operations on the chest or heart and no thyroidectomies.

Sir Ian Fraser in his Robert Campbell Oration of 1973 records the first operation performed in the new hospital:

> When the Royal Victoria Hospital opened its doors in 1903 to admit the first patients after their transfer from the old hospital in Frederick Street it was arranged that the first operation would be done with suitable pomp by the senior surgeon Dr John Walton Browne, but in the early hours of the morning a patient with a strangulated hernia was admitted requiring an immediate operation. This was done by Robert Campbell, and although gloves were available there were no gowns, all that could be found being a shroud from the mortuary. This was looked on by those with a superstitious mind as a bad omen for the future welfare of the new hospital.

By 1913 the annual number of surgical operations had more than doubled to 1,731; there had also been some changes in the pattern of general surgery, with an increase in the number of abdominal operations, so that these now occupied 20 per cent of the operating lists compared with 10 per cent in 1903. This increase probably reflects increasing worldwide confidence in effective suturing of the intestine, drainage of infection, and aseptic technique generally. By 1913 the number of deaths following surgery was 56, giving a similar surgical mortality of 3.2 per cent.

In 1912, Dr J. Walton Browne retired and was replaced by Mr Robert Campbell. Campbell had been Assistant Surgeon to the Belfast Children's Hospital since 1897 and Assistant Surgeon in the Royal Victoria Hospital from 1900 but was generally dogged by ill health having had acute nephritis in childhood. When he died in September 1920 of uraemia at the age of fifty-four it was said that 'despite his own ever-present ailments he did his best for his patients in any emergency'. He is remembered particularly as the pioneer of aseptic surgery in Belfast, though the idea of keeping infection out of the patient's wound rather than simply killing bacteria had been coming in since the days of Macewen (see page 40). Campbell quickly adopted the American novelty of wearing rubber gloves when operating, and he was the first in Ulster to advocate the use of a face mask, which the French surgeons had suggested to keep their beards in check. His surgical interests were wide. He wrote on club hand, on the operative treatment of hernia in children, and on the development of outpatient surgery. Shortly after his death, a fund was established in conjunction with the Ulster Medical Society to establish a memorial oration in his honour with a presentation medal. This lecture has been given every two to four years since 1922 by some of the most distinguished physicians and surgeons of the UK and elsewhere in the world.

The impact of the 1914–18 war on the hospital was as great as on Belfast generally, with large numbers of staff away on active service, and shortages of almost everything. Not only Professor Sinclair and Surgeon Kirk joined the RAMC but many of the younger doctors, sisters and trainee nurses. In 1915, reflecting the absence of many staff, for the first time in its history a woman doctor was appointed as House Surgeon to the hospital; she was Dr Margaret Purce, sister of Mr G.R.B. Purce (see pages 114–15). Mr A.B. Mitchell and Dr H.L. McKisack lost their elder sons in the Royal Irish Rifles and the Royal Flying Corps respectively.

The hospital took in many patients with residual problems from their active service in France. Wards 5 and 6 were set aside for wounded soldiers, and by late 1914, fifty-four more beds were reserved for them in wards that had hitherto been empty. An unlikely source of work for the surgeons was the need to operate on men excluded from serving in the forces because of hernia, varicose veins, et cetera, though who paid for these operations is not recorded. These men were admitted for operation and after surgery and convalescence were considered fit to enlist for active service. The total number of operations each year continued to rise during the war years in spite of the absence of senior staff, amounting to 2,062 in 1918. The number of gunshot wounds treated rose from 11 in 1913 to 207 in 1915 and 1916, falling off thereafter.

SURGERY IN THE TWENTIES AND THE THIRTIES

As mentioned in Chapter 3, the troubles of 1920 and 1922 had a considerable impact on the Royal Victoria Hospital, but there was relatively little civil violence during the late twenties and thirties.

When Professor Sinclair retired in 1923 he was replaced in the chair of Surgery by Andrew Fullerton. He had qualified from Queen's College in 1890 with first-class honours and obtained the FRCSI in 1901. He progressed slowly, being appointed Assistant Surgeon to the Belfast Hospital for Sick Children in 1898 but Assistant Surgeon to the Royal Victoria Hospital only in 1902, and Attending Surgeon in 1918. He joined the RAMC during World War One, which developed further his interest in genito-urinary surgery and in early trials of blood transfusion by the artery-to-vein method. He was a great innovator with the electric cystoscope and used to practise with a water-filled rubber ball standing in as a bladder. With it he learned to touch any point inside it and was able to cauterise papillomata and also to assess the function of each kidney separately by catheterising each ureter. He had a wide circle of surgical colleagues from the UK and America who came to Belfast to teach. His note-taking was meticulous and he was known for his special consideration for hospital patients and students, who always took precedence over his private practice. He was president of the Royal College of Surgeons in Ireland from 1926 to 1928 (the first from Belfast) and we are fortunate in having a fine portrait of him in his gown painted by William Conor. He retired in 1933 at the age of sixty-five and died a year later.

Mr Howard Stevenson graduated with an MB at Queen's College in 1900 and obtained the FRCSI in 1904. He was one of the last of the surgeons who worked as a junior in the old Frederick Street hospital; subsequently he was on the staff of the Ulster Hospital before being appointed Assistant Surgeon to the Royal Victoria Hospital in 1911 and Attending Surgeon in 1920. In 1938 he was elected MP for Queen's University. Although he retired from his surgical practice in 1941, Howard Stevenson returned from retirement to help during World War Two. According to Allison, 'He had a sureness of touch and economy of manoeuvre which gave a phenomenal operating speed and his excision of a gall bladder seemed to occupy seconds rather than minutes.'

Surgery during the 1920s and 1930s was so different from that in the 1990s that it is worth recalling the procedures as described by Sir Ian Fraser.

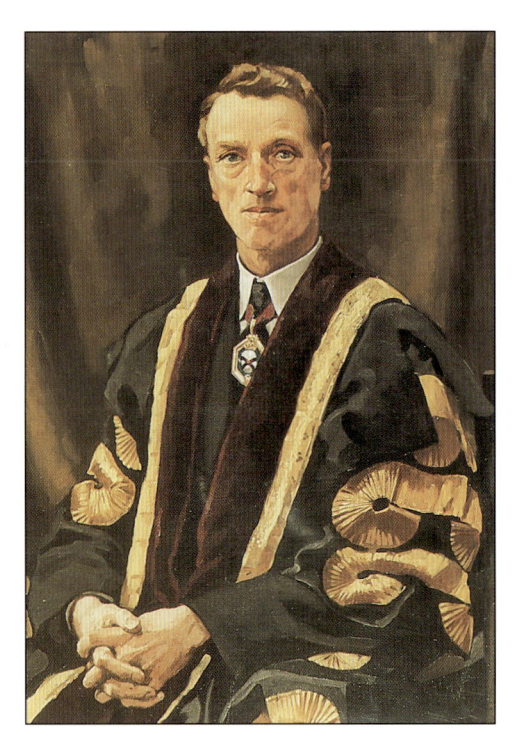

Professor Andrew Fullerton FRCSI, Professor of Surgery at Queen's University Belfast, 1923–33, Visiting Surgeon to the Royal Victoria Hospital, 1902–33, and president of the Royal College of Surgeons in Ireland, 1926–28; portrait by William Conor
ROYAL VICTORIA HOSPITAL

First, almost everything was reused. Bandages had to be washed and rolled afterwards by the nurses (with any help from students and House Surgeons that was available). Plaster of Paris bandages were prepared by rubbing the dry powder into crinoline or book muslin. At least rubber gloves in the UK were thinner than those used in Paris, which could better be described as rubber gauntlets. When damaged, however, the thinner gloves had to be repaired with patches and rubber solution. Catgut for internal stitching was bought plain and in bulk, rolled round a pair of forceps into a ball and dropped into a hardening solution containing iodine or bichromate of potash. Finally the catgut would be boiled for sterilisation. For sewing the skin, genuine silkworm gut was pulled from the mouths of silkworms; for the same purpose, Barbour's linen thread, made in Lisburn, was first introduced in Ulster before becoming a part of surgical practice elsewhere.

Surgical instruments posed a major problem of maintenance. Scalpels were usually blunt and had to be sharpened – in the Royal Victoria Hospital scissors and scalpels were taken away twice a week to be sharpened by a retired police sergeant. Stainless steel was not in use and instruments had to be oiled to avoid rust. Swabs were used over and over again after washing, as were the marine sponges used for mopping up blood. Red rubber was used for tubes and catheters as well as gloves, and frequently caused irritation.

Surgical technique was, of course, governed by the equipment available and by the likelihood of infection. Surgeon Kirk repaired all hernias with Japanese silkworm gut, a nonabsorbable predecessor of our nylon and Dacron. Wounds were only closed loosely to allow the inevitable pus to drain externally. He had a particular liking for introducing urea, which was packed into the wound by the tablespoonful. Another of his personal quirks was that he would make patients with abdominal drains lie face downwards so that pus could drain out more easily. Yet another of his curious ideas was treatment of chest infections with subcutaneous oxygen forced in from a cylinder via a needle.

With no antibiotics, recovery from infection depended on a patient's natural resistance, and Surgeon Kirk believed this could be boosted by the administration of serum. This had to be taken in the abattoir from blood from an old cow or horse that had built up a strong resistance. The blood was separated into plasma and cells, and the plasma was then administered to the patient by mouth, usually after some days' delay and smelling horrible.

By 1923 the annual number of surgical operations had risen to 2,676 (an increase of 55 per cent over the decade) with 92 deaths – a mortality of 3.44 per cent, still very good for its time. A useful picture of the changes going on comes from Mr A.B. Mitchell's address that year to the annual general meeting of the hospital. He reported an increase in cases of appendicitis from approximately 250 a year in 1908, with a mortality of 15

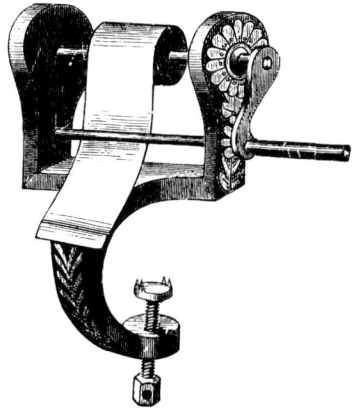

Bandage roller, with clamp for attaching it to a table
MAYER AND PHELPS CATALOGUE, 1931

per cent, to 428 cases in 1923 with a mortality of 4 per cent:

> this was largely due to the fact that the medical profession was now thoroughly alive to the necessity of operating on these cases at the earliest possible date. The cause of the heavy mortality in earlier cases was due to the fact that a very large number only arrived at hospital when peritonitis was present, or an abscess had already formed. These complications are now practically always due to delay on the part of the sufferers in sending for competent medical advice. They do not realise their condition and they continue to apply poultices or other homely remedies till the disease is already in an advanced condition.

A.B. Mitchell also pointed out that this delay caused more patient suffering, longer stays in hospital, and longer times off work.

It is interesting to read a bitter complaint, as far back as 1927, in the hospital's annual report at the number of traffic accident patients and the cost to the hospital. It appears that at the time few drivers of cars or motor cycles were insured; certainly none made any effort to help with the cost of their treatment. The accident figures are not large by current standards, however, amounting to 202 patients admitted, of whom about 25 per cent were motorists, 25 per cent were motor cyclists, and 50 per cent were pedestrians. There were 16 fatalities, resulting from head injuries (50 per cent) and multiple injuries. Seventeen beds were constantly occupied by these casualties; this figure reflects the long stay in bed then needed by patients with compound leg fractures.

Changing patterns of surgery are reflected in the purchase in 1929 of two new operating tables that could be raised or lowered and tilted in all directions. Better-quality theatre lamps were also installed at this time. Another feature of this period was the introduction of radium treatment into the surgical management of cancer. In 1925 Mr A.B. Mitchell commented that the only method of complete and permanent cure was surgical removal, but that the tumour must be treated early. Purchase of a supply of radium is mentioned in 1927, and in the 1930 report it received much prominence. Mr S.T. Irwin talked about the very encouraging results, with no operative mortality and neither deformity nor disfigurement. He did also point out, however, that results were dependent on the type and stage of the disease, the skill of the operator and, as always, the question of supplies of radium which was so tied up with cost, and carefully controlled.

This cost was eventually covered by a Radium Fund which was opened in 1931 with a donation of £1,000 from Lady Pirrie and a special overdraft facility of £4,000. At this time the radium was usually inserted into the tumour in hollow needles or applied to its surface, but the use of radon gas in suitable containers was also coming in as a more convenient alternative. The types of cases treated included breast cancer in particular, but also tumours of the skin, mouth, bone, bladder and rectum.

By 1933 the annual number of surgical operations (all fields) had risen to 4,071, including 448 patients who had been treated with radium. In 1937 the pressure on beds was eased by the extension of the surgical and other wards. This was necessitated at least in part by the continuing rise in road casualties.

Mr Samuel Thompson Irwin was appointed Attending Surgeon in 1923. He had graduated with an MB with honours from Queen's College in 1902 and was awarded an M.Ch. in 1906; he was appointed to the staff of the Ulster Hospital in 1911 and served with the RAMC during World War One. His particular interests were in orthopaedics and the surgery of the peptic ulcer; he was a quiet, expert and intellectual surgeon in the tradition of Thomas Sinclair and subsequently Cecil Calvert. He retired in 1942, was elected an MP for the University seat at Stormont (like Howard Stevenson), and was knighted in 1957. He is perhaps best remembered for his involvement with the Irish Rugby Football Union and the Royal County Down Golf Club, and for the wonderful parties he gave, one of which (for the British Orthopaedic Association) went on so long that it caused a delay in the sailing of the Liverpool boat.

The next appointment to the Attending staff was Mr (later Professor) P.T. Crymble. He graduated at Queen's College in 1904 and from then until his death in 1970 he always had considerable involvement in the Department of Anatomy, undoubtedly stimulated by the dynamic Professor Johnson Symington. He was appointed Assistant Surgeon in 1918, Attending Surgeon in 1929, and Professor of Surgery in Queen's University Belfast in 1934. He had produced the celebrated series of cadaver transections known as Man 50, used for teaching surgical anatomy; he used their strong anatomical basis throughout his career, particularly in the fields of thyroidectomy and abdominal surgery. He continued working throughout World War Two, retiring from the medical staff in 1945. Even after this retirement he continued to lecture in radiological anatomy and chaired clinico-pathological conferences.

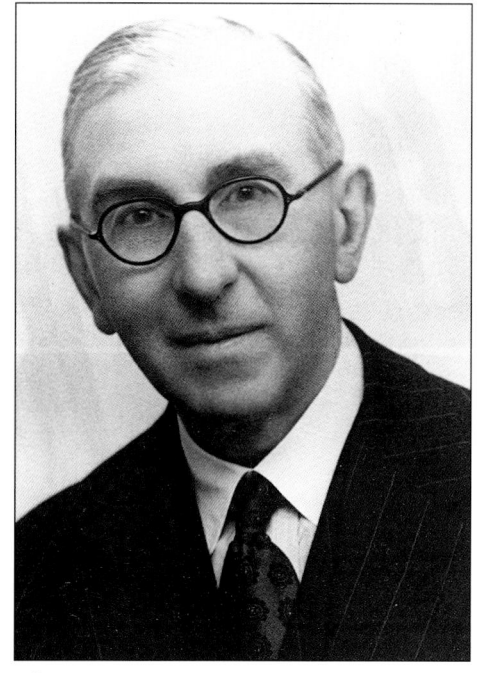

Sir Samuel Irwin MP, FRCS Edin, Visiting Surgeon to the Royal Victoria Hospital, 1918–45
ROYAL VICTORIA HOSPITAL

The two key figures on the surgical side, Professor Fullerton and Surgeon Kirk, retired in 1933 and 1934 respectively. They were replaced as Visiting Surgeons by Mr Robert John McConnell and Dr Henry Price (Harry) Malcolm. The former had graduated at Queen's University in 1912, had served in the RAMC in World War One, and had been appointed Assistant Surgeon at the Royal Victoria Hospital in 1920. He retired in 1950. He was greatly loved and respected for his teaching and friendship to all colleagues. Dr Malcolm also graduated at Queen's in 1912 and served in the RAMC; he was appointed Assistant Surgeon to the Royal Victoria Hospital in 1923. He carried on the interest in orthopaedics established by

A.B. Mitchell, and gained the degree of M.Ch. by a thesis (1920) on treatment of fractures of the shaft of the femur with the Thomas splint. (This was a light, padded metal frame easily carried to scenes of disaster, but later criticised as coming in only three sizes – large, too large, and much too large.) His base in the hospital was wards 9 and 10, which R.I. Wilson later noted always smelt strongly of infected bedbound patients and Sinclair's glue, a concoction of glue, water, thymol and glycerine used in the application of the Thomas splint. As well as looking after convalescent orthopaedic patients at the Throne Hospital, he had a lifetime involvement in the Graymount long-stay hospital and in the Greenisland Hospital. He retired in 1950.

Until World War Two, orthopaedic surgery and the management of fractures were the province of the general surgeon; patients were cared for in general surgical wards. A.B. Mitchell was certainly the pioneer worker in this field in Belfast, his work spanning two centuries. The first truly specialist orthopaedic surgeon was Robert James Wilson (Jimmy) Withers who graduated with an MB and first-class honours at Queen's University in 1930 and with an MD and gold medal in 1933. He was already running a fracture clinic as a surgical registrar in 1938; it was formally opened in 1942 and called after Mr A.B. Mitchell. R.J.W. Withers was appointed Surgeon in Charge of the new Orthopaedic Department in 1945. His major contribution was in building up a specialised orthopaedic service for the whole of Northern Ireland; he also pressed successfully for the establishment of a long-stay orthopaedic unit in 1945 using the wartime Musgrave Park Hospital. He was a popular teacher with a fund of stories suitable or otherwise, and an unbiased opinion in the law courts; he was a convivial and well-read member of the surgical travelling clubs. He died in 1965 at the height of his powers and activity at the age of fifty-six.

Overall, the decades between the world wars saw great advances in surgical technique, in that abdominal surgery became safe and routine and orthopaedic surgery was becoming a specialised field. But with both, infection in abdomen or fracture site was still disastrous. Surgery close to the body surface was the safest field, and the brain and lungs were only approached if there was no alternative.

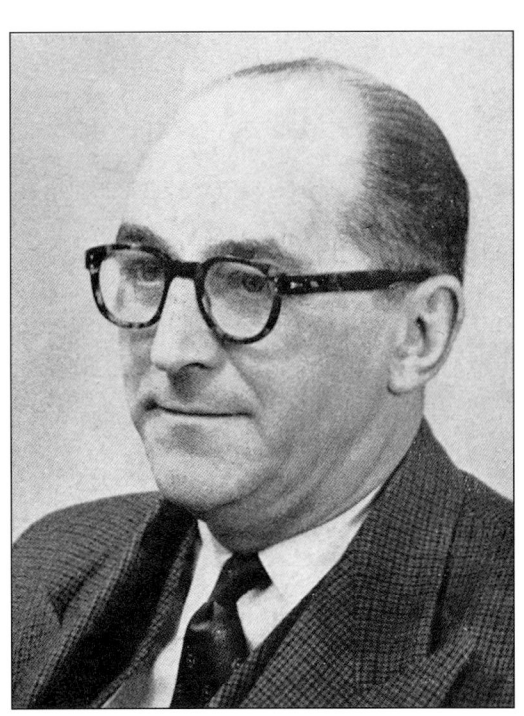

Mr Robert James Wilson Withers FRCS Edin, Visiting Surgeon to the Royal Victoria Hospital from 1945 until his death in 1965, and founder of the fracture clinic in the hospital
ROYAL VICTORIA HOSPITAL

WORLD WAR TWO

World War Two brought its inevitable troubles to the hospital – loss of skilled staff of all kinds, even less money and no hope of enlargement of facilities. Again the younger doctors of all grades went off to the war, including the surgeons Cecil Calvert, Ian Fraser and Eric McMechan, while Howard Stevenson and S.T. Irwin continued to work after retirement age. Altogether forty-eight medical graduates and undergraduates from Queen's University were killed, including the sons of Professor Thomson, Mr 'Barney' Purce and Dr Robert Marshall, who had been housemen in the hospital. At least five ex-RVH nurses were killed by enemy action or died on active service: Ruth Dickson, Ellen Lowry, Ida Nelson, Beatrice Dowling and Doreen Pedlow of Queen Alexandra's Military Nursing Service and the corresponding Naval Nursing Service. Unlike the situation in World War One, many of the medical staff who joined up were imprisoned, including Mr J.S. Irwin in Germany and Mr T.B. Smiley in the Far East; Professor J.F. Pantridge, in particular, has written of his experiences under the Japanese.

In September 1939 over two hundred beds were allocated for possible air raids but by the end of the year this precaution seemed to be unnecessary and the beds were freed again. Certain precautions were taken, however, to protect the patients in the event of a raid, such as provision of brick shelters under the wards, strengthening of the clerestory windows of side wards and the main corridor, and the building of brick walls in three of the operating theatres, the telephone exchange and the extern department. Two hundred students were enrolled as fire watchers, sleeping on paliasses in the King Edward Building hall. The nurses, in particular, were severely stretched between fire watching, taking patients to the safer parts of the wards, and caring for the injured. Day nurses could also be working at night if required, and lack of sleep became a major concern. Fire pumps and hoses were bought and a 45,000-gallon water reservoir was constructed in the open area between the hospitals.

The government of Northern Ireland comes out less than creditably for its handling of the war effort and appears to have drifted through the first twenty months of the war with few air-raid precautions or defences for the population. Certainly the government was quite unprepared when the first bombs came on 7–8 April 1941, but though they caused industrial damage they caused few casualties. However, the raid on Easter Tuesday (15–16 April 1941) devastated the residential areas in the north of the city. Some 180 German bombers rained down incendiaries, high-explosive bombs and parachute mines, and in the end about 900 people were killed (figures vary) and about 450 were seriously injured, altogether a very high figure for a single raid in the UK. The fire service was overwhelmed and many of the fire and emergency services gave up. On the other hand Peggy Donaldson in her *Yes, Matron* records that in spite of the pressure of work the hospital was relatively calm:

> Throughout the night a succession of ambulances delivered up the dead and wounded. The former were identified (if possible) and sent to the mortuary. The living were treated on the spot or admitted to the wards. Those with chest and less severe head injuries were sent to Wards 5 and 6. The severely shocked, but otherwise apparently uninjured, were put in Wards 7 and 8,

which also had the sad responsibility of caring for those near death, for whom nothing more could be done. Any whose lives were at risk were operated on as soon as possible in one of the reinforced theatres. With lighting provided by Tilley lamps and the anaesthetics administered by dripping a highly inflammable mixture of chloroform and ether on an open mask, there were times during prolonged operations when those working in theatres during the air raids felt they were in greater danger of injury from their own equipment than from the bombers overhead.

The city and hospital mortuaries were filled, and the dead were taken to such places as the Falls Road baths, where the pool was drained to accommodate 150 corpses, and St George's Market where they had 255 corpses. Emma Duffin was a nurse at the latter and recorded in her diary that she had seen 'death in many forms, young men dying of ghastly wounds' during World War One but while Death in hospital beds had been 'solemn, tragic, dignified … here it was grotesque, repulsive, horrible' (quoted by Barton, 1989). There was another large raid on the night of 4–5 May, with 191 deaths, a low figure explained by the facts that the bombs fell in the city centre and on a Sunday night people were largely at home or had fled the city.

The air raids of 1941 presented a considerable burden on the hospital, but over the year fewer inpatients and outpatients were seen because of the reserving of beds for emergency cases. A bomb fell in the grounds but the hospital itself, unlike the Ulster Hospital in Templemore Avenue east of the River Lagan, was not damaged. As already mentioned, the Benn Hospital for Diseases of the Skin was destroyed; the Throne Hospital, like much of the Antrim Road area, was damaged by bombs but fortunately there were no casualties. After the period of the air raids the war had less effect than World War One on the patient population of the hospital, probably because of the setting-up of various emergency hospitals for the armed forces, such as Musgrave Park and Waringstown hospitals. In 1943 the total number of surgical operations was 4,968, that is, a further 22 per cent increase over the decade.

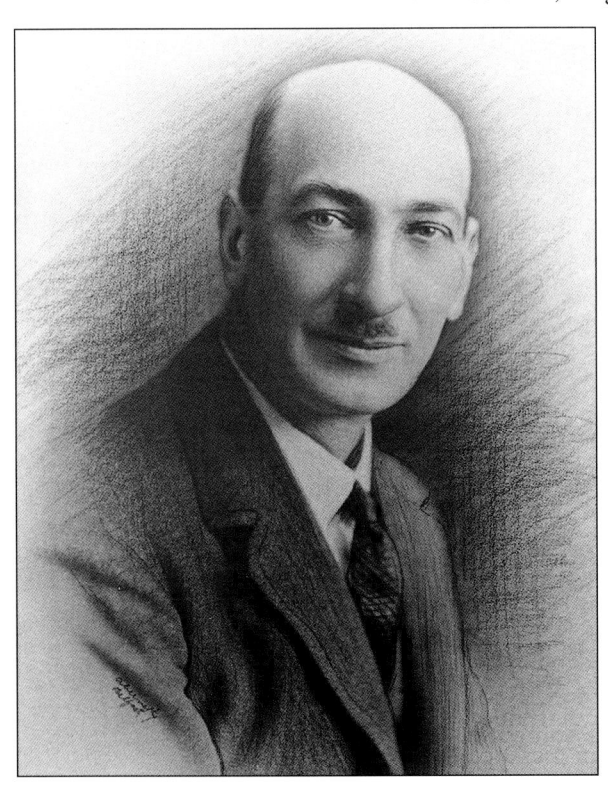

Mr Barney Purce FRCS Edin, Visiting Surgeon to the Royal Victoria Hospital from 1929 until his death in 1950, and a pioneer in both neurosurgery and thoracic surgery
ROYAL VICTORIA HOSPITAL

SURGICAL APPOINTMENTS DURING AND AFTER WORLD WAR TWO

The clinical service had to be maintained and new Visiting Surgeons were appointed. The first was Mr George Raphael Buick (Barney) Purce, who had graduated at Queen's in 1914, had served in World War One, being awarded the Military Cross, and had been Assistant Surgeon since 1929; he was appointed Attending Surgeon in 1941. Although he was a general surgeon like his colleagues, well able to remove an appendix in the home on the kitchen table when required, he made thoracic surgery his particular speciality and performed the first lobectomy (removal of a lobe of the lung) in the hospital in 1939. In addition he did the major share of the neurosurgery performed in Northern Ireland, though this amounted to only two or three cases a year, with a high mortality (see page 193). He was a generous teacher, quietly erudite and remembered for the breadth of his surgical skills; he liked to teach by example in the theatre rather than by flamboyance on ward rounds or in lectures. He was a logical thinker and a fast surgeon; outside medicine, he was also deeply involved in the more individualistic sports such as rifle shooting, fishing, golf and sailing. He is commemorated in the Purce medal of the hospital.

In 1942 Mr Cecil John Alexander (Cocky) Woodside was appointed Attending Surgeon. He had graduated at Queen's in 1917, served in the RAMC in World War One, and, having returned to Belfast as tutor and lecturer in surgery, had been Assistant Surgeon since 1933. He was mainly involved in genito-urinary surgery and was honorary secretary of the Medical Staff Committee from 1944 to 1946.

By 1945 the surgeons were returning from the war. The first to be appointed to the Attending staff was Mr Cecil Armstrong Calvert. He had graduated at Queen's University in 1922 with first-class honours and had been appointed Assistant Surgeon at the Royal Victoria Hospital in 1935. He had trained as a general surgeon and throughout the 1930s he continued to practise in all fields. When he joined the RAMC in 1939 he was invited to work with Sir Hugh Cairns in Oxford where he built up a reputation in the management of head injuries. After he was appointed Attending Surgeon in the RVH in 1945, moves were made to establish a centre for neurosurgery (later named Quin House after Senator Herbert Quin, chairman of the Board of Management, 1941–51) in the old fever wards 21 and 22; Mr Calvert was appointed its first director in 1947. The speciality of neurosurgery will be covered later but Cecil Calvert's notable characteristics of meticulous care and almost incredible slowness may be touched on here. He was tragically killed in a car accident on the way to a colleague's funeral on 4 April 1956. He is commemorated by the Calvert Room in the neurosurgical unit and by the Calvert medal of the hospital.

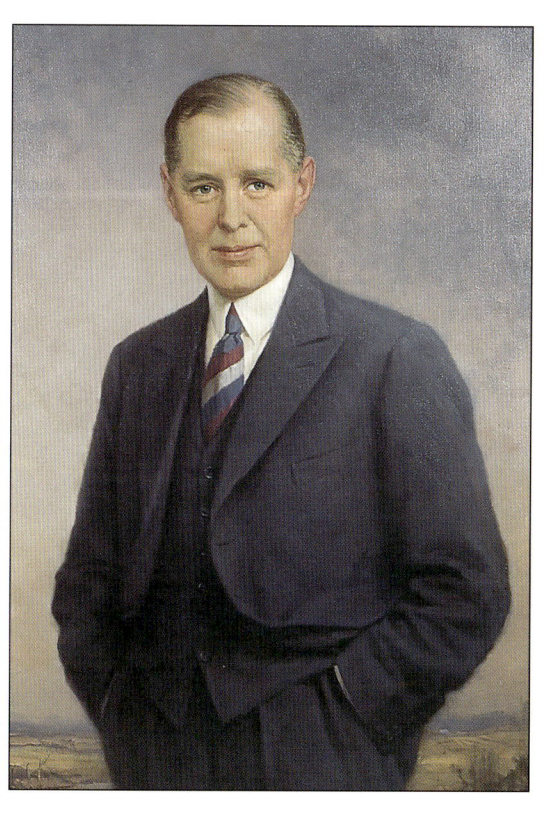

Mr Cecil Calvert FRCSI, Visiting Surgeon to the Royal Victoria Hospital from 1935 until his death in 1956, and founder of the neurosurgical unit in the hospital; portrait by Frank McKelvey
ROYAL VICTORIA HOSPITAL

In 1945 three surgeons were appointed as Assistant Surgeons (like other Assistant staff, they were termed 'Consultants' after the introduction of the National Health Service in 1948). Mr Ian Fraser DSO, OBE, had graduated at Queen's University in 1923 with first-class honours and many prizes. He obtained the FRCSI in 1926, and was appointed Assistant Surgeon to the Belfast Hospital for Sick Children in the following year. On the outbreak of war in 1939 he joined the RAMC. His service career was distinguished, and he was awarded the DSO for working for more than forty-eight hours nonstop on board the hospital carrier ship *St David* off the coast of Sicily in the face of continuous enemy bombing. Once appointed to the Visiting staff of the Royal Victoria Hospital (wards 19/20), he continued to work in all surgical fields, both adult and paediatric, until he retired in 1966. Since then he has been president of the Royal College of Surgeons in Ireland (1954) and president of the BMA (1962). He was knighted in 1962.

Mr James Stevenson Loughridge also graduated at Queen's University in 1923 with honours; subsequently he obtained an MD with commendation and the FRCSE in 1928. He was appointed to the staff of the Belfast Hospital for Sick Children in 1938 and went on to practise surgery throughout Northern Ireland during the war years. He had a lifelong connection with the physiology department of Queen's University but his principal surgical interest was genito-urinary. He was Consultant Surgeon in the Royal Victoria Hospital (wards 15/16) from 1948 until his retirement in 1967; subsequently he returned to work as part-time Medical Superintendent, 1968–73.

Mr Eric W. McMechan graduated at Queen's University in 1933 with honours, obtained the FRCSE in 1938, and joined the RAMC when war came. On returning to the Royal Victoria Hospital (wards 9/10) he developed a special interest in colo-rectal surgery but his active work was cut short by a major heart attack in the early 1960s, which led to his retirement in 1968.

Following the retirement from the chair in 1946 of the Professor of Surgery, P.T. Crymble, a new professor, Harold William Rodgers, was appointed in 1947 (to wards 11/12). He had graduated and trained at St Bartholomew's Hospital in London, and served in the RAMC throughout the war; as the first full-time Professor of Surgery he was the first to introduce surgical research to Belfast. When the new Institute of Clinical Science was opened in 1954 (see page 145) he was able to have animal accommodation installed and research facilities there were used by many of the university departments. His main surgical interest was in gastro-enterology but he contributed much to the Christian Medical Fellowship and medical care in the Third World. He retired in 1973.

General surgery in 1948 did not differ radically from that some fifty years later. One striking feature, however, was the number of operations for peptic ulcer, both elective and emergency: vagotomies, gastrectomies of various kinds, gastro-enterostomy, oversewing of bleeding ulcers, and closure of perforations. Then there were the various types of open prostatectomies, often noted for the very rapid removal of the prostate

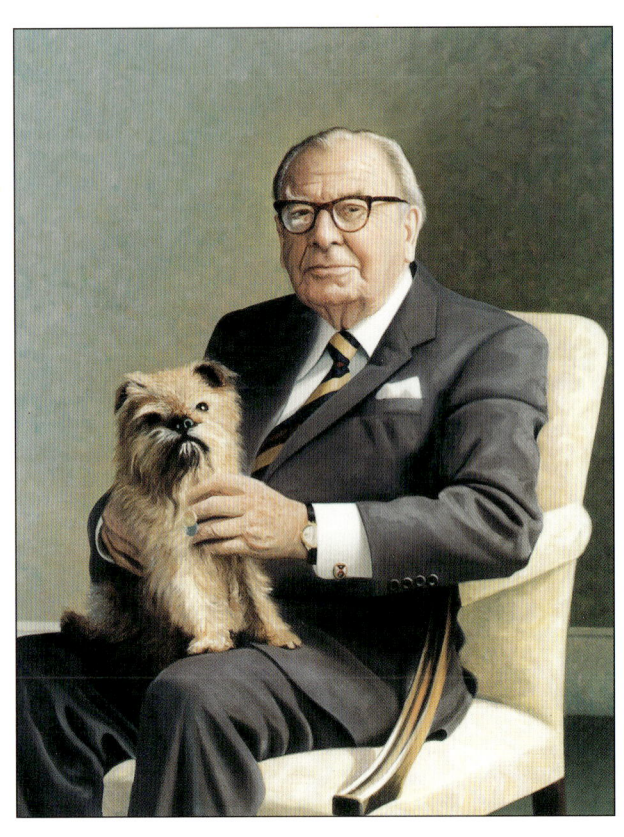

Sir Ian Fraser DSO, FRCSI, Visiting Surgeon to the Royal Victoria Hospital, 1945–66, and president of the Royal College of Surgeons in Ireland, 1954–55; portrait by Carol Graham and reproduced by permission of the artist
QUEEN'S UNIVERSITY BELFAST

(60–90 seconds!), followed by a long period spent stopping the bleeding (30 minutes), and then unpleasant open drainage which went on for many days after surgery. The trans-urethral approach, avoiding a surgical incision, was coming in with terms like 'hot-punch' and 'cold-punch' but this was still experimental. Perhaps the most unpleasant operation was the radical mastectomy, so destructive cosmetically, with considerable blood loss, and leaving the patients psychologically shattered afterwards. Thyroid surgery had been rare in 1903, but by 1948 there were many thyroidectomies for goitre, with or without thyroid overactivity. Better sedation and anaesthesia had rendered the operation for toxic goitre safer, but treatment with drugs and radioactive iodine had not yet been introduced.

Blood storage and reliable cross-matching to prevent reactions had developed during World War Two and blood was now readily available when required. The satisfactory management of severe abdominal injuries and vascular surgery was held up, however, until the problems of massive blood transfusion were understood. Antibiotics for the treatment of abdominal infection did not really come into use until the 1960s. Lessons on early invasive management would only be learnt from the Korean War because the possibilities for rapid surgical involvement were not seen in World War Two to the same extent.

GYNAECOLOGY

In 1900, 'diseases of women' were managed in the medical wards, the commonest diagnoses being endometritis, prolapsed uterus and retroversion (displacement). Such patients were often treated by surgery, however, particularly uterine curettage and perineal repair; provided the peritoneum was not opened, mortality was low. The new hospital had a ward specifically set aside for gynaecology patients (Ward 17) and this was placed with the surgical wards, and although gynaecology was still regarded as a medical speciality until 1909, the volume of surgery increased steadily.

Professor John W. Byers was the Attending Gynaecologist when the new hospital opened in 1903, with Mr R.J. Johnstone as Assistant Gynaecologist. Sir John Byers retired in 1919 and died in the following year; he was replaced as Attending Gynaecologist and Professor of Gynaecology (but not obstetrics) by Robert James Johnstone. Johnstone was born at Greenisland in 1872 and graduated at Queen's College in both Arts (1893) and Medicine (1896) with many awards and honours. He was noted as an unusually dexterous and sound surgeon but his main success seems to have been in medical politics. He was MP for the University (from 1921), president of the Ulster Medical Society (1922), foundation fellow of the College of Obstetricians and Gynaecologists (and president of its tenth congress in Belfast, 1936) and president of the BMA (1937). He was knighted in 1938. He was noted as a conversationalist, storyteller and compiler of humorous verse. He retired in 1937 because of illness and died eighteen months later. His name is commemorated in Johnstone House, the former private wing of the Royal Maternity Hospital, and there is a portrait by Frank McKelvey.

Professor Johnstone was one of many MPs who represented the University in parliament, but professors William Whitla and Thomas Sinclair were MPs at Westminster, spanning the years 1918–40. University representation at Westminster was terminated in 1950. Professor Johnstone, on the other hand, was the first of many medical MPs to the Stormont Parliament, which had four University representatives at any one time; others including Mr Howard Stevenson FRCSI, Mr A.B. Mitchell FRCSI and Mr Ian McClure FRCS Ed. While the Stormont Parliament was in existence, almost half the university's representatives were medical, a proportion probably representing the strength of medical influence within the university.

The numbers of gynaecological beds had gone up from 4 in the old Belfast Royal Hospital to 18 in the Royal Victoria Hospital (1903), and rose again to 54 in the expanded hospital in 1938. Nevertheless the numbers of medical staff involved increased only slowly, remaining at one Attending Gynaecologist with one Assistant until 1924, when Professor Charles Gibson Lowry was made a second Attending Gynaecologist. He had been born near Limavady in 1880 and was educated at Queen's College, graduating in 1903. He became interested in obstetrics and gynaecology while in general practice, and served in the RAMC during World War One. He was appointed Assistant Gynaecologist at the RVH in 1919 and Professor of Midwifery in 1921 when the chair was divided. C.G. Lowry continued to combine both disciplines throughout his life, but his great contributions were the creation of the Royal Maternity Hospital, which opened beside the Royal Victoria Hospital in 1933, and his promotion of the training and teaching of students, which had hitherto been greatly undervalued. He was a foundation fellow and vice-president of the new Royal College of Obstetricians and Gynaecologists. He was noted for his wit and for his appropriate quotations in difficult situations. ('My compliments to the Hospital Engineer, but this theatre is only fit for Shadrach, Meshach and Abednego.') He retired in 1945 and was succeeded in the chair by his son-in-law C.H.G. Macafee. There is a fine portrait of him by Sir James Gunn in the university department.

Mr Hardy Greer was appointed Attending Gynaecologist in 1937 on the retirement of Professor Johnstone. He had graduated at Queen's University in 1913, had served in the RAMC and Royal Flying Corps, and became Assistant Gynaecologist in 1924. He was a pioneer of antenatal care and, in 1962, produced the first detailed report on maternal deaths in Northern Ireland, work carried out after his retirement in 1956. He was a keen golfer and often gave his popular Saturday morning lecture in the Royal Victoria

Hospital wearing plus-fours and highly polished brown brogues.

Charles Horner Greer Macafee followed his father-in-law C.G. Lowry as Attending Gynaecologist and Professor of Obstetrics. He studied at Queen's University, graduating with first-class honours in 1921. By 1923 he was a tutor in Obstetrics, and he remained involved in obstetrics, and particularly its academic side, for the remainder of his career. He was appointed lecturer in 1925 and Professor of Midwifery and Gynaecology (the chair now reunited) in 1945. In the Royal Victoria Hospital he became Assistant Gynaecologist in 1932, later with responsibility for outpatients; he became Attending Gynaecologist at the same time as he took up the university chair, in 1945, and retired only in 1963. He was predominantly an obstetrician, and his greatest contribution to the subject was his paper and teaching on the treatment of placenta praevia. In the *Ulster Medical Journal,* he critically reviewed 122 consecutive hysterectomies he had performed and he also published jointly with Professor Sir John Biggart a definitive work on the pathology of ovarian tumours. Inevitably he was involved in medical administration, but he is best remembered for his teaching of students and for the inspiration he gave to postgraduates who worked with him. His brilliant memory of the medical history of his patients was legendary, as well as his phrases, such as 'let's sit on her' when he was condemning 'meddlesome midwifery'.

Mr H.C. (Harry) Lowry was a member of a distinguished medical and legal family and brother of Professor C.G. Lowry. Harry Lowry served in the army during World War One and then returned to Queen's University to study medicine. He graduated with an MB in 1924 and trained in Edinburgh, London and Vienna before being appointed Consultant Gynaecologist at the Ulster Hospital. He was appointed Assistant Gynaecologist in Charge of Outpatients at the Royal Victoria Hospital in 1937, but remained without beds until the advent of the NHS. He gave the annual winter oration in 1947 on 'Some landmarks in surgical technique', eventually retiring on account of ill health in 1960. His son Brian became Professor of Paediatrics and of Medical Genetics in Calgary, Canada.

Mr H. Ian McClure graduated with an MB in 1927 and with a B.Sc. in 1929 at Queen's University, and was on the staff of the Samaritan and Belfast City hospitals before being appointed Assistant Gynaecologist in charge of outpatients to the Royal Victoria Hospital in 1945. He was noted as a teacher and adviser of his younger colleagues, and he gave of his sound commonsense and foresight not only to his hospitals, but also to the Northern Ireland Hospitals Authority, the British Medical Association, the university and the Northern Ireland Parliament (as University member from 1962).

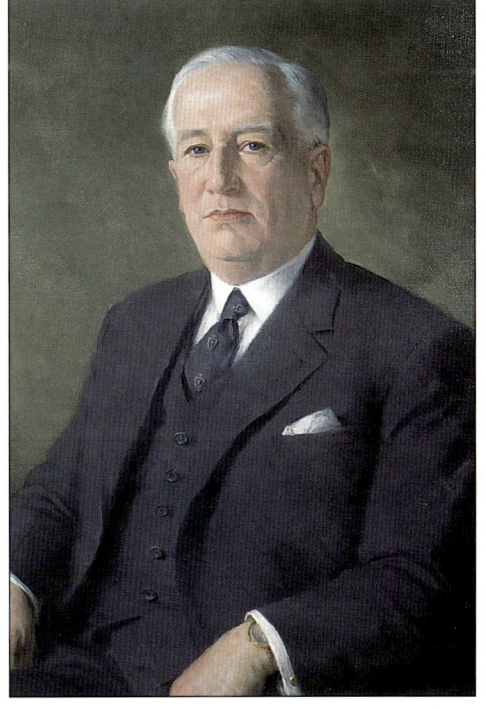

Professor Charles Horner Greer Macafee, Professor of Midwifery and Gynaecology at Queen's University Belfast, 1945–63, and Visiting Gynaecologist to the Royal Victoria Hospital, 1932–63; portrait by Frank McKelvey
QUEEN'S UNIVERSITY BELFAST

EYE, EAR, NOSE AND THROAT SURGERY

As explained in Chapter 3, the Royal Victoria Hospital opened in 1903 with a 12-bed unit for ophthalmology and otology and with an ophthalmic room in the extern department. The ward unit included an ophthalmic theatre; there was little ear, nose and throat surgery at this time. Dr Joseph Nelson was the Attending Surgeon for this department, with Dr James Craig as assistant, and in 1905, when Dr Nelson retired, Dr Craig was appointed to succeed him.

James Andrew Craig was born in Ballymoney, County Antrim, and educated at Queen's College, graduating with an MB with first-class honours in 1895. In 1902 he was appointed Assistant Eye, Ear and Throat Surgeon at the Royal and obtained the FRCSE. Throughout his career he practised in all fields of his speciality but particularly in ophthalmic surgery; one of the new advances he introduced to the Royal Victoria Hospital was the giant magnet in 1913. This had been used earlier by Dr William McKeown in the Benn EENT Hospital in 1874, and was valuable for the removal of pieces of steel from the eye – a particular problem in an industrial city in a period of minimal regard for safety precautions. He built the department up steadily until his retirement in 1937.

Mr Craig was soon joined by Henry Hanna, also a Queen's University man, educated at Queen's College and St John's College, Cambridge. His early training was as a biologist and he only obtained his medical degree in 1903. He was appointed refraction assistant to the Royal Victoria Hospital in 1907, later becoming Surgeon in Charge of Outpatients (EENT) in 1915 and Attending Surgeon in 1925. The need for a second surgeon resulted from the great expansion of work when the outpatient department moved to the King Edward Building, and from the steady growth in surgical work. Some 369 operations were performed in 1925 compared with 264 a year earlier – the increase being particularly in the removal of tonsils and adenoids, which had become a popular operation.

Henry Hanna reached retirement age in 1939 but both he and James Craig returned to work during World War Two in the absence of their younger colleagues. Hanna complemented his senior colleague by being more interested in ear, nose and throat surgery, and Hanna was a contrast to Craig in many other ways too. Whilst Craig was cool and Olympian in his aloofness, Hanna was impatient and irascible. Nevertheless, both were loyal to each other and to their department, and highly esteemed by their colleagues. In 1937 Mr James Reid Wheeler was appointed Attending Surgeon to succeed Mr Craig; like him, Wheeler had a primary interest in ophthalmology. He had graduated at Queen's University in 1923, obtained the FRCS Edin in 1929, joined the Royal Victoria Hospital as clinical assistant in 1930, and was Assistant Surgeon in Charge of Outpatients (EENT) from 1934. He retired in 1964.

The last Attending Surgeon appointed to this department before the

National Health Service era was Mr Francis (Frank) Alexander MacLaughlin. He graduated with honours at Queen's University in 1921, obtained the FRCSE in 1926, and after working as a clinical assistant was appointed Assistant Surgeon in Charge of Outpatients (ENT) in 1937. On Mr Hanna's retirement in 1939, he became Attending Surgeon for ear, nose and throat surgery, which was now firmly separated from ophthalmic surgery. He served throughout World War Two with the Royal Naval Volunteer Reserve, covering the whole field of EENT, and returned to Belfast in 1944 to be appointed lecturer in otolaryngology with the university; he eventually retired in 1964.

When Mr Frank MacLaughlin was appointed Attending Surgeon in 1939, two younger surgeons were taken on as Assistant Surgeons in charge of outpatients: Mr J. Allison Corkey and Mr Kennedy Hunter. Mr Corkey was the son of a Presbyterian minister, and graduated with an MB with first-class honours at Queen's University in 1930 and with an MD in 1933. He studied ophthalmic surgery in London and Vienna before returning to Belfast to be appointed Assistant Ophthalmic Surgeon at the Benn EENT Hospital in 1934. He progressed from his appointment as Assistant Surgeon for Outpatients at the Royal Victoria Hospital in 1939 to become Consultant Surgeon in 1948.

Mr Kennedy Hunter, the son of a Crumlin GP, had graduated with an MB with honours at Queen's University in 1930 and trained specifically as a otolaryngologist. Like Mr Corkey, he was made a Consultant Surgeon in 1948. His special interest was always in the intricacies of middle-ear surgery, a field he effectively started in Belfast. However, the extent of his interest in the whole field of otolaryngology is seen in his opening address to the winter session of 1951. Both Mr Corkey and Mr Hunter retired in 1972. A prize was founded to commemorate the work of Mr Kennedy Hunter and to encourage the study of otolaryngology; it has been awarded annually since 1973.

DENTAL SURGERY

As noted on page 58, there was no dentist in post when the new hospital opened in 1903. Dental extractions (1,915 in total during the year) appear to have been carried out by junior medical staff. It was not until 1920 that two honorary Dental Surgeons (W.M. Swan LDS RCS and Dr J.S. O'Neill LDS RCS) were appointed, with the obligation to visit the hospital twice weekly. In the same year the university initiated the LDS, BDS and MDS degrees and created four lectureships to form a new dental school within the Faculty of Medicine and Dentistry. The Working Men's Committee provided a sum of £200 to buy dental equipment, and the dental surgeons were installed in a pathology laboratory on the ground floor of the King Edward Building.

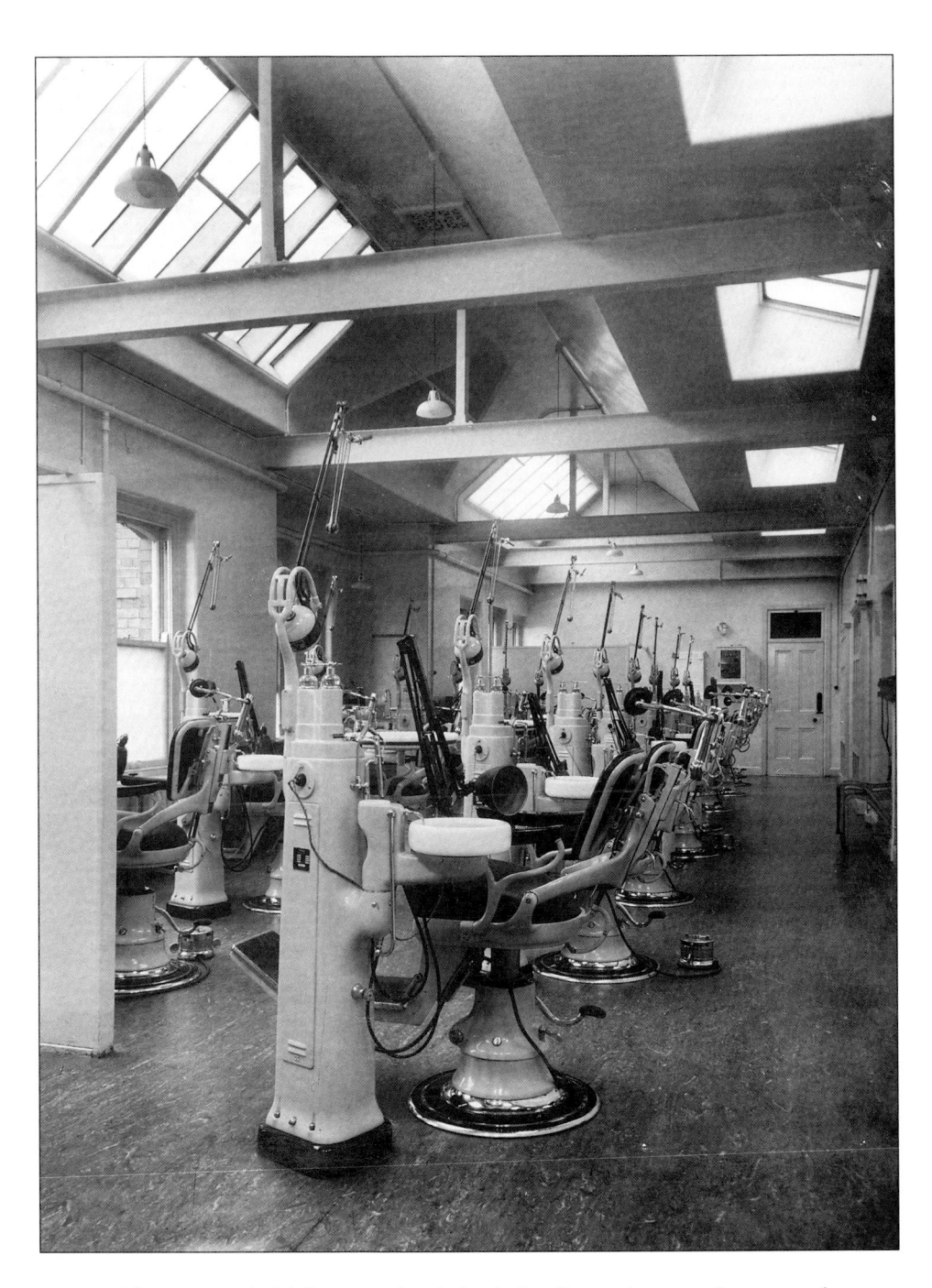

The Department of Dentistry, on the top floor of the King Edward Building, c. 1948
ROYAL VICTORIA HOSPITAL

There were initially two dentist's chairs for patients and two students, but growth in work was fast to meet the widespread demand for treatment. Three more students soon arrived and four more Dental Surgeons were appointed in 1921 (W.B.S. Andrew, H. Elwood, W.M. Hunter and J. Malone). Orthodontics was one of the earliest specialisations and Mr H.T.A. McKeag began work in this field soon after his appointment as lecturer in 1920. From this date the honorary dental staff were always listed in the hospital's annual reports. The only other appointment with this group was of an assistant anaesthetist, who gave experience and continuity to this hazardous field (first Dr D.R. Taylor and from 1924 to 1933 Dr

Dorothy Watson). Clinics were now held every morning and there were more chairs for simultaneous treatment, but patients still had to wait in the corridor. The purchase of huts followed after a Students' Dental Day in 1921 raised nearly £1,000. This provided a laboratory with a dental mechanic and a waiting room (later to be used as observation wards), but by 1924 facilities were clearly inadequate again and, after much lobbying, funds were found for a large dental department to occupy the top floor of the King Edward Building; this opened in 1926. The department now had special rooms for general anaesthesia, conservation, extractions generally, laboratories, prosthetics, and radiography, as well as a lecture room for students.

The Department of Dentistry in the King Edward Building, although large by former standards, could not accommodate all the teaching requirements of trainee dentists, and in 1929 it was agreed that Dental Mechanics and part of Prosthetics should be taken at the university. In this way the course was made comparable to the medical course, with pre-clinical and clinical elements.

In 1933 two new posts were created by the university: anaesthetic room surgeon (Dr Neil) and senior demonstrator (Mr Maurice G. Riordan). The latter became lecturer in Clinical Dental Surgery in 1938, and from this date on there were serious plans to establish a chair in Dental Surgery. Maurice Riordan was a leading figure in dental practice and teaching in Belfast but died in 1946 at the early age of forty-two. By this time there was concern in the profession and university that the whole field of dental training needed to be developed in line with changes in Britain, and in 1947 a university report strongly recommended the establishment of a five-year degree course. This did not happen immediately, but in April 1948 Professor Philip Joseph Stoy was appointed the first Professor of Dentistry.

ANAESTHETICS

In the nineteenth century, anaesthesia had been administered in the Royal Hospital by a House Surgeon or other junior member of the medical staff but from 1900, part-time, honorary Anaesthetists were appointed, Dr Victor Fielden and Mr R.J. Johnstone in the first instance. By 1902 Mr Johnstone had moved across to the field of gynaecology, but Dr Fielden remained the pillar of anaesthesia in the hospital for the rest of his working life.

Victor George Leopold Fielden had been born into a Plymouth naval family, which moved to Belfast when he was fifteen. He trained in medicine at Queen's College, graduating in 1892, and obtaining the MD with gold medal in 1912 for a thesis on ethyl chloride. After graduating he was appointed a demonstrator in Practical Pharmacy in 1893; indeed he retained this connection for many years: he had helped Dr William Whitla with the *Dictionary of Treatment* even before he graduated, and he continued to help with his *Materia Medica and Pharmacy*, at least until 1915. This very early association between anaesthetists and pharmacology in Belfast is interesting, for a strong link has remained between the two fields up to the present day, reinforced by the work of Professor John Dundee. Dr Fielden was appointed an anaesthetist at the Ulster Hospital in 1898 before joining the Royal Victoria Hospital in 1900; he became an Attending Physician in 1911, served in the RAMC during World War One, and retired in 1932. He was the only anaesthetist of his generation to devote himself solely to the field. Dr Fielden was noted as an unusually tall man (he was over six feet), of magnificent physique and with a fine beard. He was a keen cyclist and bell-ringer (at St Thomas's Church, Lisburn Road) and rang peals after the deaths of Queen Victoria and King Edward VII.

With the exception of Dr Fielden, none of the anaesthetists remained in post for more than a year or two until 1923. Many doctors, including P.T. Crymble and S.T. Irwin, gave anaesthetics as a step towards a career in surgery, and of course many general practitioners, house surgeons, nurses and medical students gave anaesthetics, even for life-threatening emergencies, as late as World War Two and into the 1950s. The anaesthetists, therefore, were not simply part-time between hospital and home but part-time in the sense that they only spent a fraction of their time in giving anaesthetics. It was the accepted practice, in smaller hospitals at least, for a patient's own general practitioner to be brought in to give the anaesthetic, though this was less common by the 1930s. It is also notable that although there was more continuity after 1923, no other anaesthetist attained the status of Dr Fielden within the hospital, and when he retired he was not replaced on the Attending staff.

Dr Olive Margery Anderson was appointed Assistant Anaesthetist to the hospital in 1923 and remained (with short breaks) until 1944, when ex-servicemen were returning. She was born in Belfast and educated at Coleraine High School and Queen's University, graduating with an MB in 1917. After a period with the Women's Army Auxiliary Corps she went into general practice in south Belfast, carrying out domiciliary midwifery and developing a pioneering interest in family planning. Her anaesthetic practice was also concentrated on obstetrics and gynaecology. She had a calm, competent manner which was not intimidated by impatient surgeons. She obtained an MD in 1932 and the Diploma of Anaesthetics in 1936. She had a strong interest in the Queen's Women Graduates' Association, the Medical Women's Federation and the British Legion, and in 1957 was the first woman president of the Ulster Medical Society in over

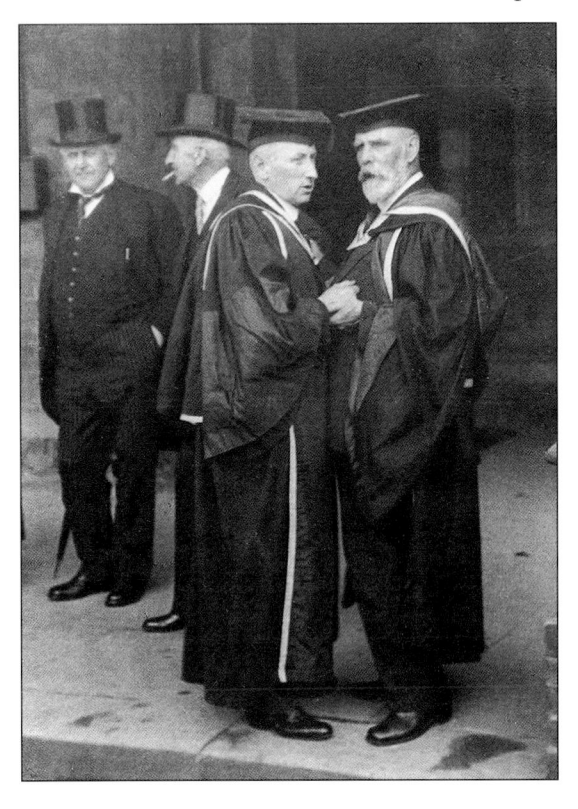

Dr Victor Fielden (*right foreground*), Visiting Anaesthetist to the Royal Victoria Hospital, 1900–32, and Dr John Morrow (*left foreground*), Visiting Physician to the hospital, 1903–30, at the Queen's University graduation ceremony in 1933
ROYAL VICTORIA HOSPITAL

one hundred years of its existence. She was awarded the OBE in 1967 for a lifetime of voluntary work. Sadly she suffered from progressive blindness.

The other part-time Anaesthetist appointed in 1923, who made a major contribution to the provision of an anaesthetics service was Dr Stafford Geddes. He graduated at Queen's University Belfast in 1915, obtained the Diploma of Anaesthetics in 1936, and in his early days was in general practice as well as being anaesthetist to the Royal Victoria and Ulster hospitals. He retired in 1956. His son Dr John Stafford Geddes was a Consultant Cardiologist in the hospital between 1971 and 1987. Dr James Wilson Heney was also an Assistant Anaesthetist, 1926–39, and was tutor in Anaesthetics from 1932. He had graduated at Queen's University in 1922, obtaining the MD in 1927; his appointment as tutor was presumably a recognition of his MD and continuing specialisation in the field even though he never had Attending status. He retired from his post in the Royal Victoria Hospital in 1940 but remained working at the ophthalmic hospital until 1942, when he was forced to retire early by ill health.

Other part-time Anaesthetists of the 1930s include Dr George Hamilton who was in business first, then graduated with an MA at Queen's in 1917 and with an MB in 1927; he combined his general practice in Great Victoria Street with the giving of anaesthetics in the Royal Victoria Hospital and the Belfast Hospital for Sick Children from 1935. He took the Diploma of Anaesthetics in Dublin in 1943, was graded as a Consultant Anaesthetist in 1948, and retired in 1952. His son Trevor Hamilton followed him in the practice but not in anaesthetics. Dr John Boyd also combined general practice with working in the two hospitals. He graduated with an MB at Queen's University in 1926 and obtained the Diploma of Anaesthetics in 1943. He was appointed Assistant Anaesthetist at the Royal Victoria Hospital in 1937, having already been an Attending Anaesthetist at the Belfast Hospital for Sick Children since 1928; he obtained his MD in 1933 for a thesis on the use of a rectal sedative called Avertin. He became a Consultant Anaesthetist at the Royal Victoria Hospital in 1948, and retired in 1969.

The practice of anaesthesia over this period is less well documented than are its practitioners. We know that in the nineteenth century chloroform was the main agent used, with sometimes methylene and the alcohol–chloroform–ether (ACE) mixture, particularly for children. As a student, Victor Fielden had used mainly the open-drop method, but in his clinical practice he used Murphy's inhaler (*c.* 1850), the Junker inhaler (1867) and finally the Vernon Harcourt apparatus (1903) which he used up to 1945. He proved that chloroform given in this way was safe and it was probably always his preferred mode of anaesthesia, though he also used ether, methylene, ethyl chloride and nitrous oxide. He thus forms a link between the original, simple method of giving ether, through the long-running chloroform, to our own increasingly sophisticated apparatus for

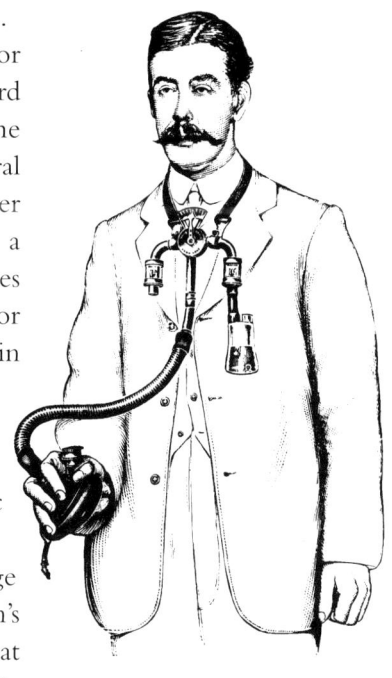

An anaesthetist with Vernon Harcourt's chloroform apparatus (1903) worn around his neck for use outside hospital, particularly in the home; it was designed to give an 'accurate' concentration of chloroform, vaporised by the patient inhaling air across the liquid chloroform.
MAYER AND PHELPS CATALOGUE, 1931

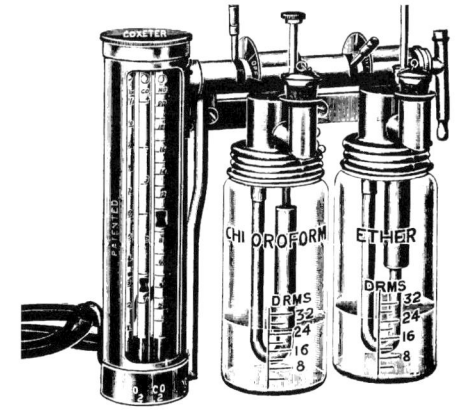

Flowmeters for nitrous oxide, oxygen and carbon dioxide gases (1929), which were directed over chloroform or ether in a measured way before passing on to the patient
MAYER AND PHELPS CATALOGUE, 1931

controlling delivery of anaesthetic, though in his day the giving of measured concentrations was never possible.

By the 1930s sedative premedication was considered desirable; both Dr James Heney and Dr John Boyd wrote about it. Dr Heney was writing in 1934 at a time when the long-acting intravenous barbiturates were coming in, but thiopentone (Pentothal) had not yet arrived in Belfast. Indeed these drugs were recommended as basal narcotics (heavy sedatives) rather than as full anaesthetics, which was at least a safe approach at the time.

RADIOLOGY

The history of radiology in the hospital is well documented. After Röntgen's discovery of x-rays in 1895, the Medical Committee of the Belfast Royal Hospital discussed it in July 1896 and the following November the necessary apparatus was purchased. Initially radiographs were taken by the firm of John Clarke and later by Lizars of Wellington Place.

Lizars apparently employed a Mr J.C. Carson, who, it is said, carried out domiciliary radiography by jaunting car at a cost of ten shillings a time. When the new Royal Victoria Hospital was opened, an Electrical Department was set up by Dr John Campbell Rankin. He had trained at Queen's College, graduating with an MB in 1900, and had spent a year in Copenhagen and Vienna studying the use of x-rays for both diagnosis and treatment, as well as the Finsen light treatment for lupus. Dr Rankin's talents were soon appreciated and he was appointed to the auxiliary staff of the Royal Victoria Hospital in 1903. In 1906 he completed his MD thesis and in 1908 produced an *Atlas of Skiagrams* (skiagrams are now known as radiographs or simply as x-rays) with Professor Johnston Symington. This is a remarkable volume, being the first to study the development of dentition from birth to adulthood using cadavers rather than dried skulls; it was a standard text in many dental schools for years to come.

The early department had problems of equipment and space. In 1904 Dr Rankin was already cramped and the replacement tube acquired that year cost £3. By 1911 when Dr Rankin was appointed to the Visiting staff, the year's new equipment (including that for the darkroom) cost a little over £400. Over the early years the use of x-rays rose steadily: from 50 plates in 1897 to 900 in 1911. By 1912 the technique was being used not only to look for fractures and foreign bodies but in one instance to investigate the cause of paralysis of certain muscles in the hand; that x-ray revealed an abnormal bony growth in the neck. The techniques of radiological screening and of stereoscopic viewing are first mentioned in 1914, in the context of finding metallic fragments in wounded soldiers. Dr Rankin continued to look after not only the Electrical Department but also Vaccine Therapy; with the surge of radiological work during World War

One, Ralph Leman was appointed radiographer in 1919; this, and the appointment of Dr Beath (below), allowed Dr Rankin increasingly to concentrate on work in the field of venereal diseases (see page 104).

Ralph M. Leman, in terms of his full-time commitment and length of service, spanned the entire early growth of the Electrical Department. He came from Norwich and had worked with x-rays in the hospital there in 1914 before volunteering his skills for Red Cross work in France. There he met Colonel Andrew Fullerton, who had left his post as Assistant Surgeon at the Royal Victoria Hospital to join the RAMC; and this contact eventually led, in 1919, to an invitation to work in Belfast with Dr Rankin. When Leman arrived, they were still using the primitive gas-filled x-ray tubes, glass photographic plates, and time exposures controlled by the time it took a weight to drop down a tube, equipment that was all very cumbersome – but then there were only six to eight patients per day. Only around 1920 was the danger of exposure to radiation being realised and protective lead aprons and gloves began to come into use. About this time x-ray films replaced the glass plates; this was a great improvement, despite the films' long exposure times and high inflammability, so that as many as 3,000 x-rays a year were taken. Mr Leman was one of the first diploma-holders of the Society of Radiographers, which was founded in 1922, and the Royal Victoria Hospital opened its own training school for radiographers in 1924. Mr Leman continued to work in the hospital until 1959, being awarded the MBE in 1951; in 1965 the many radiographers he had taught down the years presented him with a large iced cake inscribed 'Fifty Years and Still Radiating'. Fortunately he has left us a graphic picture of the scope of radiology (Leman, 1966), ranging from beautiful radiographs of flowers such as the lily (see page 94), and magnolia, to a horse with a leg fracture, x-rayed in a workshop at the back of the hospital.

The second medical appointment to the Department of Radiology was Dr Robert Maitland Beath who joined the auxiliary staff as Radiologist in 1920. He had studied medicine at Queen's University Belfast, graduating with an MB in 1914 (with first place and first-class honours) and also later at the University of London (1919). He served with the RAMC during World War One, and it was during this period that he acquired his interest in radiology. After further experience in London, he returned home to Belfast to bring new skills to the Royal Victoria Hospital. He was appointed to the Attending staff as the radiologist in 1921, and he was also on the staffs of the Belfast City, Ulster and Forster Green hospitals. He died at the early age of fifty-four, and the exceptionally warm tone of his obituaries suggests that he was held in unusual regard and affection by his colleagues. He was involved in setting up all the national radiological bodies and was president of the Faculty of Radiology in 1938. The Beath Room in the hospital's Department of Radiology was dedicated to his memory in 1964 and refurbished in 1993.

The next appointment to the department was that of Dr Frank Percivale Montgomery. He had graduated with an MB from Queen's University Belfast in 1914, playing in the university's rugby first XV from the outset and later for Ireland. Like his two colleagues in the department he had served in the RAMC in World War One (he had been awarded the Military Cross and Croix de Guerre). Then, unusually, he joined the Egyptian Medical Service, from which he was made redundant in 1923. He also studied Radiology in London and then went on to take the Diploma of Medical Radiology and Electrotherapy in Cambridge before joining the Royal Victoria Hospital as Assistant Radiologist in 1927. He was appointed Attending Radiologist in 1929 and joined forces with Dr Maitland Beath both in hospital and in private practice from the latter's home, Elmwood, opposite the university. With the inception of the National Health Service he was appointed the first chairman of the Northern Ireland Hospitals Authority and continued as its chairman until 1956. He was knighted in 1953. Like his colleagues, he also practised radiotherapy: the Northern Ireland Radiotherapy Centre (opened in 1952) was named Montgomery House in his honour. He contributed much to the Royal Victoria Hospital, and not only in the field of radiology: as well as being secretary of the Medical Staff Committee from 1942 to 1944, he was a leading force in establishing the departments of Neurology and Neurosurgery.

PATHOLOGY

In 1990 the centenary of the first pathology laboratory at the Belfast Royal Hospital was celebrated. Since 1890 this field has probably expanded and diversified more than any other in medicine. The subdivisions of morbid anatomy (the study of the appearance of tissues, by naked eye and microscope), haematology and bacteriology were so intertwined, in the early period at least, that they are best covered together. Chemical pathology became a distinct discipline somewhat later. (We are fortunate in having not only a commemorative centenary booklet edited by Professor P.G. Toner but two large unpublished histories written in retirement by Professor M.G. Nelson [1980] and Dr Margaret Haire [1993].)

When the Royal Victoria Hospital opened in 1903 it had a new mortuary, postmortem room and laboratory. The pathologist, Professor J. Lorrain Smith, left in 1904 to take up the chair in Manchester. He was succeeded in the chair by Professor William St Clair Symmers, who in the following year was appointed also to the staff of the hospital. He had been born in South Carolina but since his father came from Scotland, he was sent to be educated at Aberdeen where he graduated with an MB in 1887. He then had a remarkably varied career, working first in Banff, then in Aberdeen, Paris, Birmingham, Manchester, London and Cairo, where he stayed for seven years, before coming to Belfast for the remainder of his life.

Professor Symmers was mainly a morbid anatomist, but his published work extends into the field of bacteriology (including the bacteria content of the shellfish of Belfast Lough). He was prepared to work almost single-handedly, particularly during World War One. He was a quiet, dry man and perhaps the remark that most typifies his style is his appeal to medical students who were getting restless in one of his lectures: 'Gentlemen, I have still a few more pearls to cast.' He retired in 1929.

When Professor Symmers was appointed Hospital Pathologist, Dr Thomas Houston had already been in post since 1900 as Assistant Pathologist, and in 1905 he was appointed Haematologist. In 1911 he became Attending Haematologist. Dr Houston and Professor Symmers, both outstanding figures, set up the clinical and academic basis of the laboratory between them. Dr Houston was already heavily influenced by his fellow Ulsterman, Dr Almroth Wright, who at that time was setting up a diagnostic bacteriology laboratory and department for producing vaccines at St Mary's Hospital, Paddington.

During the 1914–18 war Dr Houston was posted to a laboratory in France, where he got to know more of Almroth Wright, his ideas and methods. There he also met Mr D. Willix who was later to be invited back to Belfast to join a Mr McWatters and Roderick McDonald Steven (Stevie) as laboratory technician. Meanwhile Professor Symmers and Dr Rankin kept the laboratory going, and by 1915 the new facilities in the King Edward Building were open, if not equipped. Dr (Major) Houston had already acquired valuable equipment in France but had been unable to get it home – a problem solved by a word to Lord Pirrie, who immediately despatched his private yacht to France and brought it back.

Over his long career Dr Houston continued to build up a modern haematology laboratory, while following his interest in the enterococcus (a common organism in the body that was blamed for a wide variety of conditions) and in vaccine therapy; it is for the haematology that we mainly remember him today. He had also gained experience of blood transfusion in France and can be credited with starting a blood transfusion service in Belfast (in the early days, though, the panel of donors consisted mainly of laboratory staff and members of the Royal Ulster Constabulary). He was awarded the OBE in 1919 and was knighted in 1927 at the relatively early age of fifty-nine. The year before his retirement in 1934, he saw the new Institute of Pathology opened as a truly joint hospital/university enterprise, its purpose being to house all the components of pathology then defined. He never married and was something of a workaholic and recluse, but he was very much liked and admired by all colleagues for his kindly human qualities.

One of the earliest bacteriologists as such was Dr Norman Clotworthy

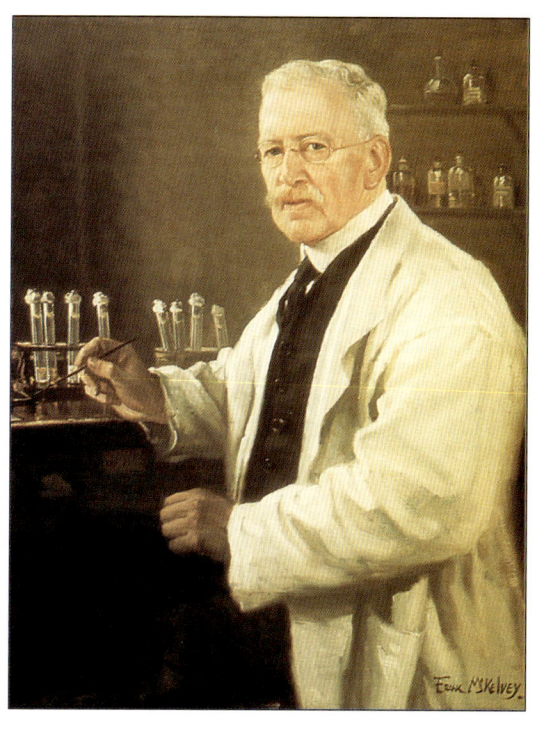

Sir Thomas Houston, Visiting Haematologist to the Royal Victoria Hospital from 1900 until he retired in 1934; portrait by Frank McKelvey
ROYAL VICTORIA HOSPITAL

Graham, 'Koch', who qualified with an MB at Queen's University in 1912 and served with the Ulster Division during World War One, winning the Military Cross in Flanders. After a period with the Belfast Public Health Laboratories, Dr Graham became a university lecturer in 1927. He remained in this post, and became Clinical Pathologist to the hospital on the retirement of Sir Thomas Houston and a hospital Consultant in 1948, retiring eventually in 1954.

Dr Eileen O. Bartley graduated with an MB at Queen's University in 1921 and with an MD in 1930, and joined the Department of Pathology in the 1920s. She was appointed to a second lectureship in Bacteriology in 1942 and became Consultant Bacteriologist in 1962. She retired in 1963.

When Professor Symmers retired from the chair of Pathology in 1929, he was succeeded by Professor Alexander Murray Drennan, also a Scot, who had graduated with an MB with honours at Edinburgh in 1906. He had already been Professor of Pathology in Otago, New Zealand, from 1914 to 1929, and two years after his appointment in Belfast he left to take up the chair in Edinburgh. His successor, Professor John Stirling Young (MB with honours, Glasgow, 1923), stayed longer but he too left for another chair, this time in Aberdeen.

Professor Young was succeeded in the Musgrave Chair by Dr John Henry Biggart; truly it can be said that, as far as medicine is concerned, he did 'bestride the narrow world like a Colossus'. He was born at Templepatrick, County Antrim, studied at Inst. and Queen's University (MB 1928, MD with gold medal 1931; D.Sc. 1937) and at the prestigious Johns Hopkins Medical School in Baltimore, USA, and in 1933 he was appointed lecturer in Neuropathology at Edinburgh. He took over the Department of Pathology in Belfast in 1937, when it was firmly settled into its new building. At that time, the main interest of the department was in providing an excellent postmortem and biopsy service, and morbid anatomy was the dominant discipline for all who passed through it. During World War Two, however, the youthful blood transfusion service had rapidly to be enlarged to provide blood for the many casualties that reached the hospital. It was only at this stage that the staff of the department handed over to House Surgeons the duty of administering blood, though they still kept the donor register and had the task of taking and crossmatching blood until eventually the Northern Ireland Blood Transfusion Service was founded in 1946. For his pioneer work in this field, Professor Biggart was awarded the CBE in 1948.

The first edition of Biggart's *Textbook of Neuropathology* had already been published while he was working in Edinburgh and he continued with this special interest, at the same time encouraging his demonstrators and lecturers to produce a series of MD theses and eventually textbooks.

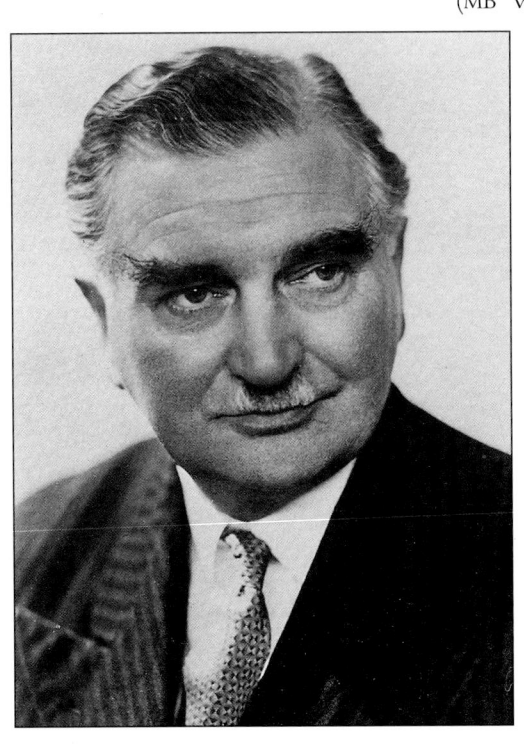

Sir John Biggart, Musgrave Professor of Pathology at Queen's University Belfast and Visiting Pathologist to the Royal Victoria Hospital, 1937–71, and dean of the Faculty of Medicine, 1943–71
ROYAL VICTORIA HOSPITAL

Professor Biggart's drive and imagination soon took him far beyond his department, however, first as dean of the Faculty of Medicine, 1943–71, then as pro-vice-chancellor and pro-chancellor of the university, 1967–79, as a member of the General Medical Council, 1951–79, and as chairman of many influential committees connected with medical education, research and the administration of the new National Health Service. The results of his work in these fields can be seen in the joint appointment system which binds together the Belfast teaching hospitals and Queen's University, and in the host of buildings and educational structures that arose in his period of office. He was made a knight bachelor in 1967, retired in 1971, and as was said in his obituary in the *British Medical Journal*, he 'accomplished more in his retirement than many do in their entire working lives'.

It is as a personality, however, that he is remembered by a generation of medical students. When a student himself he had been a prime mover in Rag Day and the student magazine *Pro Tanto Quid*; as dean he took part in the annual Dean's Birthday Party with gusto, demolishing a tumbler of Bushmills in the course of a lecture with a confidence that confirmed our belief in his omnipotence. Finally there were his brilliant Pathology and Forensic Medicine lectures and the address he gave to the staff and students of the hospital in 1967 on the Hippocratic theme of philanthropia, philotechnia and philosophia, that is, essentially, 'where there is love of Man, there is love of the Art'; what can be further removed from the present concepts of the National Health Service?

The first of Professor Biggart's trainees to take up the field of pathology as a career was Dr John Edgar Morison. He had graduated with an MB with honours at Queen's University in 1935 and joined the department in 1937, the same year as the new professor. Dr Morison was awarded the MD with gold medal in 1940 and in 1942 he moved over to the Belfast City Hospital to build up a similar department, but he returned to the Royal Victoria Hospital in 1947 as senior lecturer, becoming a Consultant Pathologist in 1948. His textbook *Foetal and Neonatal Pathology* was published in 1951 (with later editions), and he received the degree of D.Sc. in 1952. He moved back to the City Hospital in 1954 to head its Department of Histopathology and was subsequently appointed to a personal chair in pathology at the university.

Dr M. Gerald (Gerry) Nelson graduated with an MB with honours in 1937 and followed John Edgar Morison into the Department of Pathology, obtaining the MD with gold medal in 1940. After service with the RAF he returned to the Royal Victoria Hospital to take up a lecturer post in Pathology in 1946 and an assistant post in Clinical Pathology in 1947. This post at the time included bacteriology and it was not until 1962, with the appointment of Dr Eileen Bartley as Consultant Bacteriologist, that he was able to devote his time fully to haematology. He was appointed to a personal chair in Haematology in 1971, and retired in 1979.

CLINICAL BIOCHEMISTRY

Clinical biochemistry, also known as chemical pathology, developed from the simple urine and blood tests carried out in the wards. At first the doctor had only noted the presence of albumen in the urine (indicative of kidney disease) and sugar (indicative of diabetes). Later the quantitative measurement of urea and glucose in the blood gave more precise information, and clinicians came to appreciate the tests' value. It was only in 1922 that the subject was given a special laboratory within the Pathology Department in the King Edward Building. This was in fact one of the first such laboratories in the UK, and its opening coincided with the appointment of Dr John A. (Jack) Smyth with the title Assistant Physician to the Biochemical Department, which enabled him to concentrate on patients requiring laboratory diagnosis who did not need to be admitted to hospital. He had served in the army during World War One but took up medicine when he was invalided out in 1916. He graduated with an MB and B.Sc. in 1921 and was awarded an MD with gold medal in 1924. Throughout his career he was the recognised authority in Belfast on diabetes. He retired in 1958.

Mary Frances Bostock (seated *centre*), Matron of the Throne Hospital, 1887–1901, and Matron of the Royal Victoria Hospital 1901–22, with a group of sisters and nurses at the hospital, *c*.1905
ROYAL VICTORIA HOSPITAL

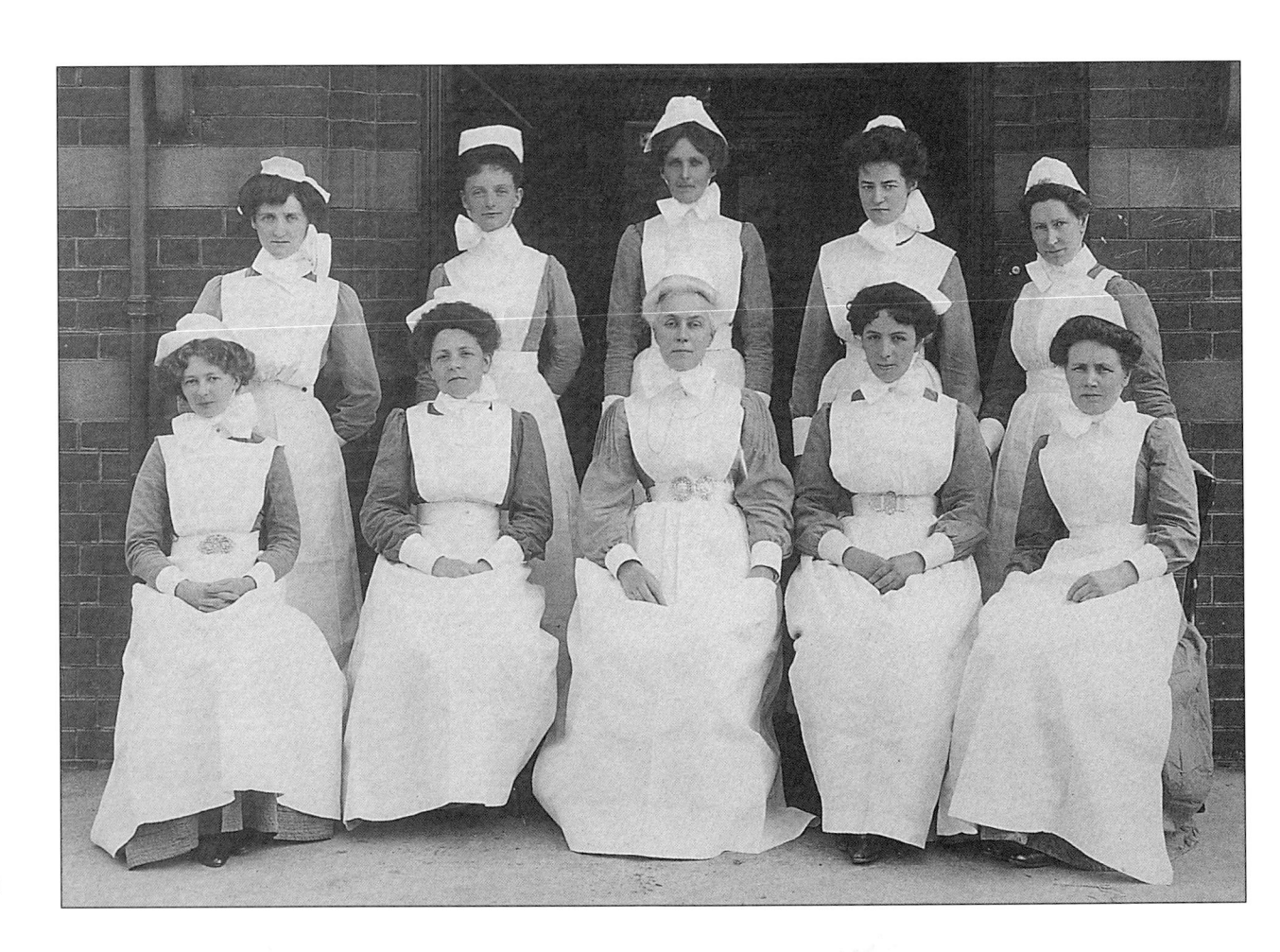

NURSING

The new Royal Victoria Hospital provided much greater integration of nurses into the hospital, since they were both paid by the hospital and under the control of the hospital's Matron. They now lived in the West Wing, even if they soon overflowed into huts where the Radiology Department was later built and into the King Edward Building. They were constantly passing up and down the corridor along with doctors and staff generally so that it was possible for everyone to know everyone. Inevitably, the person who knew most about all hospital activities was Miss Mary F. Bostock, Matron from 1901 to 1922, since she lived beside the nurses and had her office only a few yards from the hospital corridor. She was in effect Lady Superintendent of the nurses, responsible for their work, welfare and training, and also Housekeeper, with responsibility for the domestic staff, catering, supplies and laundry. Economy had to be her watchword; this was emphasised by her own salary, which started at £100 annually, though it had reached £250 by the time she retired.

Mary Frances Bostock had trained in the Leeds General Infirmary from 1880 to 1883 and subsequently worked there as a staff nurse. She then went to Barbados for a year before being appointed Matron of the Throne Hospital, where she stayed from 1887 to 1901, before serving as Matron of the Royal Victoria Hospital for twenty years. She was a firm disciplinarian, but had a sense of humour, and indisputably had the overall welfare of her nurses at heart. She died in 1950 at the age of ninety.

She was succeeded as Matron by Anne Elizabeth Musson, who trained in Nottingham General Hospital and had experience in Golders Green, Cardiff, and Newport hospitals and with the Territorial Army Nursing Service in France, 1914–19. Here she was seen by Mr Andrew Fullerton who, impressed by her abilities, managed to inveigle her over to Belfast. She came to the Royal Victoria Hospital as Assistant Matron in 1919 and served as Matron from 1922 until 1946; she was awarded the MBE on her retirement. She was regarded as rather aloof, though an excellent and fair matron. She had artistic gifts, being a frequent exhibitor at the Ulster Academy of Arts. She died on 3 February 1958. Florence Elliott replaced her on 1 May 1946 (see page 173).

The post of Assistant Matron had been created in 1903, and after 1919 a separate post of Home Sister was created; her role was to look after the welfare of the nurses and the nurses' home. The post of Housekeeper was also created early on to cope with the management of the kitchens and to look after all the resident doctors, nurses and domestic staff. The other important figure in the nursing hierarchy was the Night Sister (later known as the Night Superintendent). This post was filled from 1909 to 1953 by Sister Catherine Dynes, who was truly a legend within the hospital; she ruled it throughout the hours of darkness,

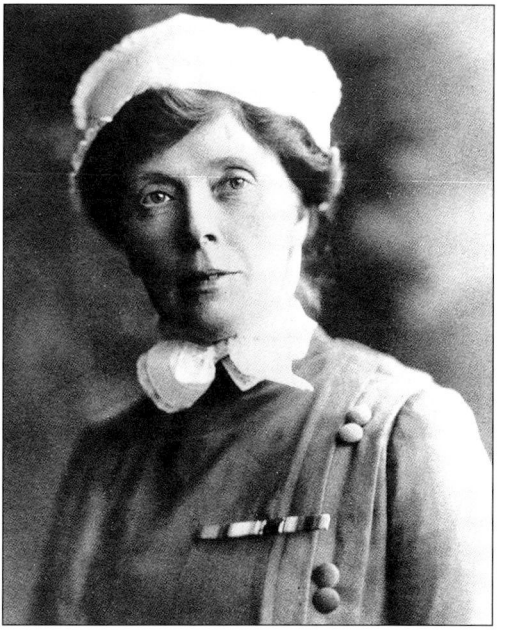

Anne Elizabeth Musson, Matron of the Royal Victoria Hospital, 1922–46
ROYAL VICTORIA HOSPITAL

not only checking up on the nurses and their doings both clinical and social, but also advising inexperienced doctors on the management of emergencies. In one ward she would appear and find the nurse in charge entertaining doctors and medical students to tea and a fry, while in another she would roll up her sleeves and help with the laying out of some badly mutilated accident victim. She was always known as Diana, and for her lifetime's devotion to the hospital she well deserved the MBE awarded on her retirement.

Ward sisters were, of course, the mainstays of the hospital with duties within their ward comparable to those of the Matron, that is, responsibility for the nursing, the kitchen and domestics, the feeding of the patients and medical matters within the ward. The ward sister was the main link between consultant and junior doctor, expected to see that the treatment was not just what the patient needed but fitted in with the particular consultant's idiosyncrasies. On the surgical wards, ward sisters were also responsible for the operating theatre. As in the hospital as a whole, the most important consideration was often economy. Stocktaking therefore loomed very large in terms both of daily counting of sheets, cutlery, basins, et cetera, and of yearly counting of everything.

The most junior workers in patient care were the probationers. Initially they had to be more than twenty-three but the minimum age was reduced to twenty-one in 1918 to help recruitment. It was reduced again, to eighteen, during World War Two. The probationers were largely young women from rural backgrounds, and the free accommodation and strict supervision of the nurses' home were two definite attractions to parents. Nurses had to be in the home by 9.00 p.m. with lights out by 10.30 p.m. in order to be up for breakfast at 6.30 a.m. They then worked in the wards from before 7.00 a.m. until 8.30 p.m. – an almost unbelievable day's work for the twentieth century in a prosperous country! The probationers had a monthly day off and a half day on Sunday plus two hours off at some time during each afternoon. The total working week was over seventy hours, on their feet, and it is surprising that some still had energy to swim in the Falls Road baths, play tennis on the hospital courts or dance in the King Edward Building. Badminton, tennis and hockey within the hospital grounds were introduced in the 1930s and not only helped to allow doctors and nurses to socialise, but also took nurses into competitive sport beyond the hospital.

As the century progressed life for the nurses improved slightly, and the building of the new nurses' home in 1937 certainly improved living conditions. Curiously, the nurse's uniform of the 1920s looks less attractive and more forbidding than that of thirty years earlier, even if the dresses are shorter. This is partly because of the 'fall' which had now come in for

Sister Catherine Dynes, Night Sister at the Royal Victoria Hospital, 1909–53
ROYAL VICTORIA HOSPITAL

trained nurses as a headdress, often coming down to the eyes.

Ill health was not unknown among the nurses, of course, but since only the fit were accepted as probationers, most nurses managed with minimal sick leave – perhaps kept going by the threat of a noxious black purgative. When early retirement was necessary from ill health, conditions were hard; nurses' pay left little over for saving, and only in 1935 was a pension scheme introduced. Married nurses were almost unknown until after World War Two; and many nurses left to get married within a year of finishing their State Registration.

The work of the nurse changed little in this period: it included the domestic work of washing and polishing for the juniors, rubbing backs for the senior probationers, preparing 'antiphlo' poultices and inhalations of friar's balsam, giving out medicines that are now seen to be of doubtful value, and the ritual of serving meals, presided over by the ward sister or senior staff nurse. Even in the enlarging hospital of Miss Musson's day it was routine for the Matron to do a complete round of all the patients. She would be accompanied by a senior sister, and she combined attention to nurses' omissions with considerable concern for individual patients' welfare and progress.

Formal teaching for nurses was nonexistent at the beginning of the twentieth century but with the introduction of State Registration in 1922, a curriculum and examinations became a necessity. The first sister tutor was appointed in 1923, and a dedicated classroom was fitted out in a redundant hut near the King Edward Building in 1925. Gradually a Preliminary Training School and study leave before exams were introduced, though lectures were still normally held during off-duty hours.

THE THRONE HOSPITAL

In 1903 this hospital consisted of three distinct parts: the Throne Convalescent Home (24 beds) which treated patients transferred from the Royal Victoria Hospital, the Martin Children's Hospital (33 beds) which treated a variety of long-term child patients, and the Consumptive Hospital (10 beds) which treated mainly advanced cases of tuberculosis. The matrons, following Miss Bostock's move to the Royal Victoria Hospital were: Miss Mildred, from Grantham, 1902–09, Miss Hilson from the Royal Victoria Hospital, 1909–36, and Miss Magee, a former sister in the Throne, from 1936 onwards. Dr Robert Reid was Attending Physician from 1900 to 1937 and Dr T. Lawrence Ross held the post from 1938. Dr H.C. Manley, Dr T.S. Kirk and Mr Howard Stevenson were surgeons from 1900 until 1944 when Mr Stevenson resigned and was not replaced. The hospital had its own Ladies' Committee which looked after the comfort and entertainment of the patients and helped to collect presents and larger donations.

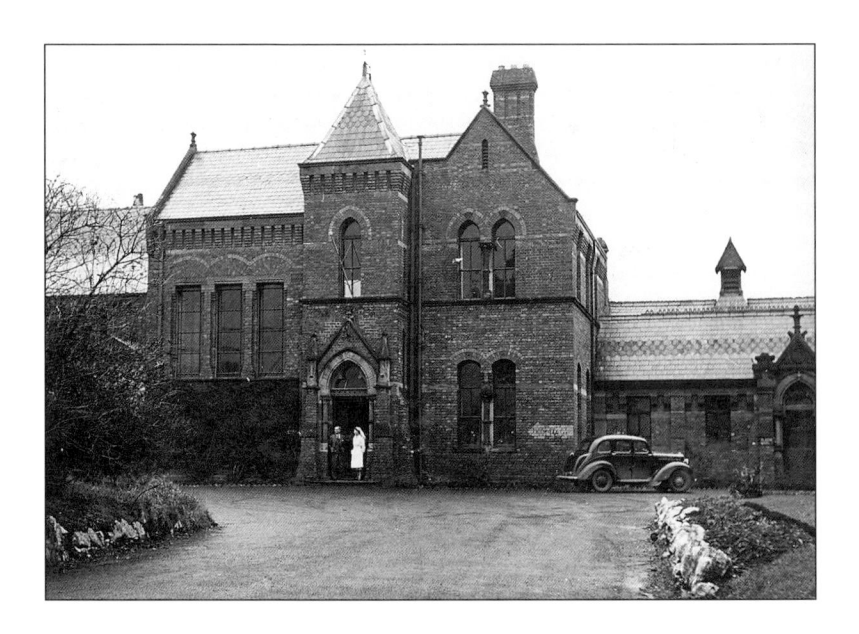

The Throne Hospital, Antrim Road, *c.* 1948
ROYAL VICTORIA HOSPITAL

Over the half-century to 1950, the pattern of admissions remained essentially similar but it was noted in 1911 that since Whiteabbey Sanatorium had opened and the Forster Green Hospital had been enlarged, the pressure for consumption beds had decreased, so in 1919 this unit was closed. In 1920 a donation of £1,000 from Mrs Wallace of San Francisco enabled many improvements to be made to the accommodation. In 1933 electric lighting was installed in place of gas. Throughout the period small numbers of operations were carried out (50 to 100 per year), but in the 1940s patients requiring hernia repair were transferred from the Royal Victoria Hospital's waiting list, and after World War Two larger numbers of these patients were operated on at the Throne Hospital by surgical registrars from the Royal Victoria Hospital.

During the half century to 1948 the Royal Victoria Hospital had expanded along the corridor and bed numbers had doubled, but the infrastructure was in constant difficulties. The King Edward Building, though a fine addition to the site, was never really suitable for the uses thrust on it, laboratory space, nurses' bedrooms or a dental hospital. Financial shortages were extreme and the major fundraising effort of the late 1930s was doomed by the advent of war. On the other hand, the Royal Victoria Hospital was the main teaching hospital of Belfast, because the other voluntary hospitals were struggling even more from shortages of funds and had little connection with the university to encourage research or attract academic excellence. In the inter-war years the Attending Physicians and Surgeons had reached a position of authority in the hospital and beyond – indeed a position far beyond what was deserved in terms of time spent in the wards or, in some cases, of academic excellence. The advent of the National Health Service was to change all this: the Royal Victoria Hospital was to gain enormously in funds for capital expenditure and a huge increase in staff, and all this would produce a more balanced expansion and a levelling-up which was of real benefit to the sick of Belfast.

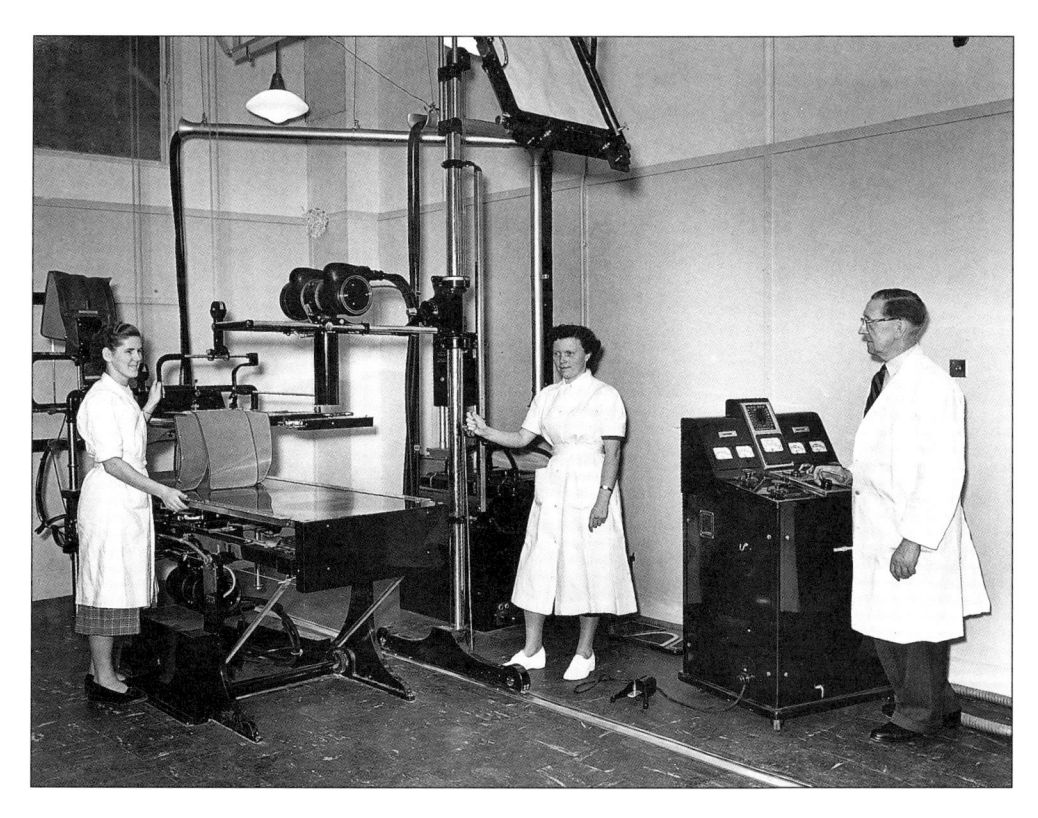

The new equipment in the neuroradiology department in Quin House, 1953, with Ralph Leman, chief radiographer, on the right
ROYAL VICTORIA HOSPITAL

5
THE NATIONAL HEALTH SERVICE HOSPITAL CHANGES AND THE MEDICAL SPECIALITIES

THE NATIONAL HEALTH ACT OF 1948 probably introduced the most radical changes in health care ever seen in the UK. In spite of changes since then and some flaws, it has given us a system that is the envy of the world. The act's conception as regards the hospital service was to take over virtually all the old voluntary and locally administered hospitals and to finance them from the state, paying all staff as appropriate.

The effects of the National Health Act on patients were many. Perhaps most far-reaching, it had a gradual effect on patients' perceptions of hospitals. No longer were they told that hospital was for the destitute and those who could afford it should go elsewhere. Instead, Lord Beveridge promised complete health care for all, from the cradle to the grave. Throughout the twentieth century, however, taxation had been steadily rising (indeed the lack of surplus funds had already reduced donations to charities such as hospitals), and it was not to be expected that the further taxation necessary to fund a 'complete' health service could go on increasing for ever, but in the middle of the century this was not apparent. Instead hospital growth was explosive, in bed numbers, in the expense of the treatments being undertaken, and in costs of administration. Patients came to feel then, and to some extent they still do, that they should receive any treatment whatever that could possibly help their condition, regardless of cost, and of course doctors always wanted the best for the individual patient.

The Health Service Act (NI) set up two main divisions – the Northern Ireland Hospitals Authority to oversee all the hospitals in its charge, and the Northern Ireland General Health Services Board to oversee general practice – as well as local Welfare Committees and the Northern Ireland Tuberculosis Authority (already established in 1946). Hospitals that joined the new National Health Service were divided into geographical groups such as those on the Royal Victoria Hospital site together with the Claremont Street (nervous diseases), Haypark (long-stay and convalescent), Lissue (children's long-stay) and Killowen (convalescent) hospitals.

The act came into force in June 1948 and to smooth over the transition period the Royal Victoria Hospital's Board of Management was replaced by a temporary committee from July 1948 until March 1949. It was then replaced by the Belfast Hospitals Management Committee (BHMC) (for what is now the Royal Group of Hospitals), with Herbert Quin MP continuing as chairman. He was succeeded in 1951 by Professor F.H. Newark, followed in 1962 by Albert Grant and in 1965 by Austen Boyd. Victor Clarendon, who had been the previous honorary treasurer, was appointed honorary secretary with F.M.R. Byers. Again there was a committee of about thirty members, of whom seven were doctors or dentists. (The doctors and dentists were soon phased out.) Reporting to it was the Finance and General Purposes Committee, also chaired by Herbert Quin. Also working with the BHMC were committees for the Royal Victoria Hospital (including the Musgrave and Clark Clinic and the Throne Hospital), the Royal Maternity Hospital, the Royal Belfast Hospital for Sick Children and Claremont Street Hospital. In general, matters of finance and senior medical staffing, which crossed the boundaries of individual hospitals, were handled by the BHMC rather than the committees, but it is often difficult to distinguish roles. This committee structure terminated at the end of 1964, after which the management committee took on all responsibilities.

It soon became clear that the problems of running the medical aspects of the hospital group required a further committee, and this role was taken on in October 1953 by a Group Medical Staff Committee. In the following year this became the Group Medical Advisory Committee (GMAC). This committee was responsible for the appointment of registrar trainees in all specialities and for all medical problems affecting the group as a whole. It was small, comprising only a few representatives of each of the main specialities, and soon became the most powerful committee regarding medical matters within the hospital. Subcommittees reported to it on matters relating to anaesthetics, the control of infection, laboratory services, pharmacy, radioisotopes and the various hospital medical staffs.

The major change that the National Health Act produced for all voluntary hospitals was that they lost their independence and all funding for running costs and new building was now provided and controlled by the Northern Ireland Hospitals Authority (chaired by Dr Frank Montgomery). A requirement was that all voluntary hospitals had to be handed over free of debt, but in return they were allowed to keep and (up to a point) control their endowment funds or investments from voluntary donations. They were no longer allowed to appeal for funds, but gifts were treated as endowments and the Ladies' Committee and the Working Men's Committee continued to raise funds, though on a reduced scale. The naming of wards and erection of plaques were frowned on in 1949 because they suggested that hospitals were still appealing to the public for donations, but gradually all the prohibitions relaxed. All hospital staff were now salaried, and in particular the old Visiting staff were taken on as part-time consultants and paid according to the number of their 'sessions', up to eleven per week; the consultants of all specialities were paid at the same rate. This greatly increased the involvement of the senior medical staff and, as younger men came in, undoubtedly led to an improvement in the quality of medical care. At the same time the number of secretarial and administrative staff began steadily to increase.

One of the questions which now arose was how best to use the substantial interest flowing from the hospital's endowment fund. From the outset the BHMC had no doubt that it should be used for additional purposes not funded by the NHS; the two that emerged were to fund members of staff to travel to conferences (which was easily implemented) and to fund young doctors wanting to undertake research. A research committee was therefore set up in 1954 under Dr R.S. Allison to select suitable research fellows, and in August 1955 Dr John Weaver was appointed as the first. Funding has enabled about eight fellowships to be awarded each year, though the term of the fellowships and the method of selection have varied. From the early years the committee was concerned with commemorating the two distinguished surgeons Mr Cecil Calvert and Mr Barney Purce, and for a period there were named fellowships for each. More recently the arrangement has been that after completion of their work one of the fellows is selected to give a Calvert Lecture and one a Purce Lecture, each receiving an appropriate medal. After 1971 a new committee was formed to represent the whole Royal Group, allocating also the interest from the free funds of the Royal Maternity Hospital and the Royal Belfast Hospital for Sick Children, so that additional fellowships could be awarded. The success of the scheme is illustrated by its survival through so many subsequent hospital changes.

The day-to-day running of the hospital continued in the hands of Brigadier Thomas Davidson as Superintendent, Leonard Reid as secretary and Florence Elliott as Matron, so the upheavals in administration were not as great as might be supposed. For the period 1957–62 Brigadier Davidson took on the additional responsibilities of group secretary and Leonard Reid became accounts officer. In this period of expansion, Robert T. Spence was appointed deputy secretary (1957); he became secretary in 1962. He was to prove a particularly powerful and effective secretary until he resigned in 1974 to become director of the Northern Ireland Housing Executive.

In 1965, Brigadier Davidson retired as group medical superintendent, to be replaced by Colonel T.E. Field; Florence Elliott retired in 1966 and was replaced by Kathleen Robb. Colonel Field resigned in 1968 and was replaced by J.S. Loughridge (1968–73) on a part-time basis. From 1957 the senior full-time administrators attended the BHMC meetings, and it is probably from this period that they began to have more influence in decision making as opposed to simply carrying out the instructions of the management committee.

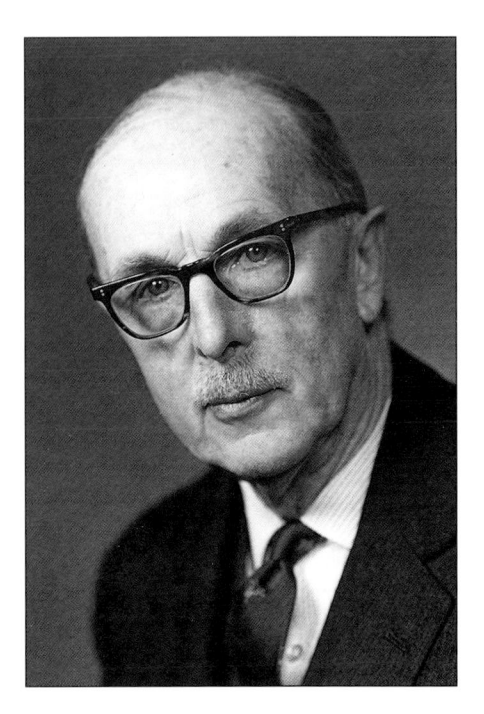

Brigadier Thomas Davidson MD, Medical Superintendent of the Royal Victoria Hospital, 1946–65
ROYAL VICTORIA HOSPITAL

THE 1972 REORGANISATION AND THE EASTERN HEALTH AND SOCIAL SERVICES BOARD

The management structure outlined above lasted for almost twenty-five years and gave the hospitals on the Royal Victoria Hospital site a measure of autonomy as well as considerable influence with the Northern Ireland Hospitals Authority. In 1972, however, it was decided to divide Northern Ireland into four area boards, each with its own independent budget, and to abolish the BHMC. Greater Belfast was now covered by the Eastern Health and Social Services Board (EHSSB) which had various district committees including the North and West Belfast District Committee covering the hospitals on the Royal Victoria site, the Mater Infirmorum Hospital (which now entered the NHS) and the social services for the whole district. The hospitals in the North and West Belfast District Committee area were administered by a Medical Executive Committee (set up by Professor M.G. Nelson, its chairman, after visiting centres in England) and no less than twenty-five subcommittees representing staff of the component hospitals, the medical specialities and other fields such as planning, finance and pharmacy. The eleven speciality committees were known as 'cogwheel' committees or divisional committees, and this system of cogwheel committees, although very cumbersome, gave a large measure of democracy within the hospital structure.

The administrative personnel of the hospital and district also changed at this time. Robert T. Spence carried on with the new title District Administrative Officer until 1974. He was replaced by Mr J.C. Girvan Jackson who had been involved in the building committee in Queen's University Belfast, and he filled the District Administrative Officer post for ten years in all. Mr J.S. Loughridge retired from the part-time post of Medical Superintendent in 1973 to be replaced by Mr Bertram Leslie Ardill FRCSE under the new title District Administrative Medical Officer (DAMO). Kathleen Robb changed from being Matron of the Royal Victoria Hospital to being District Administrative Nursing Officer (DANO) for the group. May McFarland effectively became Matron of the Royal Victoria Hospital, 1973–75, followed by Heather Barrett, 1975–84. Dr Ardill died in 1977 at the early age of thirty-nine, and was succeeded as DAMO from 1979 to 1984 by Reginald A.E. Magee FRCSI, a retired obstetrician and gynaecologist and former Stormont MP.

The year 1984 saw yet another reorganisation of hospitals within the area: the North and West Belfast District was replaced by the Royal Group of Hospitals and a separate Community Management Unit for the North and West Belfast area, plus the Mater Infirmorum as a separate unit. These changes were heralded as improving services and making them more efficient and responsive to public need, but in retrospect it is unlikely that any of these effects followed; this was probably the beginning of the period of stringent cutbacks in government funding of the health and social services.

The senior administration within the Royal Group all changed in 1984. Girvan Jackson moved to the area headquarters and was replaced by Samuel C. Haslett as Group Administrator who himself was replaced in 1988 by William McKee, who later became Acting Unit Manager. Dr Harold Love, a retired anaesthetist, was Medical Administrator (1984–87), succeeded by Dr George A. Murnaghan, who continued to work part-time as an obstetrician. Kathleen Robb, having retired, was replaced by Elizabeth Duffin with the title Director of Nursing Services for the Royal Group.

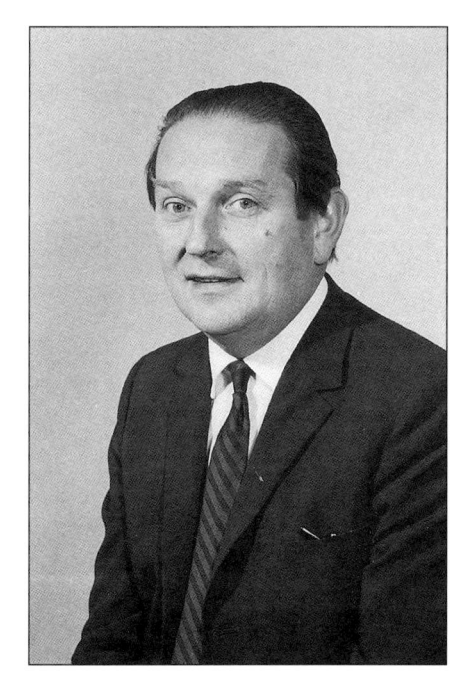

Robert T. Spence, deputy secretary and later secretary of the Belfast Hospitals Management Committee (after 1972, the North and West Belfast District), 1957–74
ROYAL VICTORIA HOSPITAL

POST-1945 BUILDING CHANGES

The first structural change made to the hospital after the end of World War Two involved no new building and was a desperate expedient to provide space economically. In 1947 the old extern hall was split horizontally leaving most of the outpatient facilities unchanged at ground level, but

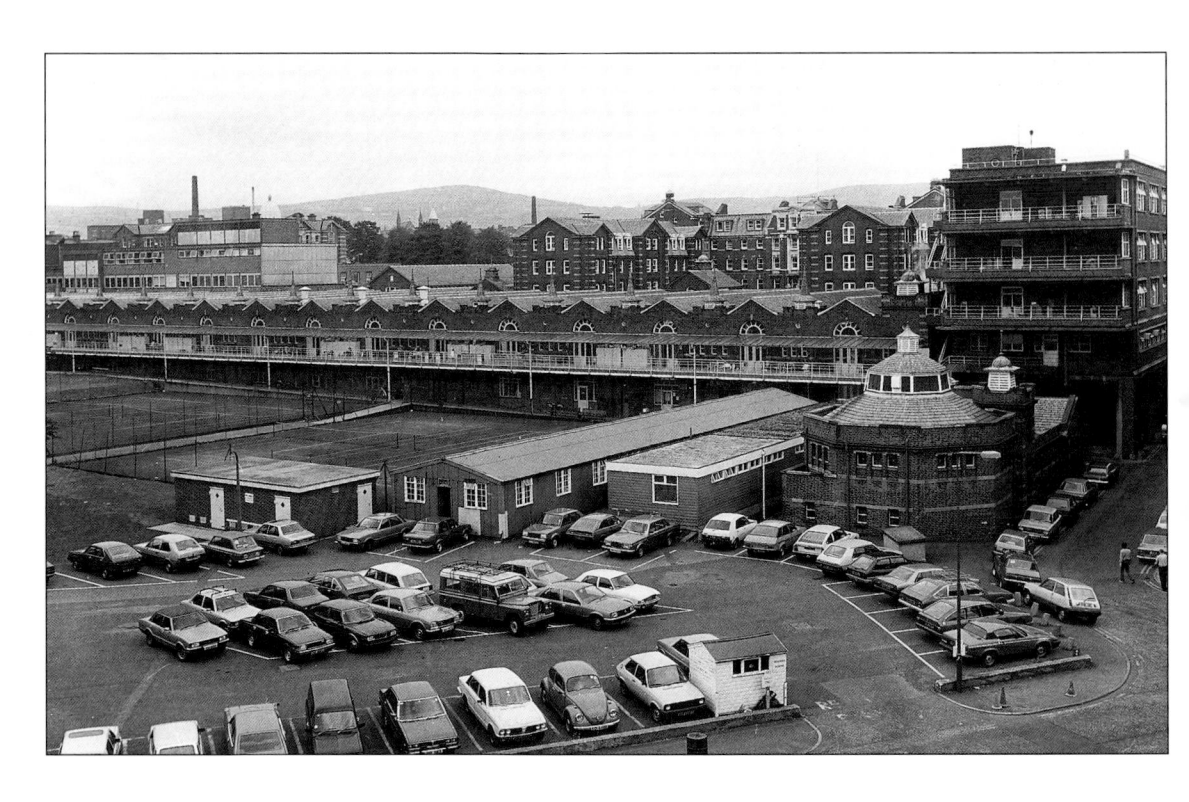

View from the Dental Hospital of the Royal Victoria Hospital, c. 1970, showing the main row of wards with the block containing the new operating theatres and x-ray department (*left background*), the old administration block (*centre background*) and the metabolic and skin wards (*right*). In the foreground are the tennis courts, the huts which provided residential accommodation for junior medical staff and students for many years, and the mortuary.
ROYAL VICTORIA HOSPITAL

moving surgical and gynaecological outpatients to the new upper floor. The Central Registry for patients' records was also housed in the upper floor. At the same time the Good Samaritan window was moved from the extern hall to the lower end of the main corridor. (All these functions were to be moved to the Austen Boyd Outpatient Building after it was completed in 1969, and the ground floor was subsequently adapted for the Ganymede catering system and expanded cardiac catheterisation facilities in 1973.) The wards were refurbished in 1947 in a further move to help staff and patient morale. This involved removing the old marble dedicatory tablets above each bed, with their overtones of death, and replacing them with small brass plates. Anglepoise lamps and wireless installations were also supplied for each bed (there had been some wireless installations in the hospital since 1936).

The money for new projects became available only slowly after 1948, and even projects that had a large amount of funding from voluntary sources were delayed for the government's contribution. The first building work therefore consisted in modifications and enlargements, and it was five years before a major new building (Bostock House) was completed. Progress thereafter continued to be slow; many man-hours were wasted by committees, and plans were drawn up only to be scrapped, over the next decades.

In 1951 another economical change made to reuse space already available was the move of the pharmacy from its site on the hospital corridor into the archways below wards 4 and 5. This made room for an ECG department – which was now providing an important diagnostic service for the whole hospital, but this was only the first of many cardiological expansions. A restaurant and staff sitting room was constructed below wards 6 and 7. This area, known as 'the caves', did much to bring together students, junior doctors, nurses and other staff, even when it was partially replaced by the Bostock House restaurant. Until about 1970, when the Dining Club in the King Edward Building opened, the restaurant also included a fenced-off area with waitress service for senior staff. Also in 1951, a fourth floor was added to the Institute of Pathology to give much-needed space for laboratory medicine.

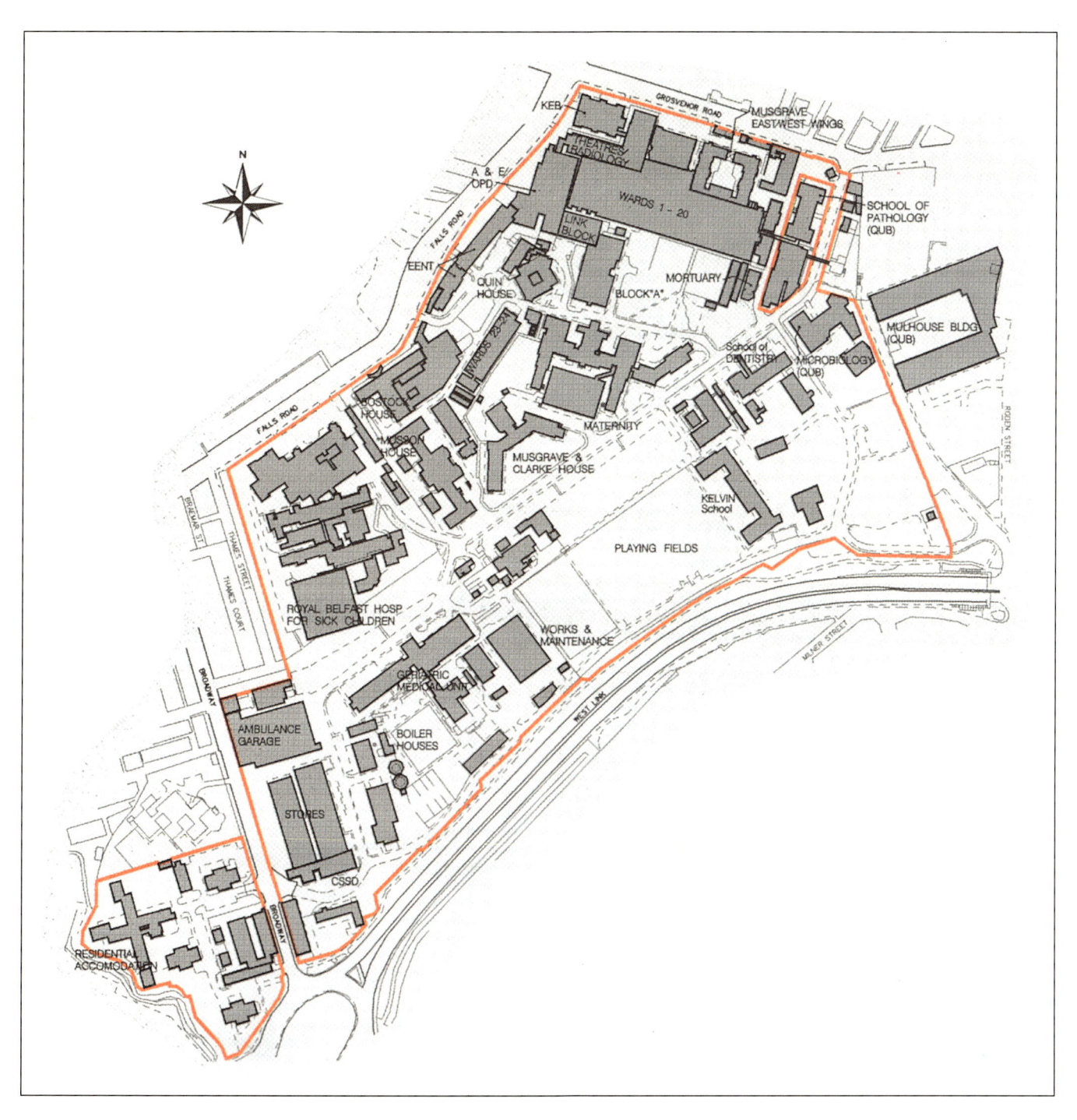

In 1952–53, the pre-war septic and isolation wards (wards 21 and 22)

Map of the Royal Hospitals site, *c.* 1980, bounded by the Grosvenor Road, Falls Road, Thames Street, Broadway and the West Link: the post-war development includes Quin House, the Outpatient Building, EENT building, A Block, Bostock House, extensions to the Royal Belfast Hospital for Sick Children, the ambulance garage, stores and maintenance areas, the Geriatric Medical Unit, conversion of Kelvin School into laboratories, and the School of Dentistry
ROYAL VICTORIA HOSPITAL

were converted into a neurology–neurosurgical unit. This involved doubling the bed numbers to about 70 and building on an operating theatre and electro-encephalogram unit. The whole block was now named Quin House after Herbert Quin. The new unit's circumferential corridor linking the four-bed and single wards meant that, unfortunately, the greater privacy for patients was more than offset by difficulties in nursing supervision.

Musson House had seemed spacious before the war, but since then additional accommodation had had to be found for nurses in the former Medical Superintendent's house (now known as Riddel House). There were also prefabricated huts built in 1946 for ninety-four nurses alongside the covered way leading to the nurses' home. These inevitably provided much less supervision than a true nurses' home of that time and were a popular social asset in the life of nurses and medical students. Nurses were also accommodated further afield, in the Throne Hospital and Lennoxvale, but at last in 1953 a new building was completed, appropriately named Bostock House. It included a large hall, to be used for nurses' prizegivings and many hospital functions, notably the Jubilee Ball of its opening year. In 1960 the building was expanded and four years later a large restaurant was added.

As far back as 1936, Sir George Clark and his brother Captain H.D. Clark had left £25,000 to the hospital, £15,000 of which was to go towards private accommodation (see page 93). The remaining £10,000 was to provide accommodation for the investigation and treatment of metabolic disorders. This unit had not been built when war began and was further delayed for various reasons, but in 1957 the Sir George Clark Metabolic Clinic (based on Ward 25) was finally opened. It consisted of an outpatient clinic (later converted into a laboratory) at hospital corridor level (Level 2), above which were two floors for patients with endocrine diseases (Ward 25). The top floor (Ward 26) was named the Purdon Skin Ward and bore a plaque to the dermatology pioneers of the nineteenth century who had founded the Benn Skin Hospital (the latter having been destroyed in an air raid in 1941). In 1972 the metabolic and dermatology outpatients were moved to the new Austen Boyd Outpatient Building (see page 147) and replaced by the expanding endocrine section of the biochemistry laboratory, to be named the J.A. Smyth Endocrine Laboratory. The whole unit was always rather cramped structurally, though the closing in of its balconies made some bright day rooms.

The other development in 1957 was the move of the gynaecology wards from their old position on the corridor (wards 17 and 18) to new single-storey wards to the west of Quin House and conveniently beside the Royal Maternity Hospital. The new unit, known as wards 23 and 24, with 48 beds was rather smaller than wards 17 and 18, but its theatres and day room made it more convenient and the layout gave much greater privacy to the patient. Wards 17 and 18 were swiftly converted into a new fracture unit, bringing together patients who had formerly been scattered throughout the surgical wards of the hospital.

The post-1945 period saw the construction of major new buildings by the university along the hospital road. First there was the Institute of Clinical Science, in two parts joined by a bridge, which opened in 1954 and housed the departments of Medicine, Surgery, Obstetrics, Child Health, Social Medicine and (later) Anaesthetics, as well as providing two spacious lecture theatres and a medical library. The Microbiology Building, funded by a large grant from the Poliomyelitis Society and perhaps the most architecturally distinguished post-war building on the site, was designed by Sir Hugh Casson, and opened in 1964. In 1966 the hospital bacteriology and biochemistry laboratories moved into 'temporary' accommodation in wooden huts; they were only moved into buildings of bricks and mortar twenty-eight years later.

Increasing pressure on hospital accommodation was felt particularly acutely in the area of radiology. The demand for x-rays was increasing and equipment was getting larger, yet there was no room for expansion in the King Edward Building. Moreover, it was relatively remote from the hospital corridor. A new block was therefore started in 1961, situated where the old EENT wards and theatres had been, and completed in 1964. Radiology was on the ground floor and now had adequate space not only for taking x-rays but also for developing films, reporting, typing, et cetera. Shortly afterwards, in 1966, work began on a new School of Radiography where the Department of Dentistry had been housed in the King Edward Building.

On the first floor of the new block were four spacious operating theatres and a recovery ward, and on the second floor were changing rooms, workshops, et cetera. These catered for the four surgical units 9–10, 11–12, 13–14 and 15–16, leaving 17–18 (orthopaedics) unchanged and likewise 19–20, which already had a larger-than-average operating theatre. When this Main Theatre Block opened in 1964 the benefits of the change were immense: quiet, dedicated space for induction of anaesthesia, large theatres, rooms for scrubbing up, laying out of trolleys and cleaning of instruments and, what was relatively advanced at the time, a large recovery room with a one-to-one nurse–patient ratio. Changing into theatre clothes was no longer an optional luxury to be carried out in cramped space under the extern waiting-hall. Instead it became compulsory, and adequate changing rooms and a coffee room were provided on the top floor. One theatre, used by the Professor of Surgery, even had an observation dome and intercom arrangements for teaching students (soon to be abandoned as too remote!).

It was not all gain, however, and whereas in the old theatres a nurse or medical student could push a patient the short distance from the ward down to theatre, now special portering and nursing arrangements were required, with all the risks of patient mix-up (fortunately very rare!). Time was certainly lost in the changeover of patients, and the new arrangements only worked because more nursing and portering staff were made available – as was typical of this less cost-conscious era. Nevertheless, the gains far outweighed the losses, and the extra space enabled new techniques such as open-heart surgery, in particular, to be introduced and carried out for many years without significant need for alterations.

Once the four theatres on the corridor had been abandoned, yet another refurbishment of the old wards took place, providing much-needed office and teaching space. The continually criticised toilet–sluice area was again upgraded, an improvement later extended to all the wards.

The Royal Victoria Hospital Act, passed by the Parliament of Northern Ireland in 1947, had amalgamated the Ophthalmic Hospital, the Benn EENT Hospital and the EENT department of the Royal Victoria Hospital, and referred to the need for a single larger and better-equipped hospital for Belfast for this whole field. A committee was set up in 1949 to plan a new joint hospital, but again with pressure from other projects only in 1953 was a decision made regarding the exact site, that chosen being between Bostock House and the Outpatient Clinic. Indeed the first two committee chairmen, Sir Milne Barbour and Dr William Anderson, died (in 1951 and 1956 respectively) before the plans were finalised and G. Lennox Cotton, followed by John E. Sayers, took over. Delays resulted from indecision regarding a site, fears of a third world war and general shortage of funds, but pressure finally came from the demolition of the old EENT wards on the Royal Victoria Hospital corridor in 1960. Foundations were laid in that year and the building opened in 1965. It consists of seven floors above the basement: the ground floor is for offices, patient reception, et cetera, and above this are five floors of wards (wards 27–31, for ENT and ophthalmology, designed to accommodate about 150 patients, both adults and children), and an operating theatre floor. The first of the ward floors

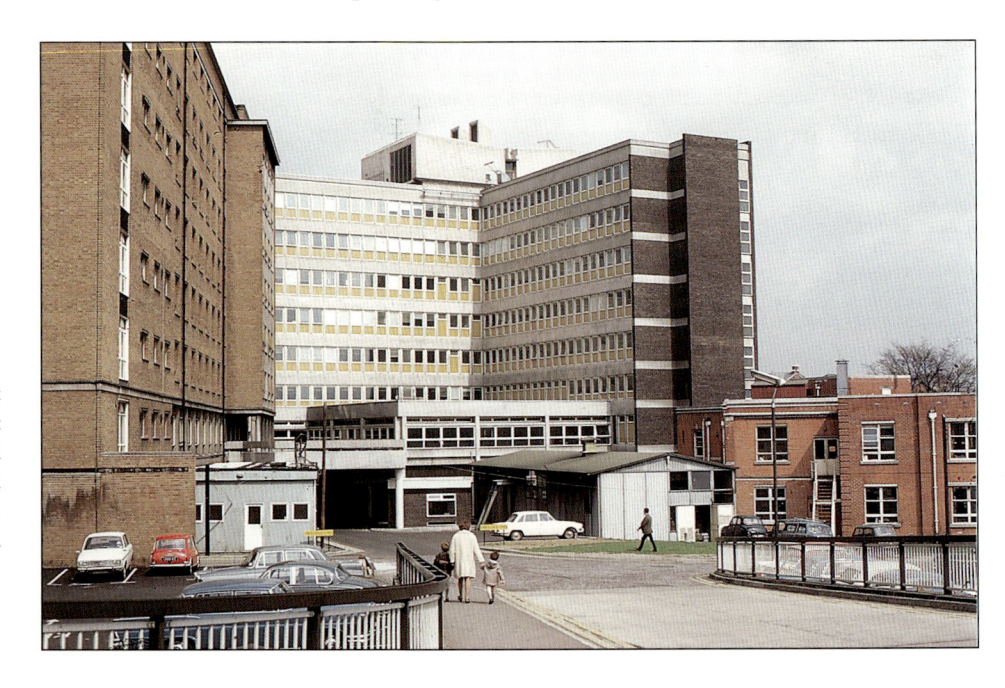

Eye, Ear, Nose and Throat Hospital (*left*), Outpatient Building with Accident and Emergency entrance (*centre*) and Quin House (*right*) in 1971
ROYAL VICTORIA HOSPITAL

has dedicatory plaques to Dr Samuel Browne and Sir John Walton Browne; on the floor above there is a plaque to Mr Edward Benn, founder of the Benn EENT Hospital. The building is severe externally but contains only single-bed, and four- and six-bed wards, with a considerable attempt in the internal decor to make surroundings attractive to the patients.

These hospital buildings were followed, as a joint enterprise, by the new Dental Hospital and Dental School. It had long been needed, and pressure was on from the appointment of Professor Stoy in 1947, as the old department in the King Edward Building was becoming increasingly cramped. A site was identified in 1953 but with pressure of all the other developments, work did not begin until 1963 and the new building was only opened in 1965. It consists of four floors housing the various subspecialities above a basement and for many years it appeared spacious, though eventually pressure to expand the Dental School necessitated an extension in 1993.

Soon after Bostock House was completed it became evident that a much larger amount of independent accommodation was required for staff wishing to live close to the hospital. The Broadway Housing Association was therefore formed in 1964 to fund the building of blocks of flats specifically for such staff – largely, trained nurses. The first twelve-storey apartment block, known as Broadway Tower, was opened in 1966 on an old allotment area on the west side of Broadway. It was followed by Victoria Tower in 1969 and a smaller block (Biggart House) of single rooms for medical students and short-term junior doctors in 1971. The three blocks on this site were sold to the Ministry of Health and Social Services in 1972 but continued in their original role. A further block, named Grosvenor Tower, was opened in 1979.

All the major new building projects on the site naturally made heavy demands of the existing heating system, and a new boiler house and chimney were built in the Broadway area; they opened in 1969. At about the same time, plans for the Belfast urban motorway (the Westlink) which was to run along the southern edge of the site, beside the Blackstaff River, necessitated redeployment of administrative and maintenance services. The administration moved into the King Edward Building, the School of Physiotherapy moved into the Broadway area, and new maintenance workshops constructed beside the boiler house opened in 1972.

The construction of the new Outpatient Building went on from 1965 to 1969, but the formal opening and naming by Mr Austen Boyd did not take place until 1971. It was an ambitious project including the photographic department on Level 9, all the hospital outpatient clinics on Levels 5 to 9, medical records on Level 4, physiotherapy and the

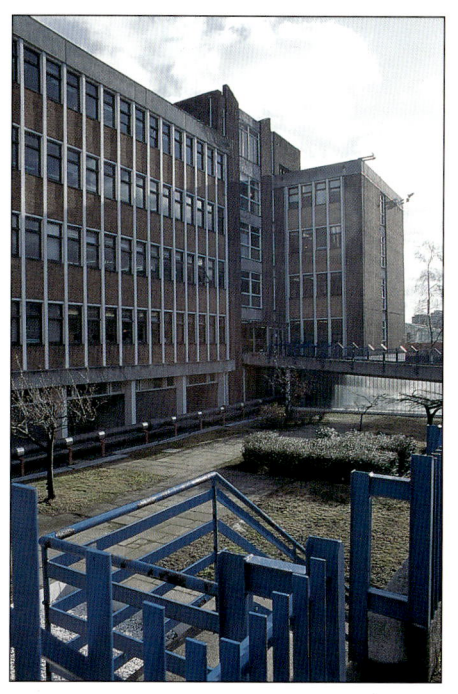

The Dental Hospital, which opened in 1965
ROYAL VICTORIA HOSPITAL

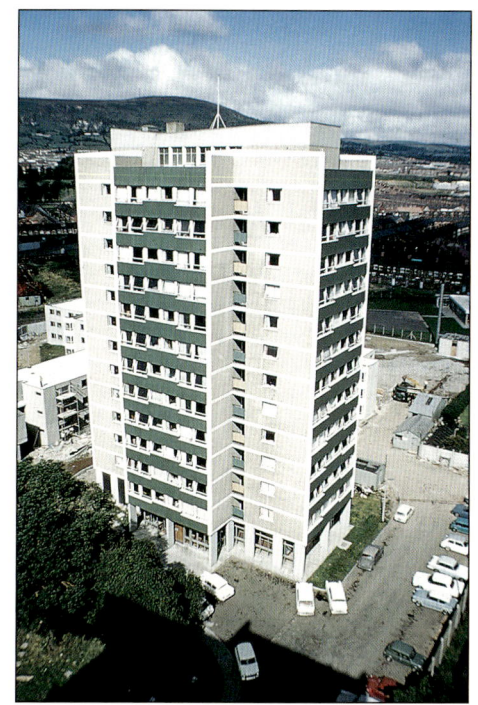

Broadway Tower, the first of the apartment blocks, was opened in 1966, to provide accommodation mainly for trained nurses.
ROYAL VICTORIA HOSPITAL

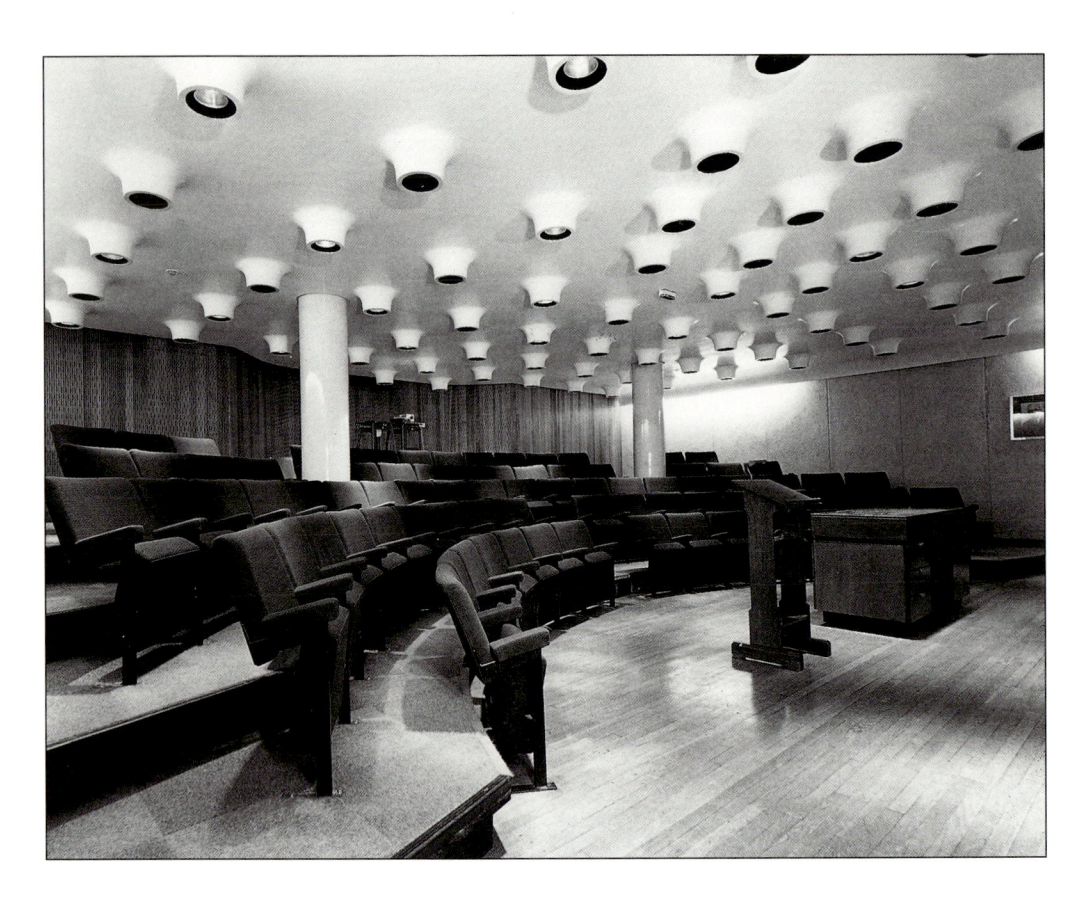

The Sir Samuel Irwin Lecture Theatre in the basement of the Outpatient Building, used for small professional meetings
ROYAL VICTORIA HOSPITAL

A Block (*left*), built 1971–75, with the fire escape and clock tower that were added in the mid-1980s
ROYAL VICTORIA HOSPITAL

swimming pool on Level 3, accident and emergency and orthopaedics on Level 2 (ground floor), together with the Sir Samuel Irwin Lecture Theatre and various services in the basement. The ventilation of the building was unsound, however, and by 1990 it had been decided that major work would be needed to maintain it in working order.

Planning for the main clinical facilities in the sixties envisaged an A Block for various regional surgical specialties, a 'link' block for neuroradiology and intensive care, eventually a B Block for other wards, and indeed many further blocks. The completion of the Outpatient Building was therefore immediately followed by the two-storey link block in 1970. Neuroradiology had formerly been squeezed into space beside the neurosurgical theatres in Quin House, and was now moved to be nearer the planned neurosurgical facilities of the A Block. Intensive care had been in 'grace-and-favour' accommodation in Ward 22 of Quin House, but now had a 12-bed unit with a bedroom for the doctor, laboratory, workshop, rest room and offices (Ward 32). Its proximity to the accident and emergency department of the Outpatient Building and the forthcoming A Block was to prove invaluable during the long years of the Troubles.

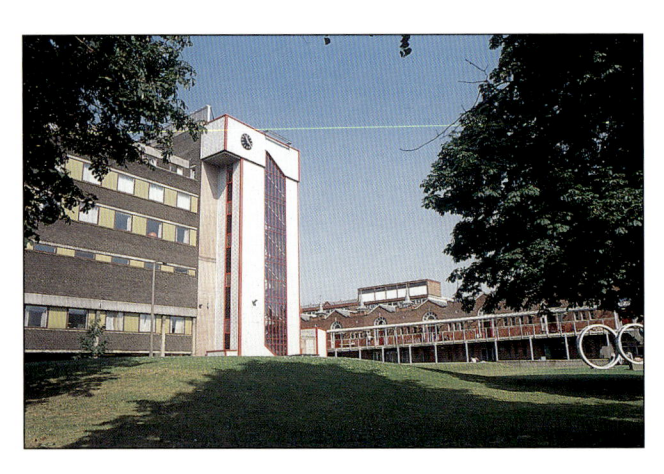

Construction work on the A Block started in 1971 and was completed in 1975. Its plan was straightforward, with a private wing (wards 43 and 44) on Level 6, fracture wards on Level 5 (wards 41 and 42, 60 beds), neurosurgical wards on Level 4 (wards 39 and 40, 40 beds), six operating theatres on Level 3, a night admission unit (Ward 37, 28 beds) and burns unit (Ward 38, 14 beds – not opened until 1979), on Level 2, and a sterile supplies department (CSSD) and plant room on Level 1. The building was to accommodate approximately 142 NHS patients in six-, four- and single-bed rooms. The additional private accommodation of 38 rooms, named the Heron Clinic in recognition of a bequest of £132,000 from Francis Adams Heron, proved to be too large with the opening of the Ulster Independent Clinic on the Stranmillis Road, and half has regularly been used for overflow of patients from the cardiac wards. The operating theatre suite consisted of the six individual theatres plus a plaster room, recovery room, et cetera; it has always proved rather cramped compared with the spacious accommodation of the main theatre block.

Simultaneously work was going on near Musson House for a new geriatric unit to serve north and west Belfast. It was opened in 1971 with four wards of 36 beds each. Wards 33 and 34 were named Florence Elliott House after the former Matron (1946–66), and wards 35 and 36 were named Catherine Dynes House after the former Night Sister (1909–53). These wards from the outset had an emphasis on rehabilitation and were well provided with their own physiotherapy and occupational therapy departments, and some limited garden space including a bowling green.

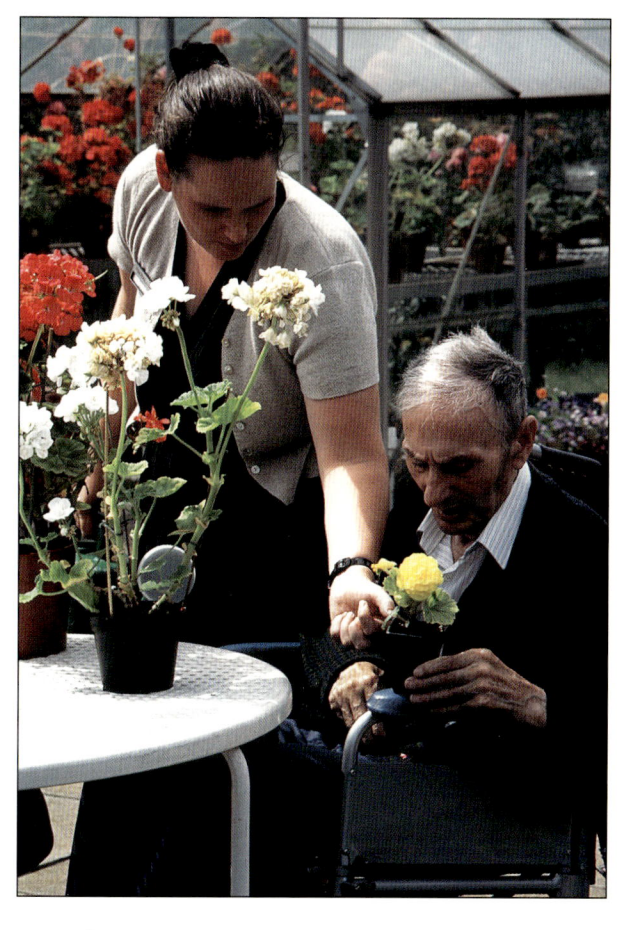

Activity nurse Rae Doherty with one of her patients in the conservatory of the geriatric ward, 1996
ROYAL VICTORIA HOSPITAL

THE MEDICAL STAFF COMMITTEE AND MEDICAL ADMINISTRATION

Following the National Health Service changes, the Medical Staff Committee of the Royal Victoria Hospital continued to meet essentially as before. It consisted only of the former Attending staff (amounting to about thirty in number) and replacements, plus a few new Consultants of distinction with beds in the corridor wards (for example, Professors) but not the so-called auxiliary or dental staff even though they were graded as Consultants by the Northern Ireland Hospitals Authority. The number of medical staff styled 'consultants' and of specialist doctors and dentists grew steadily after 1948, but the proportion having a voice on the Medical Staff Committee actually fell. This was already a problem by 1950, but by 1961 the total Consultant staff numbered 119, of whom only 49 were members of the staff, as the committee was known; the remainder were other Consultants (42), senior hospital medical officers (13) and dentists (15).

The largest block of the 'other consultants' consisted of 10 anaesthetists, and all these groups were getting more and more restless at their lack of representation. In 1962 the committee chairman, Mr J.R. Wheeler, expressed the feeling that if the staff did not 'put their own house in order it might be done for them at a higher level'. The issue of enlarging the staff was strongly contested and the decision to open up the staff to all who provided specialist services on the site was carried by 25 votes to 10. The effect of this decision was to decrease the influence of physicians and general surgeons and to increase the say of EENT surgeons, gynaecologists, various diagnostic groups and a large block of anaesthetists. The large body of dentists was not added to the Medical Staff Committee until 1983.

A feature of the medical staff as individuals (noted by John Dundee in his paper 'The last of the fifty – a time of change' [1986]) has been the number of father-and-son groups. He suggests that this reflected family traditions in medicine rather than family cliques, and it is much less obvious today than in the 1940s, for example. The great majority of hospital Consultants in the first half of the twentieth century had been born in Northern Ireland, reflecting some degree of political isolation of the area. The university in the 1950s made a strong move to appoint professors from Britain, and soon five of the main clinical chairs were held by Englishmen (and there was Professor Graham Bull – see page 153 – who came, via England, from South Africa); all of the professors were, of course, on the Medical Staff Committee. Many of them did not remain long, however. Moreover, once the Troubles began in 1968, it became very difficult to attract outside graduates to any posts, and there has been a gradual swing back to recruitment of more locally born staff. It should be said that even when locally born graduates have been appointed to chairs and Consultant posts, they have always done at least some of their training outside Northern Ireland.

GENERAL MEDICINE

Undoubtedly the great changes we have seen in general medicine since the middle of the twentieth century have been pharmacological. A look at the British Pharmaceutical Codex (BPC) for 1949 reveals many substances that Sir William Whitla would have recognised. Typical of the host of laxatives in regular use was the fruit of the cassia plant; it was abandoned soon after this, leaving the senna pod as the only botanical laxative now in use. Substances such as chloroform, chrysarobin (an anti-fungal) and cinchona have all been replaced by better alternatives. However it is from the introduction of antibiotics that the revolutionary changes have followed. Penicillin was in the BPC in 1949, and indeed doctors in the Royal Victoria Hospital had been involved in clinical trials in 1945–46, but streptomycin was still under trial at this time. The effectiveness of the antibiotics era has been helped by the steady stream of new drugs introduced as strains of bacteria developed resistance to the older agents.

The second big group of drugs that emerged was the beta blockers which act on some of the receptors in the nervous system to control hypertension. Their discovery was the work of James Black (later Sir) while working with the chemicals giant ICI; propranolol, the first of the group, was introduced into clinical use in the mid-1960s. The potent diuretic frusemide, which contributed much to the management of cardiac failure, came in at about the same time. Other groups of cardiac drugs have followed, but they have represented improvements rather than fundamental changes in the management of hypertension and heart failure.

The drugs based on endocrine hormones or modifications of them were introduced in the 1950s. Before this time there had been preparations of the adrenal cortex for the treatment of Addison's disease, and of the posterior pituitary for diabetes insipidus. However, the 1950s saw the introduction of a host of steroids which changed the prognosis of rheumatic diseases, asthma and major allergic problems. Inevitably there was delay in appreciating their true place and limitations, and these preparations were misused, but they still represent one of the great advances of the second half of the twentieth century.

The final group worth highlighting is the so-called H_2 blockers, that is, drugs acting to block the nerve endings responsible for the secretion of hydrochloric acid in the stomach. These drugs have reduced the number of patients with gastric and duodenal ulcer to a mere trickle and, since hospitalisation is now rarely necessary, have removed a large group of patients from both medical and surgical wards. Interestingly the role of these drugs also was demonstrated by Sir James Black. His contribution to medical research has since been recognised by an honorary MD from Queen's University Belfast.

GENERAL PHYSICIANS

In 1947 many of the doctors who had served in the armed forces during the recently ended war joined the Royal Victoria Hospital as registrars under the Government Rehabilitation Scheme. These included Dr J.M. Beare, Dr G. Gregg, Dr J.S. Logan, Dr J.H.D. Millar, Dr D.A.D. Montgomery and Dr J.F. Pantridge, who all subsequently became Consultant Physicians at the hospital; Mr J.A.W. Bingham, Mr W.S. Braidwood, Mr N.C. Hughes, Mr V.A.F. Martin, Mr E. Morrison, Mr T.B. Smiley, Mr H.M. Stevenson and Mr R.I. Wilson, who subsequently became Consultant Surgeons; and Dr J.F. Bereen who became a Neurosurgical Anaesthetist.

The post-1945 era saw the break-up of general medicine into many subdivisions. For convenience they will be discussed separately here, even though, for instance, cardiologists were not regarded as a separate type of physician for many years.

One of the first NHS appointments in 1948 was that of Dr George Gregg as physician in charge of the new Department of Physiotherapy. He had qualified with an MB at Queen's University Belfast in 1938 and after his houseman's year joined the RAMC. For his services he was awarded the Belgian Croix de Guerre and was a Chevalier of the Order of Leopold II. After the war he obtained the MD in 1946 and trained in Physical Medicine at Guy's Hospital, London. He remained associated with the Territorial Army medical units in Northern Ireland for the rest of his life, being awarded the OBE and TD. Although he never was given inpatient beds, he contributed greatly to the hospital by his energy and enthusiasm for his department, and he gave a memorable winter oration in 1963 on 'The state of medicine at the time of the Crusades'. He retired in 1977.

Dr William Lennon was a part-time clinical assistant physician in the Royal Victoria Hospital in the 1930s; he served in the RNVR during World War Two and was Consultant Rheumatologist in the hospital from 1948 (with a rheumatic clinic in the Royal Victoria Hospital and beds in the Throne Hospital) until his retirement in 1966.

Tuberculosis was still a killing disease in 1948, even though the death rate had fallen from 300 per 100,000 population in 1906 to 80 per 100,000 in 1946. The Northern Ireland Tuberculosis Authority had been set up in 1946 and one of the essentials was to establish diagnostic chest clinics to identify early cases. Some of these were run by the authority but one was set up in the Royal Victoria Hospital in 1948, attended by Dr Brice R. Clarke MC, who was Director of Tuberculosis Services in the authority and Consultant Chest Physician at Musgrave Park Hospital. Because of the success of the anti-tuberculous drugs the authority was wound up in 1959; Dr Clarke was awarded the CBE, before retiring in 1961. The Tuberculosis Authority's chest physicians also saw inpatients with tuberculosis, on request. Other Consultant Physicians attended the clinic throughout the 1950s and 1960s, particularly Dr Charles Campbell, who was appointed to the Medical Staff Committee in 1962 when it was enlarged; he retired in 1977. Dr Campbell was followed as a respiratory physician by Dr C.F. Stanford.

Dr John Logan graduated at Queen's University Belfast in 1939, served in the RAMC, obtained his MD in 1946 and MRCP in 1947, and was appointed Consultant Physician to the hospital in 1951. He is the son and grandson of general practitioners and himself the father of two physicians. He gave the annual winter oration in 1973. His main interest has always been in the field of gastroenterology and occupational diseases of all kinds, but when he retired in 1982 he took on the role of honorary hospital Archivist, which he held until 1993. His wife Mary was a niece of Sir Samuel Irwin.

Sir William Thomson retired and died in 1950 but was not replaced as Professor of Medicine until Dr Graham MacGregor Bull was appointed in 1952. Professor Bull's was certainly a revolutionary appointment for he was not only an outsider but had graduated with an MB as far away as Cape Town in 1939. He was an active research worker, having obtained his MD in Cape Town in 1946 and worked from 1947 to 1952 at the Postgraduate Medical School at Hammersmith Hospital, London. He was a world authority on renal failure and as the first full-time physician and professor, receiving a salary and not needing to keep up a private practice, he continued to advance this field in Belfast. He resigned in 1966 to become Director of the Medical Research Council Unit for Clinical Research at Northwick Park Hospital, London.

In 1954 Dr Thomas Terence Fulton was appointed consultant physician. He was the son of Dr Thomas Fulton of Great Victoria Street, Belfast, and graduated with an MD with honours in Cincinatti, and subsequently at Queen's University with an MB with honours in 1945. As a postgraduate he trained in the RAF, in Hammersmith and Belfast, taking his MD (QUB) in 1951. He was Consultant Physician in the Banbridge, Dromore and South Armagh Group of hospitals, 1951–54. His major interest has been in liver disease and its management, on which he published many studies in conjunction with his surgeon and pathologist colleagues. He gave the winter oration on 'The making of a doctor' in 1979, was chairman of the Medical Staff Committee, 1981–83, and retired in 1986, to be awarded the OBE. Having a deep interest in art in general, he gave a presidential address to the Ulster Medical Society entitled 'Through the artist's eyes' (1982).

Another physician of this era was Dr John Andrew Weaver, who had served with the Gurkha Parachute Regiment in the Far East for four years during World War Two. He then studied medicine at Queen's University Belfast, graduating with an MB in 1950 and with an MD in 1954. He was the first Royal Victoria Hospital Research Fellow in 1955; subsequently he had a travelling fellowship to Baltimore before being appointed Consultant Physician to the Royal Victoria Hospital staff in 1959. While in the Royal Victoria Hospital he took a special interest in endocrinology and diabetes, but throughout his working life he has always remained a general physician of wide interests. He gave the 1983 annual winter oration.

Dr Richard Arthur Womersley, who came to Belfast in 1953 as a lecturer with Professor Graham Bull, became senior lecturer and Consultant Physician in the Royal Victoria Hospital in 1954. He was a graduate of Cambridge, and had worked in the Middlesex Hospital and Yale Medical School. His major interest throughout his career was in general medicine with special emphasis on electrolyte imbalance, and he started the lipid clinic. In the latter part of his career he had a major road

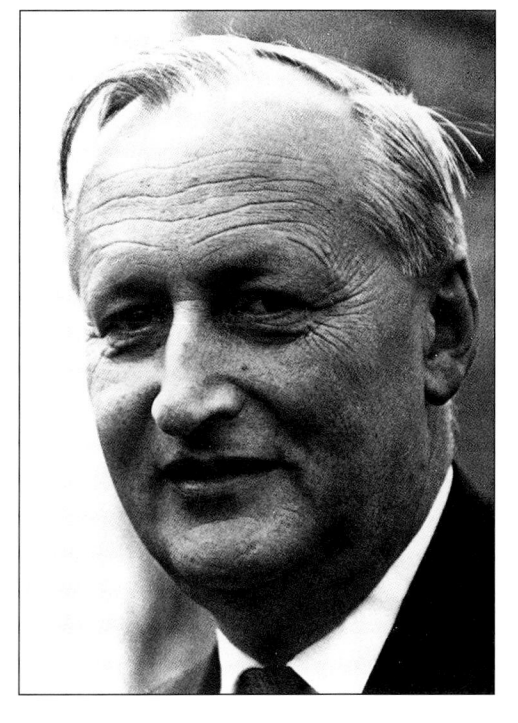

Professor Graham MacGregor Bull, Professor of Medicine at Queen's University Belfast, 1952–66, and a leader in the field of renal medicine
ROYAL VICTORIA HOSPITAL

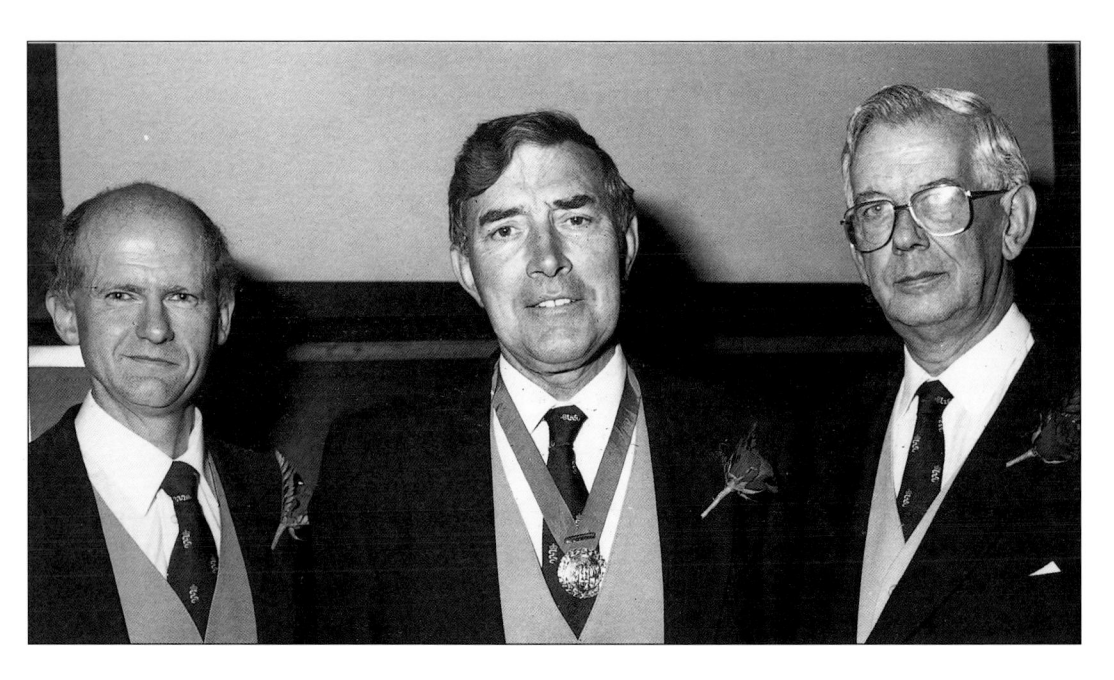

Left to right: Dr Norman Campbell, secretary of the Medical Staff, Professor John Bridges, chairman of the Medical Staff, and Dr Teddy McIlrath, pictured after Dr McIlrath had given the annual winter oration in 1992
ROYAL VICTORIA HOSPITAL

accident, and he moved into medical administration before retiring in 1984.

Dr Andrew Henry Garmany (Gary) Love worked in the university departments of both Physiology and Medicine before being appointed Consultant Physician in the Royal Victoria Hospital in 1963. He was appointed to a personal chair in Gastroenterology in 1973 and to the chair of Medicine in 1983. He has also been dean of the Faculty of Medicine, 1981–86, and he gave the 1988 annual winter oration.

Professor John Vallance-Owen was appointed to the chair of Medicine and Consultant Physician in 1966. Like his predecessor G.M. Bull he was not a Belfast graduate (MB Cambridge 1946; MD 1951); he had trained in the Hammersmith Hospital and Philadelphia, and had been a Consultant Physician and lecturer in Durham (1958–64) and Consultant Physician and reader in Newcastle upon Tyne (1964–66). His major interest was in diabetes. He resigned at the end of 1982 to take up the chair of Medicine in the Chinese University of Hong Kong (1983–87) and retired in 1988 to live near Cambridge.

In 1966 Dr Stanley Desmond Roberts was appointed Consultant Physician to the Royal Victoria and Musgrave Park hospitals with a special interest in rheumatology. A graduate of Queen's University, he was a research fellow at the MRC Research Unit in Taplow, Buckinghamshire, from 1964 to 1966 and was president of the Royal College of Physicians of Ireland from 1994 to 1997. He gave the annual winter oration in 1994 and in 1997 he was awarded the OBE.

Dr Keith Deans Buchanan, a Glasgow graduate, joined the Royal Victoria Hospital in 1969 as senior lecturer and Consultant Physician, with an interest in diabetes and gastrointestinal hormones. He has remained heavily involved in the academic research field ever since, and was appointed to a personal chair in Metabolic Medicine in 1976.

From this period onwards the physicians appointed with a main involvement in this hospital have been the following: Dr Kenneth Irvine, physical medicine, Consultant (1968–88); Dr Thomas Ryan, geriatrics, Consultant (1969–82); Dr C.F. (Fred) Stanford, respiratory diseases, Consultant, 1978 until he resigned in 1990 to take up a post in Saudi Arabia; Dr Michael E. Callender, gastroenterology, Consultant (1982–); Dr David McCluskey, clinical immunology, Consultant (1984–); Dr D. Paul Nicholls, heart disease, Consultant (1984–); Dr Timothy R.O. Beringer, geriatrics, consultant (1985–); Dr Patrick Bell, metabolic diseases, Consultant (1986–); Dr Brendan Collins, gastroenterology, Consultant and senior lecturer (1987–90), when he resigned to take up a post in Perth, Australia; Dr John S.A. Collins, gastroenterology, Consultant (1990–); Dr Robert Watson, internal medicine, Consultant (1991–).

DERMATOLOGY

As in medicine generally, the great advances in dermatology have been connected with new drugs. The first group, the steroids, has been mentioned already (see page 151); the advent of topical steroid ointments in the 1950s provided an anti-inflammatory remedy for a variety of skin diseases which also avoided the mess and odour of tar-based ointments.

The other great advance in treatment was in the anti-fungal preparations; this is particularly associated in Belfast with the work of Dr John Martin Beare, who graduated with an MB with first place and honours at Queen's University Belfast in 1942 and with an MD in 1946 and was appointed Consultant Dermatologist at the Royal Victoria Hospital in 1953. He published widely on skin diseases of all types, but it was on fungal infections of children and adults that he was a world authority. He saw the introduction of griseofulvin in the 1960s, which quickly pushed out the much more dangerous radiotherapy in treatment of diseases such as ringworm. Dr Beare gave the annual winter oration in 1977 on 'Industrial dermatitis and the law in Northern Ireland' and retired in 1985. Another Queen's graduate, Dr David Desmond Burrows, was Consultant Dermatologist from 1961 until his retirement in 1995. He gave the 1987 annual winter oration. Like his colleague he had a wide interest in all types of skin problems and published copiously, but his special field was in contact dermatitis caused by such substances as nickel, chromium, mercury and rubber.

The next appointment in dermatology was that of Dr Roger (Rory) Corbett in 1978 as Consultant and senior lecturer; his work was divided between the Royal Victoria and Belfast City hospitals. When Dr Martin Beare retired in 1985 he was replaced by Dr Ann Bingham.

After Dr Ivan McCaw (see page 103) died in 1961 his colleagues decided to endow a prize in his name, and this was awarded over the years

1972–76. In 1975 Dr Maureen E.M. Taylor, a well-loved trainee dermatologist, died suddenly in Chicago and her family contributed to a prize to commemorate her name. This incorporates the earlier McCaw Prize and has been awarded every year since 1977.

CARDIOLOGY

Until 1954 when Dr Marshall and Dr Campbell retired, there were two senior physicians specialising in cardiology and while they required special equipment, notably the ECG and x-ray screening equipment, they remained general physicians. Increasingly, however, wards 5 and 6 were seen as wards with special expertise in this field, and a coronary care unit was set up in 1963. The emphasis overall was on disease of the heart, rheumatic and later coronary arterial, rather than the whole sweep of cardiovascular medicine. The objection to this specialisation arose not from any concept of the desirability of having broadly experienced physicians, but from the need to have four general medical wards taking in emergencies in rotation; this practice persisted into the 1980s.

The moving force pushing specialisation forward was Dr James Francis (Frank) Pantridge. Born near Hillsborough, County Down, he graduated with an MB at Queen's University Belfast in 1939, and within three months had volunteered for the RAMC along with ten of his colleagues. Almost immediately he was sent out to Singapore and like so many was captured with its fall in February 1942. His period in Japanese prisoner-of-war camps was etched in his memory; he was awarded the Military Cross and survived to return to his medical career in 1946, obtaining the MD in the same year. After taking his MRCP in London (1947) he spent a year at Ann Arbor University, Michigan, then returned to Belfast as a committed cardiologist.

He was appointed Consultant Physician to outpatients in 1951 with six beds in wards 5 and 6, working with Dr Marshall, and when the latter retired, Pantridge became the main cardiologist in the hospital, though sharing these wards with Dr Smyth and Dr Weaver. From the outset he was involved in investigation of the function of the heart by cardiac catheterisation, mitral valvotomy (see page 196) and (later) open-heart surgery. His main interest gradually became the electrocardiograph and coronary artery disease, however, and this culminated in his advocacy of pre-hospital coronary care (the cardiac ambulance) and the Pantridge defibrillator (1965). He was awarded the CBE in 1979 and retired in 1982. He was a pioneer and an enthusiast and inevitably met with much resistance. In addition he did not suffer fools (or those he considered to be fools) gladly and fell out with many of his colleagues, but he laid the foundations of specialist cardiology in Belfast and influenced treatment all over the world. His life is entertainingly described with much outspoken

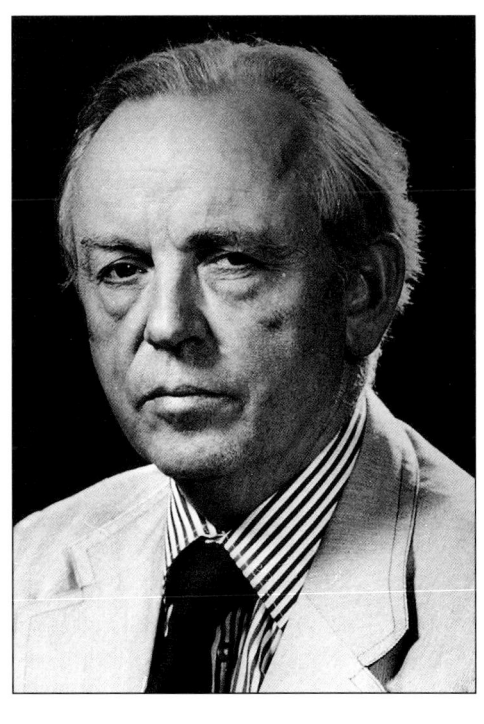

Professor James Francis Pantridge, Consultant Cardiologist, 1951–82, and an enthusiastic advocate of the cardiac ambulance and pre-hospital coronary care
ROYAL VICTORIA HOSPITAL

comment in his autobiography *An Unquiet Life* (1989).

The mainstay of the cardiac catheterisation unit from the 1950s was Dr George Charles Patterson, who was appointed Consultant Physician in 1969. He had a physiological training and took over the diagnostic aspects of heart disease in the unit, successively introducing improvements in blood gas analysis, contrast injection, rapid sequence radiography and cine-radiography and coronary artery angiography (see page 162). He retired in 1991.

A succession of cardiologists have worked in the hospital, the first additional Consultant being Dr Dennis Boyle, who was appointed in 1965 and worked also in the Ulster Hospital. He was followed in 1971 by Dr Jennifer Adgey (who was appointed to a personal chair in Cardiology in 1993); also in 1971 by Dr John Stafford Geddes (the son of the anaesthetist Dr Stafford Geddes, see page 125); in 1976 by Dr Connor Mulholland (who had a major interest in paediatric cardiology); in 1978 by Dr Samuel Webb; in 1979 by Dr Norman Campbell; and in 1982 (following the retirement of Professor Pantridge) by Dr Mazhar Muhammad Khan. Following Professor Pantridge's retirement, cardiologists at the hospital held differing views on automatic external defibrillators and the administration of the medical cardiology unit, and although Dr Geddes resigned in 1987, this was a period of very rapid growth which corresponded with increasing development in the out-of-hospital resuscitation and management of patients with heart attacks.

This period of growth corresponded with the introduction of the cardiac ambulance. The implanted cardiac pacemaker had been introduced

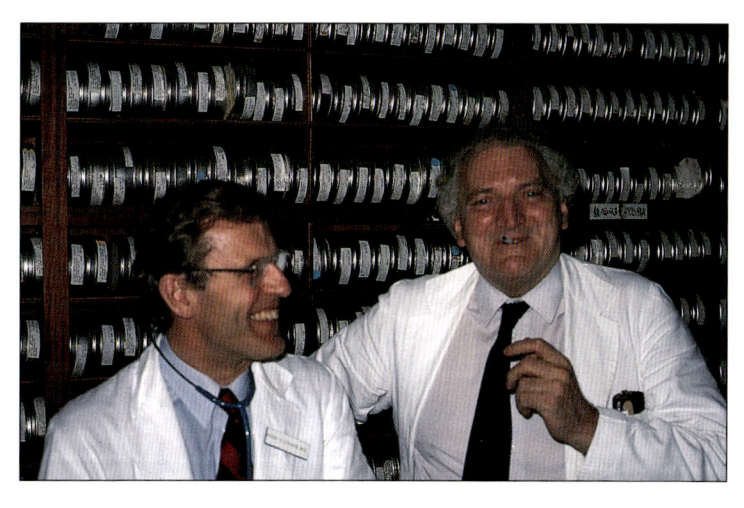

Dr George Patterson (*left*), Cardiologist, and Mr Hugh O'Kane, Cardiac Surgeon, in the angiogram store, 1989
ROYAL VICTORIA HOSPITAL

Below:
Coronary angiogram with radio-contrast medium outlining the coronary arteries in a patient with angina. X-ray (*left*) shows a short area of narrowed artery and X-ray (*right*) the same area after dilation with a cutter and balloon catheter
DR M. KHAN AND ROYAL VICTORIA HOSPITAL

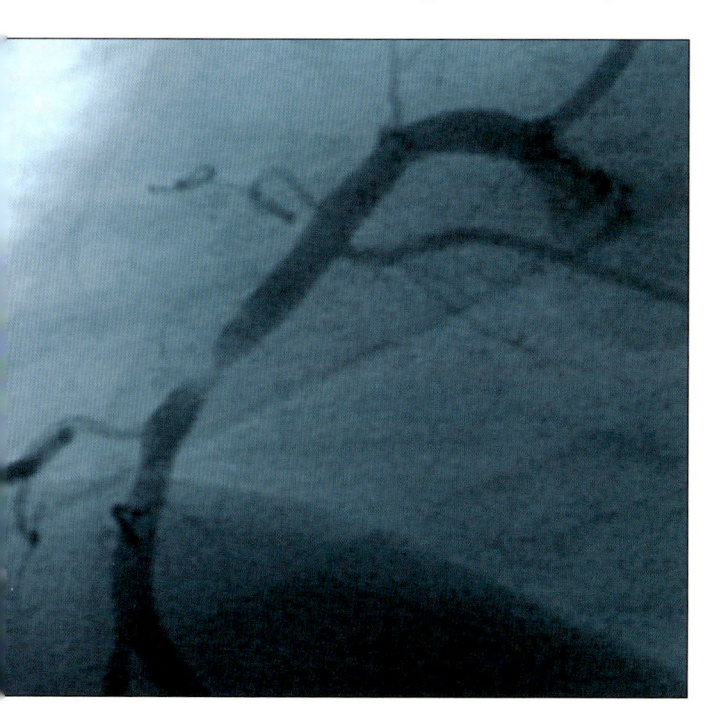

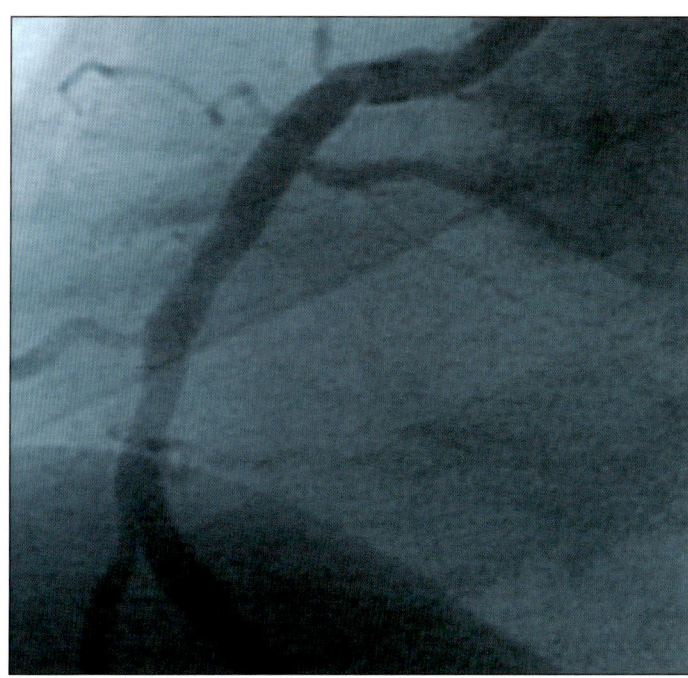

in the 1960s and its use for heart block continued to expand in the 1970s. Angiocardiography developed as a technique in the early 1970s but concerns about its hazards led to the Goodwin Report in 1974, and its development was slow.

Progress in the Royal Victoria Hospital had to await the Dugdale Report which advocated many more beds (132 altogether) on the main corridor for medical cardiology, surgical cardiology and thoracic surgery. In order to increase capacity, overflow facilities were provided in the Musgrave and Clark Clinic, and in 1977 in part of the Heron Clinic (Ward 44), but the most satisfactory solution found was the use of wards 5 and 6 solely for medical cardiology and in 1981 the bringing of Ward 7 into the unit. This expansion was delayed by a shortage of trained nurses in the 1970s and 1980s which led to an increased waiting time for cardiac surgery (Chapter 6). A second angiocardiograph theatre was opened to speed up the investigation of the surgical patients and the number of cardiac catheterisations had reached 1,000 per year by 1983.

This resulted partly from the introduction of coronary angioplasty in 1982 as a method of opening up the channel in the arteries without surgery. Since then, as the capacity for undertaking coronary arterial surgery has increased, so the medical investigative side has continued to expand.

METABOLIC MEDICINE

The speciality of metabolic medicine, in the Royal Victoria Hospital at least, may be said to have developed from the work of Dr J.A. Smyth (see page 132). He was appointed in 1924, at about the time that treatment of diabetes became an effective reality, and he wrote a paper on 'The Royal Hospital experience with insulin' as early as 1923/24. He was also treating thyrotoxicosis in the 1930s, and his responsibility covered the laboratory and the whole field of laboratory medicine. His retirement in 1958 came just after the opening of the specialist metabolic unit in 1957.

Dr Desmond A.D. Montgomery was appointed Consultant Physician with an interest in endocrine diseases in 1951. He had graduated with an MB at Queen's in 1940, served in the RAMC in India and had done postgraduate training in Hammersmith Hospital, obtaining his MD with gold medal in 1946. By this time the number of endocrine diseases that could be treated had expanded greatly to include phaeochromocytoma (tumour of the adrenal medulla), Cushing's syndrome, Addison's disease, and insulinomas; a more precise management of endocrine disease in pregnancy was also possible. His work culminated in the writing, with Professor R.B. Welbourn, of *Clinical Endocrinology for Surgeons*, published in 1963; several foreign editions were to follow. Dr

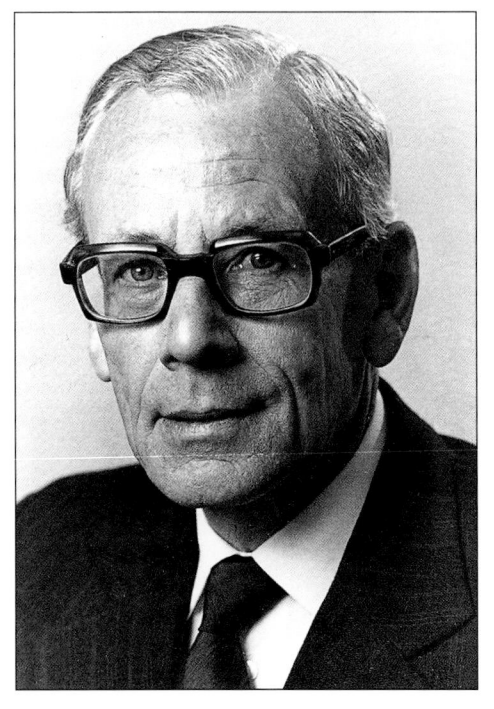

Professor Desmond Montgomery, Consultant Physician in Charge of the metabolic unit, 1958–79
ROYAL VICTORIA HOSPITAL

Montgomery was made Physician in Charge of the metabolic unit in 1958, gave the annual winter oration in 1972, was given a personal chair in 1975, and retired in 1979 with the CBE. He continued to chair both the Northern Ireland Council for Postgraduate Medical Education and the Northern Ireland Distinction Awards Committee until 1987.

Dr David R. Hadden was appointed Physician to the metabolic unit in 1967. He is married to Dr Diana Hadden, an accident and emergency specialist. His particular field has been diabetes, and indeed both in the metabolic unit and in the university Department of Medicine work on this disease has shown how simplistic the original 1920s concept of diabetes in fact was. He was appointed to a personal chair in Endocrinology in 1991 and in 1996 he gave the annual winter oration, entitling it 'Health and education: the metabolism of a teaching hospital'. Dr A. Brew Atkinson was appointed Consultant to the unit in 1980 and honorary Professor in the School of Clinical Medicine in 1993; he had a major interest in hypertension. Dr David Robert McCance was appointed Consultant in 1993.

VENEREOLOGY (GENITO-URINARY MEDICINE)

The outpatient clinic established in 1919 in the King Edward Building had not greatly changed by 1948; for most of that time it had been under the charge of Dr John Rankin and Dr Hugo Hall.

Dr John Sydney McCann graduated with an MB at Queen's University in 1936 and with an MD with gold medal in 1940. He was unable to serve in the armed forces during World War Two on medical grounds and took up the speciality of venereology in the Royal Victoria Hospital. Dr Frederick Bonugli (1913–67) graduated with an MB at Queen's University in 1937, served in the RAMC and graduated with an MD in 1946. He joined Dr McCann on the auxiliary outpatient staff of the Royal Victoria Hospital in 1947 and both were given consultant status in the hospital in 1948. Both published much on syphilis in the early years of their appointments, but with the decline in the incidence of both syphilis and gonorrhoea since the 1960s, the work of the speciality has changed to concentrate on other, more recently recognised bacterial and viral sexually transmitted diseases. Chlamydia is now seen to be a major cause of female infertility, and the department's work also includes investigation of the papilloma viruses which cause ano-genital warts and lower genital tract cancers, and HIV, the cause of AIDS.

Dr Bonugli died in mid-career in 1967 and Dr McCann was joined first by Dr John Mahony who was appointed Consultant in 1968 and resigned in 1972 and then by Dr Thomas Horner, who had first gone into general practice in Belfast, but in 1973 was appointed consultant in the Department of Venereology; he retired in 1993. Dr McCann retired in

1977 and the next appointment was Dr Raymond Maw, who was appointed Consultant in the unit in 1979. The most recent appointments have been those of Dr Wallace Dinsmore, who was appointed Consultant in what was now called the Department of Genito-Urinary Medicine in 1987, and Dr Michael McBride, who was appointed in 1994. In recent years the research profile of the department has been greatly raised; it has received major research grants and a much greater emphasis has been placed by staff on academic publication.

NEUROLOGY

The idea of neurology (and electroencephalography) as a separate department of the hospital dates from 1947 when Dr Sydney Allison returned from war service. At this time he was also a prime mover in pressing for a Neurosurgical Department, with the result that when wards 21 and 22 were enlarged in 1952, a valuable double unit was created. The Hospital for Diseases of the Nervous System, Paralysis and Epilepsy in Claremont Street had since its opening in 1896 served as a subacute hospital for neurology and Dr Allison and Dr Hilton Stewart were already on the Visiting staff before 1939. It had gradually become less suitable for acutely ill patients, and it was finally closed in 1985.

Dr Harold Millar joined the new department as Consultant in 1952. He had graduated with an MB at Queen's University in 1940 and an MD in 1946, served in the RNVR from 1914 to 1946 in minesweepers in the North Atlantic, destroyers in Arctic convoys, and finally in the Far East before returning to Belfast in 1947. His main academic interests were multiple sclerosis, on which he wrote a monograph (1971), and epilepsy; he was a prolific publisher in the field, and was made honorary reader in Neurology by Queen's University. He gave the 1975 annual winter oration. He was an enthusiastic and benign teacher and a caring and active supporter of patients in the community and of the neurological charities. He retired in 1982 and continued to live life to the full though disabled by chronic illness.

Dr Hilton Stewart was the son of A.W. Stewart, editor of the *Belfast Evening Telegraph*. He studied medicine at Queen's University, and after various posts in Belfast and Maida Vale, London, he returned to Belfast in 1929 as Assistant Physician at Claremont Street Hospital and the Ulster Hospital. He built up Claremont Street during the 1930s and fostered a major expansion in 1939 with the opening of departments of Radiology and Electroencephalography there, so that at its peak the hospital had sixty-one beds. He was appointed to a third Consultant post in neurology at the Royal Victoria Hospital in 1956, but died only five years later.

Dr Lewis Hurwitz was a brilliant and legendary figure in the

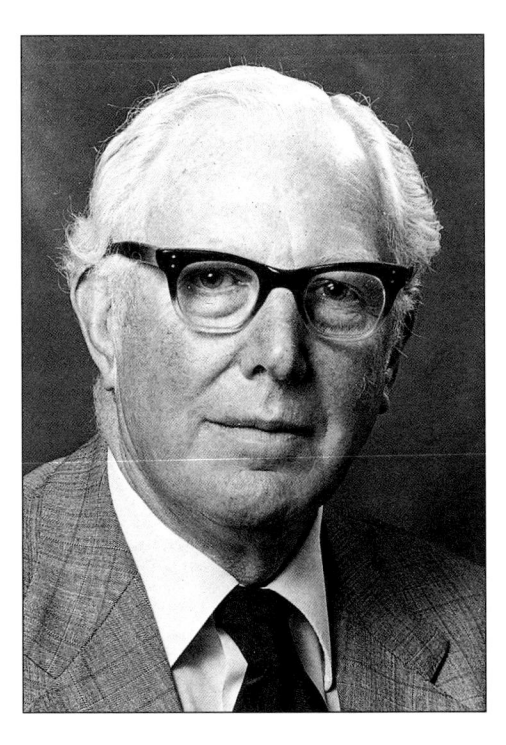

Dr Harold Millar, Consultant Neurologist, 1952–82
ROYAL VICTORIA HOSPITAL

Department of Neurology. He graduated with an MB at Queen's University in 1949 and immediately devoted himself to neurology, taking a B.Sc. (1952) and MD (1953) in pathology to further his specialism, and training in Liverpool, Bradford, the National Hospital, Queen Square, London, Bellevue Hospital in New York and La Salpêtrière in Paris. He was appointed Consultant Neurologist at the Royal Victoria Hospital as well as at Claremont Street and the Belfast City Hospital in 1962. The extent and depth of his work can be seen in the memorial volume of his papers edited by Michael Swallow (1975), which covers such topics as the mental processes in ageing, the mechanisms and treatment of Parkinson's disease, and the causes of various types of muscle paralysis.

Dr Michael William Swallow was born in London, studied medicine at King's College and the Westminster Hospital and graduated with an MB in 1952. He trained further at Queen Square and University College Hospital, London, before being appointed Consultant Neurologist at the Royal Victoria Hospital in 1964 on the retirement of Dr Sydney Allison. He had wide neurological interests, particularly in the fields of neurological disability, Parkinson's disease and rehabilitation; these, coupled with his skills as a musician, led to his involvement with music therapy. For instance, he promoted the first Share Music course in Northern Ireland in 1985 at a centre in County Fermanagh, which attracted both people with physical disabilities and a wide range of musicians and care workers. Similarly, he was one of the first to introduce the visual arts into the Royal Victoria Hospital, both as therapy for patients and to give pleasure to the staff. He has continued working in these fields even after he retired in 1989.

Dr J.A. (Joe) Lyttle was appointed Consultant Neurologist in 1970; he retired in 1996. Dr Bharat Bhushan Sawhney has been a Consultant from 1978 with a special interest in neurophysiology. Dr Stanley Hawkins was appointed as a Consultant in 1981. Dr John Mark Gibson, son of the first Professor of Mental Health at Queen's University and a graduate of Trinity College Dublin, became a Consultant in 1988. Dr Victor Patterson was appointed Consultant in 1984, and Dr James Morrow was made a Consultant in 1989.

Neurology has always been one of the more intellectual branches of medicine, with a strong emphasis on the esoteric diagnosis. This aspect is still seen in the writings and television programmes of Oliver Sachs. However, new drug treatments are now being introduced for a range of diseases such as multiple sclerosis and epilepsy, even before the causes of the diseases have been fully understood. Surgical treatment is again coming to the forefront, but much more precisely focused than before. The diagnostic side has not been abandoned, but it has left the bedside and moved to the laboratory, where collaboration with medical geneticists has allowed us to understand much more precisely the causes and transmission of nervous diseases.

RADIOLOGY

If the first half of the twentieth century saw radiology established as a single independent discipline, the second half saw its development and division into many subspecialities. For instance the use of barium for outlining the alimentary tract had become well established during the decade following 1910, but the technique of adding air to give the double-contrast barium enema, which did not come into use in the hospital until 1967, in expert hands gave really detailed pictures of any colonic tumour. The first subspeciality of the post-1945 era, however, was neuroradiology, which established angiography (the outlining of blood vessels with a radio-opaque material) as a primary role of the radiologist. This technique spread to coronary artery angiography in which much faster sequential pictures were necessary, including cine-radiography.

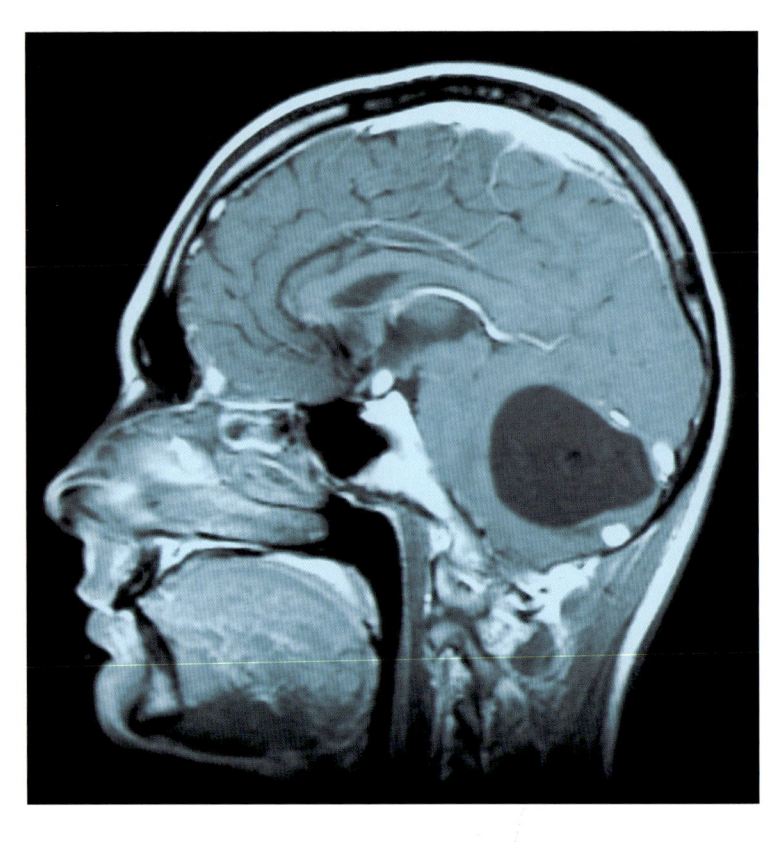

The idea of Computed Tomography (CT) scanning dates back to 1972 and must be credited to an Englishman, G.W. Hounsfield. The Royal Victoria Hospital first acquired the EMI scanner for the neuroradiology department in 1977; this was replaced by a faster mode scanner in 1982. In 1994 the most sophisticated model was added, allowing three-dimensional assessments to be made. Essentially it enables the radiographer to take x-ray 'slices' through the body with (unlike ordinary x-rays) a remarkable degree of differentiation of different types of tissue, normal or abnormal. In the 1970s, also, ultrasound (using the principle of the German physicist Doppler) was introduced to assess the flow along blood vessels (qualitatively and later quantitatively), particulary the carotid arteries and the vessels of the lower limbs. Also to this era can be traced the various developments in nuclear medicine, again assessing blood flow but by means of radio-isotopes such as thallium and technetium – particularly applicable to bone scanning for tumours, and lung scanning to detect clots that have lodged there. The Royal Victoria Hospital obtained its first gamma camera in 1971.

These techniques have been essentially noninvasive – that is, not involving cutting or needling – but from the same period can be dated the advance of the radiologist into the surgical realm, or 'interventional radiology'. This consists in the insertion of catheters through the skin into peripheral arteries and bile ducts and then threading up progressively wider catheters and 'stents' or expanding sheaths, which can be used to close off

Magnetic Resonance Image (midline sagital) of a patient with a tumour of the cerebellum, the large dark area in the lower posterior part of the brain; no other type of x-ray could identify its size and shape as clearly. The densely black areas are air-filled spaces and the white areas are blood vessels.
DR S. McKINSTRY AND
ROYAL VICTORIA HOSPITAL

aneurysms (swellings) or fistulae (abnormal openings) in vessels.

The National Breast Screening Programme conceived of by Sir Patrick Forrest is not yet of proven efficacy as a cost-effective way of detecting breast cancer. However mammography, leading where necessary to fine-needle cytology and breast biopsy for selected cases, has a very high detection rate and was certainly an advance of the 1980s.

The most recent arrival on the hospital site has been the Magnetic Resonance Imager (MRI), paid for by the Carrickmannon Appeal and housed, rather inconveniently, in the lower car park. The idea for this device came originally from the USA and those responsible won the Nobel Prize as far back as 1952. Although magnetic resonance imaging was potentially much less harmful than the use of ionising radiation, the huge cost of an MRI delayed the acquisition of one by the Royal Victoria Hospital until 1993. The instrument, using yet another different physical principle, permits even finer distinction than CT scanners between different soft tissues of the body.

The first NHS consultant radiologist to be appointed at the Royal Victoria Hospital was Dr David Cuthbert Porter, who had graduated with an MB with honours at Queen's University in 1933 and with an MD in 1936. He had served in World War Two with the RAMC and had trained as a radiologist at the Middlesex Hospital, London, from 1942 to 1946. After a further period as a trainee at the Royal Victoria Hospital he was appointed Assistant Radiologist in 1947 and Consultant in 1948, being later appointed Consultant to the Ulster Hospital, both of which appointments he held until his retirement in 1975. He was a founder fellow of the new Faculty of Radiology of the Royal College of Surgeons in Ireland in 1961, and in 1962 gave the annual winter oration on the topic 'The new photography'. Probably his main local contribution was to establish gastro-intestinal radiology on a firm basis.

Dr W.H.T. (Harry) Shepherd, another Queen's graduate, served in the RAF and graduated with an MD in 1950. He took up the new discipline of neuro-angiography and was appointed Consultant Radiologist at the Royal Victoria Hospital in 1950. He soon became expert at the difficult skill of direct puncture of the carotid and vertebral arteries, and set up the subdepartment beside the neurosurgical theatre in Ward 21; he gave the annual winter oration in 1966, and eventually retired in 1979. He was joined in the same field in 1959 by Dr F.S. (Fred) Grebbell, who not only pressed forward the technique of angiography, but was an enthusiast for the new technology of CT scanning, as seen in his 1986 winter oration. Dr Grebbell retired in 1988. Dr Roslyn (Ros) Hutchison joined this speciality as a Consultant in 1981, but resigned in 1986 to take up a post in Canada. Dr Steve McKinstry was appointed Consultant Neuroradiologist in 1987, as was Dr Kathleen Bell in 1988.

Dr J.O.Y. Cole followed Dr Shepherd in the field of general radiology.

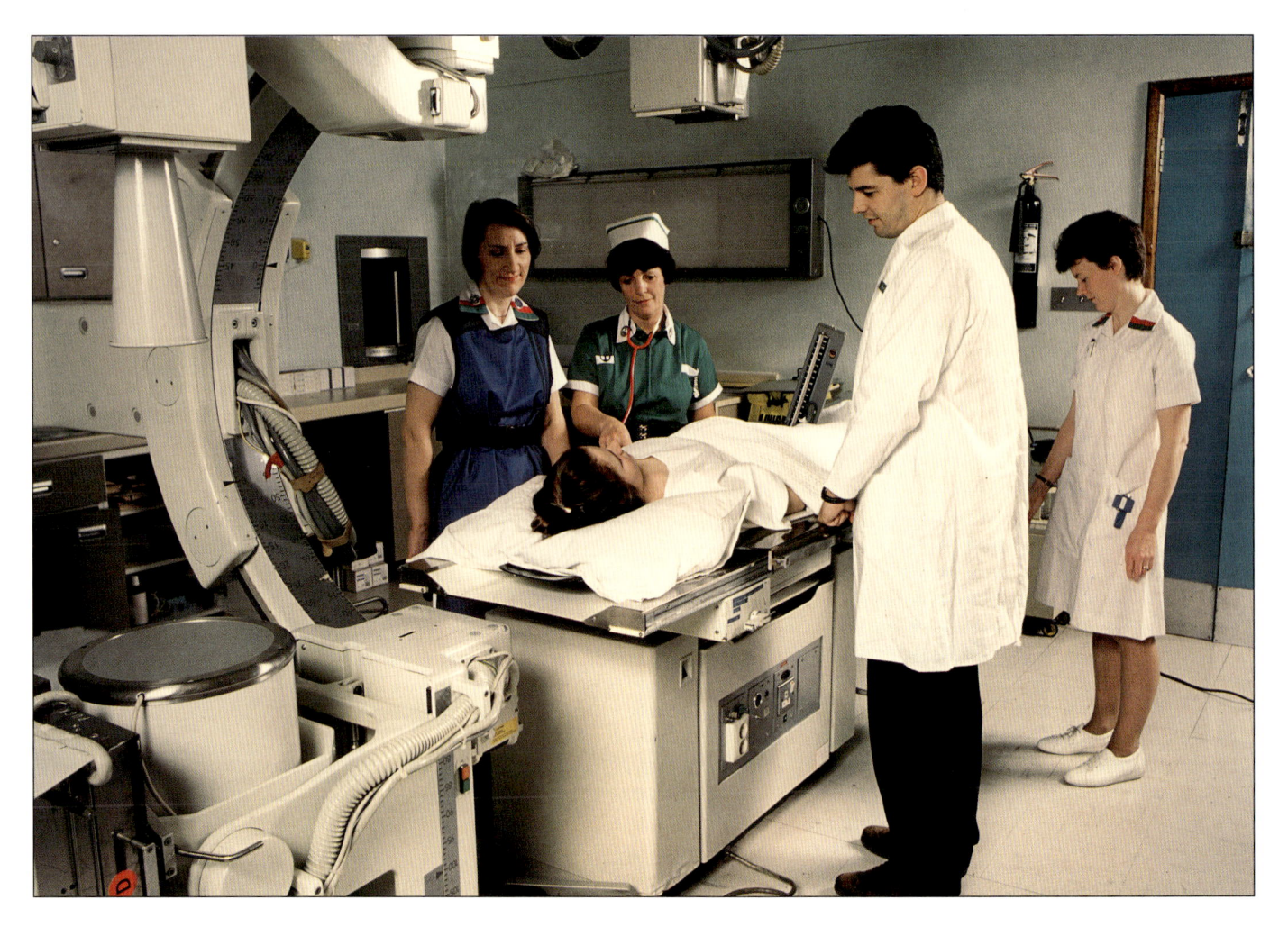

Angiographic equipment of the 1990s: *left to right*: Katherine Grant, Muriel Robinson, Dr Patrick Lowry and Mandy Weathers
ROYAL VICTORIA HOSPITAL

He had graduated at Queen's University in 1938, trained in Manchester and Cambridge, served with the RAMC in France, North Africa, Italy, India and Burma, and returned to St Thomas's Hospital, London, to train further and prepare an MD thesis. He was first a Consultant at Altnagelvin Hospital in Londonderry, and then was appointed Consultant Radiologist at the Royal Victoria Hospital in 1960, where his main field was industrial chest disease; he was also involved in early work on mammography. He was on the Council of the Faculty of Radiology of the Royal College of Surgeons in Ireland and was dean of the faculty, 1977–79. He retired in 1979, settling finally in Victoria, Australia, where he died in 1991.

Dr Richard Stanley Crone graduated with an MB in Dublin in 1949 and with an MD in 1954, trained in Oxford and Belfast and was appointed Consultant Radiologist to the Royal Victoria, Belfast City and Musgrave Park hospitals in 1959. He resigned on grounds of ill health in 1989.

Dr E.M. (Teddy) McIlrath, a graduate of Queen's, trained as a radiologist at University College Hospital, London, and in Sweden, and was appointed Consultant Radiologist to the Royal Victoria Hospital in 1965. His interests have spanned most aspects of radiology and he has also been chairman of the Medical Staff Committee, 1989–91; he gave the winter oration in 1992. Subsequent Consultant appointments have

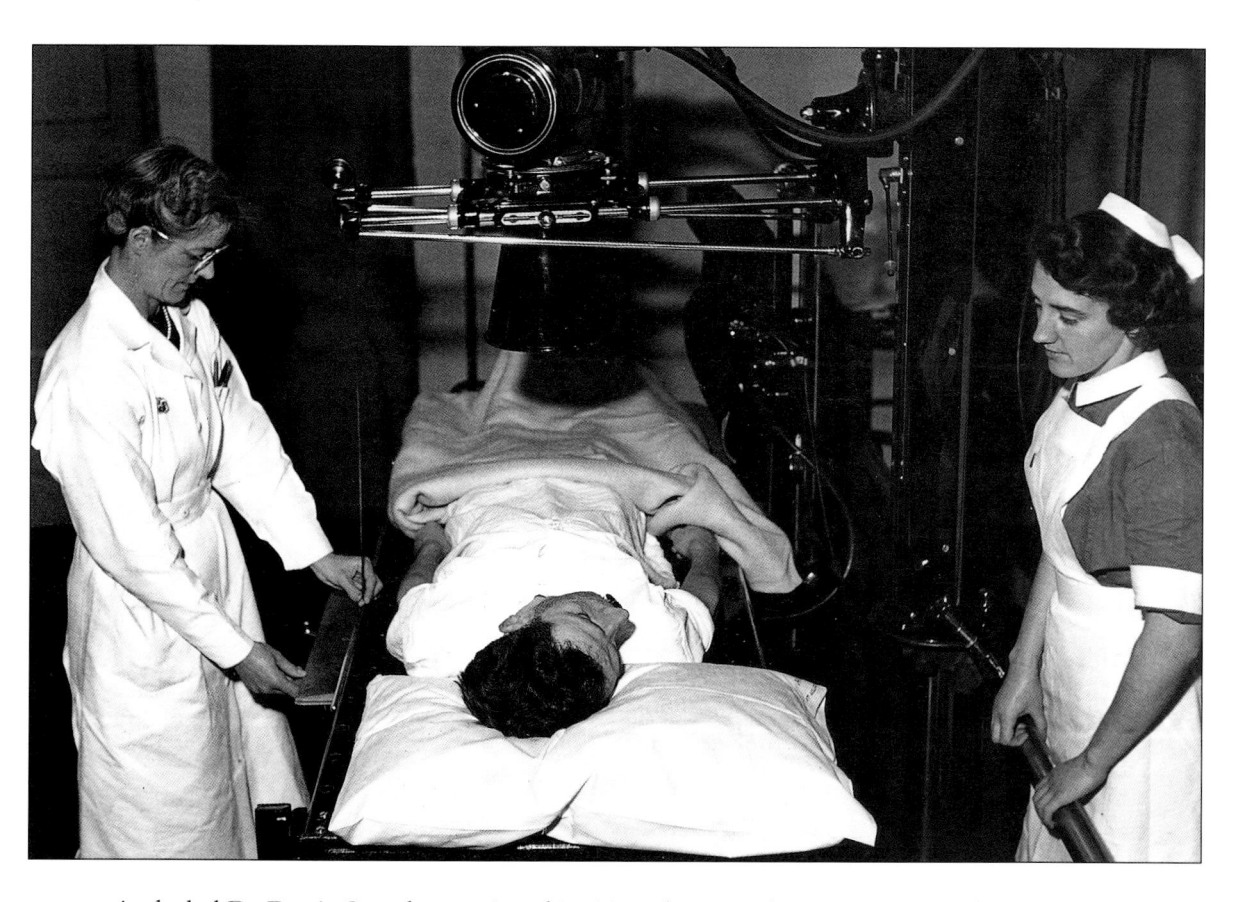

Radiology department, c. 1960: on the left is Belle Dickson, the first Superintendent Radiographer.
ROYAL VICTORIA HOSPITAL

included Dr Denis Gough, appointed in 1966 (he retired in 1993); Dr Paul Thomas, appointed in 1968 (he gradually moved to being involved wholly in the Royal Belfast Hospital for Sick Children); Dr J. Craig Hunter, appointed in 1971 (he resigned in 1976 to take a post in Australia); Dr Manton Mills, appointed in 1973; Dr James Laird, appointed in 1979; Dr J. Graham Crothers, appointed in 1985; Dr Ann O'Doherty, appointed in 1989; Dr Martin McGovern, appointed in 1994; Dr Barry Kelly, appointed in 1995; and Dr Ian Kelly, appointed in 1995.

Following the retirement of Ralph Leman in 1959 his deputy, Belle Dickson, became Senior Radiographer. She was involved in commissioning the new department on the main corridor which centralised four previous departments. With her successor, Lesley Irwin, the accident and emergency (A & E) department of radiography was planned; it opened in 1968, almost synchronously with the start of the Troubles. The standard of planning was reflected in the department's ability, to this day, to cope with unprecedented numbers of severe injuries. Lesley Irwin died prematurely in 1990; by a combination of character and professional skills she left a legacy of technical performance in the department unchallenged within the UK. She was succeeded by Maureen McMillan, the present unit radiographer.

The School of Radiography, which had existed in cramped conditions in the King Edward Building since 1924, moved into new, purpose-built accommodation beside Musson House in 1975, while Gwen McCullough was principal; it moved to the University of Ulster at Jordanstown in 1991.

RADIOTHERAPY

Radiotherapy developed during the late 1920s in the form of radium and x-ray treatment as described in Chapter 4, and until 1952 was carried out in the King Edward Building. At that time Dr Frank Montgomery and his colleagues combined an interest in diagnostic radiology and radiotherapy. It was Dr Montgomery in his role of chairman of the Northern Ireland Hospitals Authority who was responsible at the end of 1952 for setting aside one of the buildings of the fever hospital at Purdysburn for radiotherapy; this was to be named Montgomery House in his honour. From this time onwards, radiotherapy was not carried out in the Royal Victoria Hospital (except for treatment of skin diseases), but the radiotherapists visited patients in the wards and were later involved in some treatments.

Dr C. Abernethy and Dr Frank Benton are recorded as Radiotherapists in the early 1950s. Then came Dr John Millen who graduated at Queen's University in 1935 and gained an MD in 1939; after serving with the Indian Army Medical Corps and training in the Physiology Department at Queen's University Belfast and at the Christie Hospital, Manchester, he was appointed Consultant Radiotherapist at the Royal Victoria Hospital in 1953. Dr Arnold Richard Lyons graduated from Queen's in 1940 and after service with the RAF and training at Edinburgh Royal Infirmary was appointed Consultant Radiotherapist in 1960. He retired in 1983 and was awarded the OBE in the following New Year Honours. He was followed by Dr 'Gerry' Lynch, another Queen's graduate, who was appointed Consultant Radiotherapist in 1962. Dr George Edelstyn was appointed Consultant Radiotherapist in 1966. He was an enthusiastic pioneer in the introduction of chemotherapy in Northern Ireland and a founder member of Action Cancer, himself dying of a form of the disease at the age of forty-nine. More recent consultant radiotherapy appointments are Dr Brian Burrows and Dr William Paul Abram, both appointed to the Royal Victoria Hospital from 1983.

PSYCHIATRY

Dr Norman Graham was appointed Assistant Physician for psychiatry in 1927. He was Medical Superintendent of the Belfast Asylum at Purdysburn and his successor there, Dr Charles Booth Robinson, followed him as Consultant Psychiatrist to the Royal Victoria Hospital in 1948, although he was not appointed to the Medical Staff Committee until 1962. The psychiatrists have also been involved in consultations about inpatients, particularly about patients who have taken a drug overdose. Other Consultant Psychiatrists have been Professor John Gibson, appointed the first Professor of Mental Health in the university in 1957 and on the Consultant staff of the Royal Victoria Hospital from 1957 until his early death in 1974; Dr William Norris, a Consultant from 1962 until he retired in 1990 when he

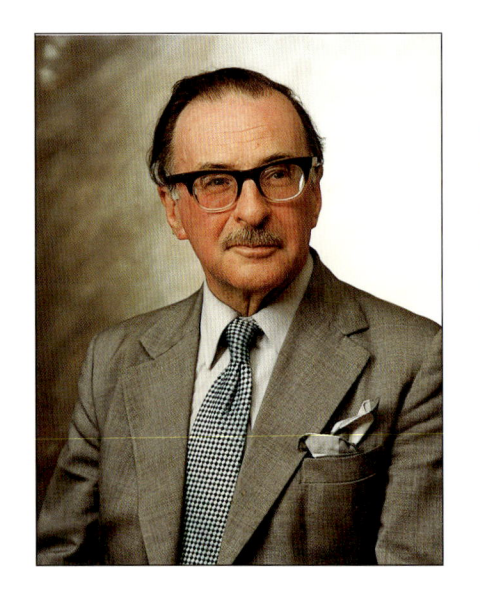

Dr Arnold Lyons, Consultant Radiotherapist to the Royal Victoria Hospital, 1960–83
ROYAL VICTORIA HOSPITAL

was awarded the OBE; Dr Gordon MacCallum, a Consultant from 1970 until he retired in 1989; Dr Arthur Kerr, a Consultant from 1983 until he retired in 1991; Dr Graeme McDonald, appointed in 1990; and Dr Philip McGarry, appointed in 1991.

PATHOLOGY AND ITS SUBDIVISIONS

In the first half of the twentieth century, pathology had become subdivided into morbid anatomy, haematology, bacteriology and clinical biochemistry, and nearly fifty years later each of these has undergone further division. Unity is preserved, however, by the concept of a Directorate of Laboratory Services; this is currently led by the Professor of Pathology.

Professor Sir John Biggart retired in 1971 and was followed in the Musgrave chair by Professor Dugald Lindsay Gardner, another Scot but a graduate of Cambridge and Edinburgh. He had held research posts in Edinburgh, Ohio and London, and always retained his London address while in Belfast. He resigned in 1976, moving to Manchester and later Edinburgh. Professor Elizabeth Florence McKeown succeeded him in the chair. Having graduated with an MB with first-class honours at Queen's University Belfast in 1942, she had joined the Pathology Department in 1943, completing a thesis for the MD with gold medal in 1945. Her main interests were cardiac pathology and the pathology of the aged, the subject of a book and a D.Sc. study in 1965. She retired in 1984.

Professor Peter Toner, who succeeded her in 1984, was a graduate of Glasgow University and had already been a Visiting Professor in Denver, Colorado, 1977–78, and Professor of Pathology in Glasgow for a year before his move to Belfast. His wife, Professor Katherine (Kate) Carr, is Professor of Anatomy at Queen's. Other general Pathologists appointed to the department were: Dr Denis Biggart, son of Sir John Biggart, appointed senior lecturer and Consultant in 1970 but who soon moved to the Belfast City Hospital; Dr Hoshang Bharucha, appointed 1974, whose wife Chitra is a Consultant Haematologist and deputy director of the Blood Transfusion Service; Dr James Sloan, appointed in 1974; Dr Denis O'Hara, appointed in 1975; Dr Claire Hill, appointed in 1980; Dr Maureen Walsh, appointed in 1986; and Dr Patrick Watt, author of *Pathology for Surgeons* (1986), appointed in 1988; he died in 1990 at the age of thirty-seven.

A branch of the Pathological and Bacteriological Laboratory Assistants' Association had been founded in Belfast in 1926 by David Willix, R. McDonald (Stevie) Steven and J. Bell to carry out some informal training; the status of this was considerably strengthened by the granting of a charter in 1944 under the title of the Institute of Medical Laboratory Sciences. It had the strong support of Professor Biggart and organised teaching in the department, though this was taken over by the College of Technology in the 1960s and later by the University of Ulster. One of the pillars of the bacteriology–haematology field was Albert Lamont, who joined the department in 1933 when he was only thirteen (receiving special dispensation to leave school early). He worked with all the great figures of the department and retired as recently as 1984, having been awarded the MBE in 1983. Robert (Bert) Russell joined the staff in 1940, when Stevie, who had been there it is said since 'the turn of the century' was still there; Stevie retired in the mid-forties and died in 1947. Bert Russell had as an assistant Louis Bell, with a withered arm, who was particularly kind and supportive to generations of medical students in terror of 'John Henry'. Cecil Bennett joined the department in 1941 and both he and Russell had almost as long a reign in the department as Stevie before they retired.

Neuropathology has been recognised as a separate clinical service since 1967 and Dr Ingrid Victoria Allen was appointed Consultant Neuropathologist in that year. She had studied medicine at Queen's University Belfast, and she was appointed to the newly created chair of Neuropathology in 1979; she was awarded the CBE in 1993. She gave the annual winter oration in 1995. Dr Meenakshi Mirakhur was appointed Consultant Neuropathologist in 1988. The department is widely recognised as an active research centre and has a total research funding to date of well over £2 million.

Cytology as a concept can be traced directly to the work of George Papanicolaou in the USA as far back as 1928, though its active use was delayed in the UK until after World War Two. In 1962 a cervical cytology service for Northern Ireland was set up, based in the Department of Pathology of the Royal Victoria Hospital. It started by taking cervical smears from women over forty years of age attending the gynaecological outpatient clinics of the hospital, but was extended to embrace greater Belfast and the whole of Northern Ireland. Having started with cervical smears, it developed in the 1970s to the more refined technique of fine-needle aspiration of cells, a method suitable for other tissues particularly the breast. In 1966 Dr Jacob Willis was appointed as a Consultant Pathologist to establish the new service; he retired in 1995. Dr Linda Caughley was appointed Consultant Pathologist in the service in 1986.

Dental pathology as a separate subdivision was established by Dr Harold Jones, who had both medical and dental qualifications; he was only on the Consultant staff for a few months in 1966–67 before moving on as senior lecturer to Cardiff, and then to Manchester as Professor of Oral Medicine and pro-vice-chancellor. Dr Frank O'Brien was also doubly qualified, though he had achieved his dental qualification before his medical one. After more training at the Eastman Dental Hospital, London, and further experience of life on the SS *Canberra*, he was appointed senior lecturer and Consultant Dental Pathologist. He was later appointed to the chair of Dental Surgery; he retired in 1991, and was sadly missed for his entertaining and thought-provoking wit. His field has been taken over by

Seamus Napier BDS FFD.

Forensic pathology was for long the province of Professor Sir John Biggart within the university, but in 1958 a separate state pathology service was set up with Dr T.K. (Tom) Marshall at its head. He had been a clinical pathologist in Aden (1949–50) with the RAF and lecturer in Forensic Medicine in Leeds (1950–58) before coming to Belfast. He was appointed senior lecturer and Consultant on the staff of the Royal Victoria Hospital in 1963 and honorary Professor of Forensic Medicine of Queen's University in 1973. He was a prolific writer on many aspects of forensic medicine, and his works include a textbook *The Disposal of the Dead* (1958) and writings on many aspects of the Troubles. Dr Derek Carson was appointed to the Department of State Pathology and honorary Consultant in 1968. Dr Marshall retired in 1989 and was succeeded as State Pathologist by Dr Jack Crane, who had been Consultant and special lecturer in the department since 1985. He was given the title of honorary Professor in 1993. Dr John Press of this department was appointed an honorary Consultant in 1985.

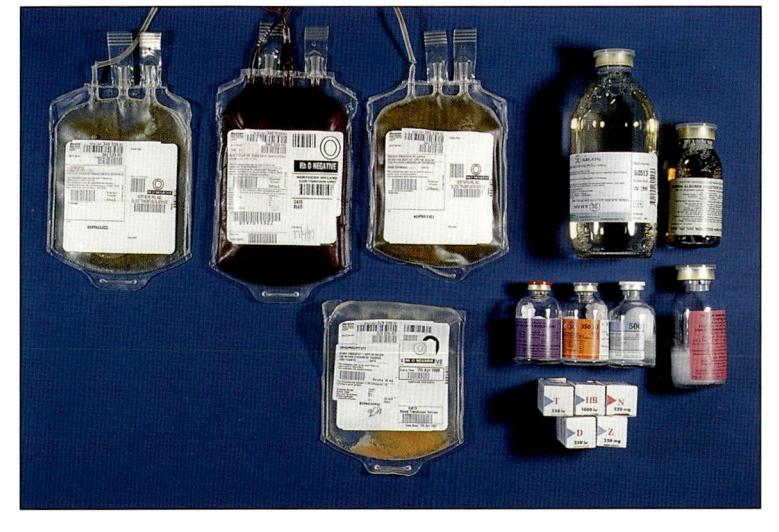

Haematology has passed far beyond its original role of looking at blood cells and counting them. Since the 1940s donor blood has become increasingly fractionated into various types of both cells and plasma. The laboratory is increasingly involved in analysing the exact deficiencies in a patient's blood and in providing the exact blood component for the patient's needs. The best-known example of this type of work is the provision of Factor VIII for haemophiliac patients, especially before surgery, but specific problems are also known in other patients (for example, during labour) who have massive haemorrhage and develop platelet, fibrinogen or other deficits. Research carried out in these fields has rapidly passed into the routine clinical field and includes work on the genetic basis for leukaemia, the production of erythropoietin (which is responsible for the formation of red blood cells), and the use of radio-isotopes to look at the way in which iron is absorbed.

A large number of products are now available that are derived from a single unit of blood: *top (left to right)* platelets, red cells and fresh plasma, which yields albumin concentrates; *below (left to right)* are cyroprecipitate, clotting factors such as Factor VIII, Factor IX and anti-thrombin, and a large number of different immuno-globulin fractions, so that the maximum use is made of any one blood donation.
ROYAL VICTORIA HOSPITAL

Dr John Moore Bridges was appointed Consultant Haematologist to the Royal Belfast Hospital for Sick Children in 1962 and joined Dr Gerry Nelson as a Consultant Haematologist to the Royal Victoria Hospital in 1966. As well as making a special study of leukaemia and bone marrow transplantation, Dr Bridges has been heavily involved in the Leukaemia Research Fund and other charities. He was appointed to the newly created chair of Haematology in 1979 and, having been chairman of the Medical Staff Committee from 1991 to 1993, was awarded the CBE in 1993; he retired in the following year.

Dr Elizabeth Mayne, a Queen's graduate, was appointed Consultant Haematologist in 1972. She has a special interest in haemophilia and was appointed honorary reader in 1991. Dr F.G.C. (Frank) Jones was appointed Consultant Haematologist in 1992, having previously been consultant haematologist to the Ulster and Ards hospitals.

BACTERIOLOGY (MICROBIOLOGY)

In 1948 Dr Norman Graham and Dr Eileen O. Bartley were in post as lecturers in Bacteriology, and until 1962 Dr Gerry Nelson covered this field as well as Haematology. Dr George Gibson was Consultant Bacteriologist from 1962 until 1970, when he resigned to become Director of the Public Health Laboratories in Leeds. The next permanent appointment in the field was Dr James Dunbar who had been Professor of Bacteriology in Khartoum and was appointed Consultant Bacteriologist and senior lecturer in 1964; he resigned in 1977. Professor Robert Gillies was appointed the first Professor of Clinical Bacteriology in 1976; he died suddenly in 1983. In the following year Professor Michael Emmerson was appointed to the chair; he resigned in 1989 to take up the chair in Microbiology at Nottingham University and since then the chair has not been filled. Dr Edward Smyth was appointed Consultant in 1984, Dr Cecil Hugh Webb became a Consultant in 1988, and Dr Kathleen Bamford became a Consultant and senior lecturer in 1990. The work of this hospital department, while still based on the growing of bacteria, has moved on to the determination of bacterial sensitivities and of antibiotic levels in the blood.

The field of virology in Belfast may be dated from the appointment of Professor George Dick in 1954 as the first Professor of Microbiology. A distinguished graduate of Edinburgh, he set up the Virus Reference Laboratory in 1956–57 in a particularly dynamic period of concern about poliomyelitis, influenza ('Asian flu') and hepatitis; he was also able to attract the large grants that led to the opening of the new microbiology building in 1964. Dr David Dane joined him in 1955 to become reader in Microbiology. They were appointed Consultants in the Royal Victoria Hospital in 1955 and 1957 respectively but both resigned in 1966 to join the Middlesex Hospital, London. Dr John Connolly joined the department in 1955 and, apart from a year in the Johns Hopkins medical school, Baltimore, he remained in this field from then on, becoming Consultant Virologist in 1968 and honorary Professor in 1991. He retired in 1993. Professor Kenneth Fraser MC was the second Professor of Microbiology, 1966–82, and was followed by Professor David Simpson, 1982–.

Dr Tom McNeill, a nephew of Dr Eileen Bartley, was a Consultant and senior lecturer in Microbiology from 1969 to 1973 and then became reader in Immunology until he retired in 1994. Dr Margaret Haire was appointed senior lecturer and Consultant in Microbiology and by the late 1970s both she and Dr McNeill were recognised as Consultant Immunologists. By the time Margaret Haire retired in 1986, strong links had been established with the clinicians on the hospital corridor, in particular Dr David McCluskey.

CLINICAL BIOCHEMISTRY

Even before the changes of 1948 the medical staff of the hospital had decided to appoint a full-time biochemist to run the biochemical laboratory on a full-time basis, to introduce technical innovations and to supervise the technical staff. The appointment was not made until 1951 and in the event the choice was Desmond Neill, son-in-law of Dr Robert Marshall (see page 101), who was a chemistry teacher without any background knowledge of hospital problems. The appointment, probably strongly advocated by Professor Biggart, achieved all that had been hoped for and starting with the equipment for sodium and potassium analysis by flame photometry, the technology moved on to include steroid analysis and, most exotic of all, the Sequential Multiple Autoanalyser with Computer (SMAC) which produced 20 different measurements on 24 samples per minute. By this time the laboratory had moved from the Institute of Pathology to the huts below the hospital road, and soon a further branch was set up in the metabolic unit. It was a period of great expansion and, while the laboratories were very expensive and probably absorbed a disproportionate amount of the pathology budget, the availability of so much

Dr Desmond Neill (*left*), the first full-time biochemist in the Royal Victoria Hospital, taking delivery of new laboratory equipment from IBM staff, *c.* 1960
ROYAL VICTORIA HOSPITAL

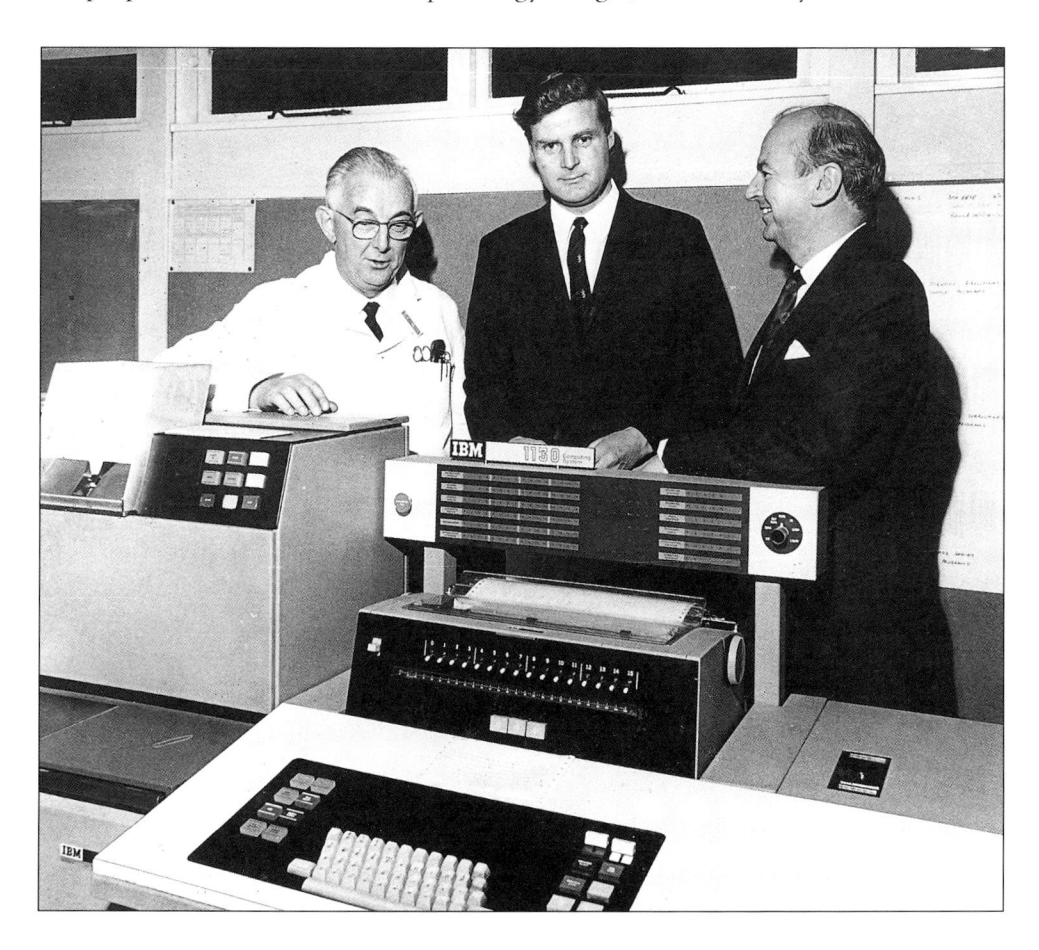

information certainly produced a steady increase in the clinician's appreciation of the usefulness of biochemistry and better patient care.

As with general pathology there have been strong links with the past, notably in Mr John Coulter who looked after the laboratory in the early days of Dr Jack Smyth, being on the staff altogether from 1934 to 1977.

Desmond Neill retired in 1986, and in 1987 Professor Elizabeth Trimble was appointed the first Professor of Chemical Pathology and Consultant Biochemist. Since then the laboratories have made yet another move – out of the 'temporary' accommodation in the huts to an attractive three-storey building on the site of the old Kelvin School. In addition to improving facilities for all, this has enabled the endocrine and paediatric biochemical laboratories to be united again with the main unit. The laboratory now handles about 10,000 separate analyses per day and employs a staff of about fifty people – certainly a great leap from the laboratory set up by Dr Jack Smyth in the 1920s with its one technician and 1,400 analyses per year.

NURSING, 1948–66

Florence Elliott had already been appointed Matron in 1946 and Nora Earls as Home Sister in 1945 and their reign dominated the next twenty years. When Florence Elliott took over, Anne Montague (Monty) was still Assistant Matron. She had been in the post since 1925, having started nursing in the days of Miss Bostock. She retired in 1950, and thirty-five years later, in 1985, she celebrated her 100th birthday at a party in England with Kathleen Robb and Doreen McCullough as well as a cake baked by Miss 'Lofty' Lowry. The Queen's telegram had to share the limelight with a letter and poem from Sir Ian Fraser.

Nora Earls became Assistant Matron in 1950 and Deputy Matron in 1952. Mary Scott was appointed a second Assistant Matron in 1950; sixteen years later it must have seemed like the end of an era when Miss Elliott, Miss Earls and Miss Scott all retired together. It has been said that Miss Elliott was very fortunate in having first-class Deputy Matrons; Peggy Donaldson's description of Nora Earls as 'a modern Monty, wise, practical and kind' was obviously intended to be the highest praise.

One of the particular interests of Florence Elliott's predecessor, Anne Musson, had been in the possibility of forming a Royal Victoria Hospital League of Nurses; in the event, this was not realised until 1949 when it was finally inaugurated and she, in her retirement, was elected president. It built up as a worldwide force with a membership of over 1,000 to keep former RVH nurses in touch with each other and with the hospital. Sadly, with changes in the training system and the dissolution of a specifically Royal Victoria Hospital School of Nursing, it and the distinctive badges all went in 1993.

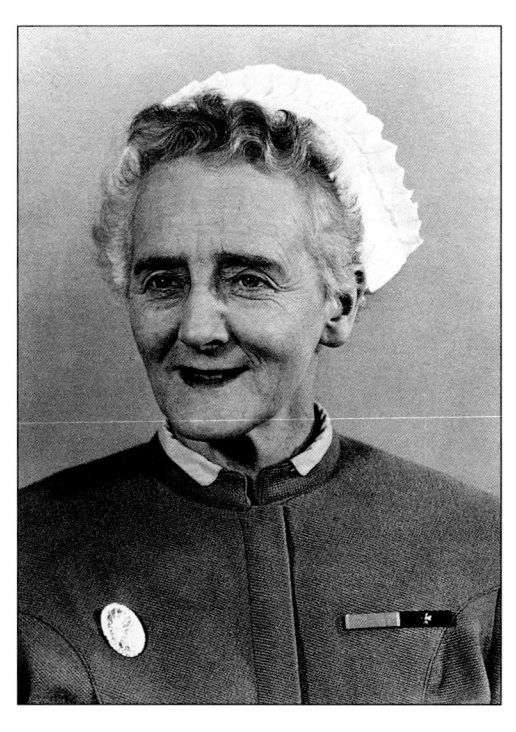

Florence Elliott, Matron of the Royal Victoria Hospital, 1946–66
ROYAL VICTORIA HOSPITAL

Florence Elliott was born in 1905 in Duneane Manse near Randalstown, County Antrim, the daughter of a Presbyterian minister. Overcoming early ill health, she trained in the Royal Victoria Hospital, 1927–30, and continued to work as a staff nurse and medical ward sister. She then took the midwifery training course in Edinburgh and remained there for a further five years before applying (reluctantly) for the troubled post of Matron of Whiteabbey Sanatorium in 1943. She went there after several enforced resignations of senior staff and the appointment of commissioners to reorganise the hospital, and having made the necessary corrective changes there and restored morale, she was the obvious choice to be Matron at the Royal Victoria Hospital to succeed Anne Musson in 1946.

At the Royal Victoria Hospital, Florence Elliott guided nursing through the difficult changes following 1948, always putting the welfare of the patient as the nurse's first concern. She was also heavily involved in the Royal College of Nursing, the Joint Nursing and Midwives' Council and various committees of the Northern Ireland Hospitals Authority. She was awarded the OBE in 1951 and retired in 1966, being awarded an honorary MA degree by Queen's University Belfast. She was remembered after retirement by the Florence Elliott Lectures (now discontinued) and by the geriatric wards of Florence Elliott House, and died in 1996.

The other great figure of the past, Sister Catherine Dynes, the Night Superintendent, retired after forty years in 1953 at the age of seventy-five, the last of Miss Bostock's nurses working in the hospital. Agnes Campbell followed her for two years and then came Hazel Gaw, who held the post for twenty-three years, making a total of twenty-eight years on night duty. Both Catherine Dynes and Hazel Gaw were awarded the MBE on retiring.

The advent of the NHS brought undreamt-of funds to the Royal Victoria Hospital which were gradually to lead to improvements in the comfort of the patients. The wards were refurbished in 1947, but small items followed such as the provision of coloured bedspreads, individual trays with cups and saucers, cruets and paper napkins plus a full evening meal, to give an approach to hotel conditions (mainly financed by voluntary bodies, such as the Ladies' Committee). A cooked breakfast followed in the 1960s. Visiting was extended from four to seven days per week and a waiting room was provided for visitors to critically ill patients. Rails for curtains were put up round the beds giving greater privacy and avoiding the horrors of a portable screen falling over in the middle of the night. Indeed, reduction of noise generally in the wards resulted from new floor coverings and soundproofing of the nurses' station – itself an innovation of this period to give better supervision of the paired wards. Lastly, in 1966, there was the opening of a night admission unit which avoided the constant interruptions of patients' sleep by new admissions, their treatment and journey to and from theatre.

There were also changes in nursing practice, such as the introduction of disposable needles, gloves, dressings, blood transfusion sets and, most acceptable of all, the introduction of the disposable sputum mug. Non-nursing duties such as scrubbing tables were reduced by covering them with Formica and by the employment of ward clerks and theatre orderlies. Timetables were reorganised to avoid patients trying to eat breakfast while their beds were being made, surely a recipe for frequent disasters. The other reorganisation of the 1960s was the change from the night nursing practice of doing three months in a run, to letting the nurses do shorter periods of night duty in the ward to which they were attached during the day. Implementation of the nursing changes was largely the work of Doreen McCullough, Assistant Matron, who moved on in 1968 to be Matron of Lurgan and Portadown Hospital, later to commission the Craigavon Area Hospital and to be Chief Nursing Officer with the Department of Health. Peggy Donaldson points out in *Yes, Matron* that some of these changes were not welcomed by all staff either among the senior nurses or the doctors (for instance the plastic doors replacing the wooden doors of wards 1 and 2), but at least they were admitted by most people to be improvements.

Changes to the life of nurses were also coming, though the forty-four-hour week, promised in 1948, took nine years to be implemented and the forty-two-hour week did not come until 1966. The nurses requested that a lady doctor be appointed for their care, and eventually Dr Margaret Campbell succeeded Dr Howard Crozier – certainly less terrifying but not necessarily any more sympathetic to those just wanting a few days' rest. She introduced the nurses' sick bay, first in the gynaecology wards and later in wards 21 and 22, and overall ensured that sick nurses actually received nursing care. There was more leisure for playing games, most of which were available in the hospital grounds, but the most memorable activity was the hospital choir founded in 1951 by Sister Rita Roulston and bringing nurses and doctors together. The highlight of its year was the annual Christmas concert.

The progression from a totally service role for student nurses to one closer to that of university students continued throughout the fifties and sixties. One of the plans introduced by Florence Elliott was to rotate the nurses through a full range of specialities during their training, which meant, of course, that as soon as they became skilled and useful to the doctor, they were moved on. The only solution to this was gradually to introduce more part-time trained nurses and more staff nurses, and to bring in junior sisters ('blue' sisters as distinct from 'red' sisters). With the object of making training more relevant, lectures and training allocations were planned in advance so that nurses had their relevant lectures immediately before their practical experience. The other change in training in the fifties was the use of the

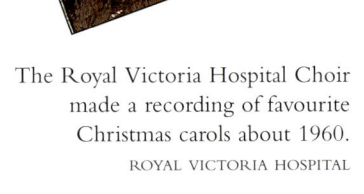

The Royal Victoria Hospital Choir made a recording of favourite Christmas carols about 1960.
ROYAL VICTORIA HOSPITAL

Beeches in Hampton Park, a large house where nurses in the Preliminary Training School (PTS) could live and enjoy a stress-free introduction to nursing, though this was given up in 1964 when Bostock House was opened and more space became available in Musson House.

NURSING SINCE 1966

Kathleen Robb took over from Florence Elliott in 1966, having trained in the Royal Belfast Hospital for Sick Children, the Royal Victoria Hospital and Western General Hospital, Edinburgh, as well as in the Agnes Hunt Orthopaedic Hospital in Oswestry, Shropshire. She was then appointed Matron in Armagh and returned to the Royal Victoria Hospital as Nurse Planning Officer in 1963, a new post raising nursing representation into a higher administrative level. She was therefore well fitted for the posts of Matron and District Administrative Nursing Officer for the North and West Belfast District, 1973–84. She held these posts during the worst part of the Troubles, and in 1973 she was awarded the OBE and in 1977 was made a fellow of the Royal College of Nursing.

M.A. (May) McFarland was appointed Assistant Matron in 1952, Deputy Matron in 1966, and Principal Nursing Officer (Matron) in 1973; she retired in 1975. She was followed by Heather Barrett who had been born and trained in Kenya, worked as a surgical sister during the Mau Mau uprisings, and was actually termed Divisional Nursing Officer. She threw herself enthusiastically into a field new to her and worked loyally for the hospital until 1984. At this stage a further reorganisation divided the North and West Belfast District into management areas, creating a Director of Nursing Services for the whole Royal Group of Hospitals and dividing the Royal Victoria Hospital into five areas in charge of assistant directors of nursing. Heather Barrett resigned, taking up a post in Saudi Arabia, and Elizabeth (Liz) Duffin was appointed the first Director of Nursing Services for the whole Royal Group of Hospitals. There was no longer a Matron of the Royal Victoria Hospital. The bare catalogue of names gives no feeling for the upheavals and stresses faced by all the senior nurses who followed Florence Elliott. They faced frequent reorganisations, the heavy nursing pressures of the Troubles and, from the mid-1970s, a steady reduction in nurses to do the work in the wards.

The Salmon Report came out in 1966, putting forward its notorious proposal for a hierarchy of nurses: Salmon 10 = matron or equivalent title, 9 = senior nursing officer, 8 = nursing officer, 7 = ward sister or charge nurse, et cetera. The report was not implemented in the Royal Victoria Hospital until after 1972; over the next ten years it resulted in a steady proliferation of nursing officers, putting more and more barriers between the ward sisters, who saw the patients, and the Matron. At the same time the paperwork (and this was not only for the nurses) also began to

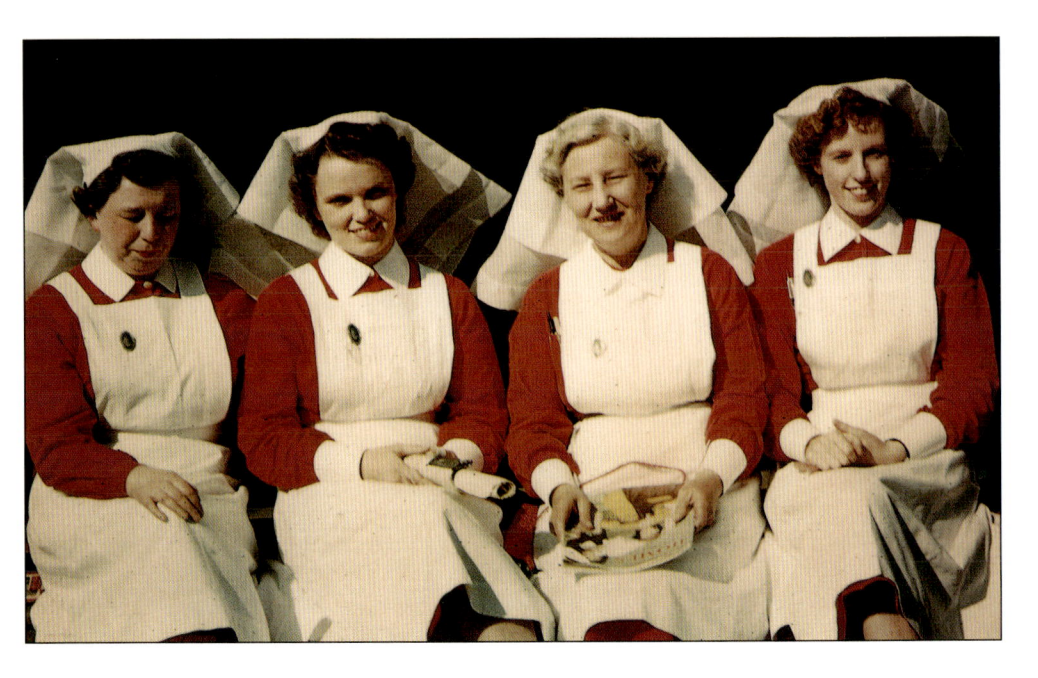

Ward sisters, *c.* 1970: *left to right:* Doreen McCullough, Florence Betty, Edna Elkin and Noel Morrow
ROYAL VICTORIA HOSPITAL

proliferate. When the changes had crystallised by 1984, there were ten Senior Nursing Officers for the group, one being for the Royal Maternity Hospital, one for the Royal Belfast Hospital for Sick Children, and the other eight for different areas of the Royal Victoria Hospital.

The Troubles are discussed in Chapter 6. Here it need only be stressed that the nurses, at all levels of seniority, bore the brunt of them. They could look out of the windows of Broadway Tower at gun battles; one nurse had to crouch down behind her boyfriend's car to avoid ricocheting bullets. Hazel Gaw bravely confronted several members of the IRA dressed in white coats as they were abducting one of their comrades from the hospital. May McFarland had to go down to casualty after a shooting incident accompanied by a priest and an administrator, to confront relatives who were trying to invade the treatment area. Kathleen Robb was given the OBE, Sister Kate O'Hanlon (A & E) and Sister Noelle Gibson (intensive care) received the MBE, and Sister Hadessa (Dessa) Dodds of the neurosurgical wards was chosen as Nurse of the Year in 1976. And overshadowing all, who can forget the death of Marie Wilson, a third-year student nurse, who was killed by a bomb at the war memorial in Enniskillen on Armistice Day 1987?

But in many ways the strikes of ancillary workers of the late 1970s and 1980s were more disruptive then the Troubles. The nurses protested but did not strike, but the other workers staged strikes and picketed; the management, doctors and nurses had to go to great lengths to keep the service going.

The other problem faced by the nursing staff of the wards has been a constant cutting of staff. It is not easy to see why the Department of Health has had the constant illusion that the wards and operating theatres were overstaffed with nurses whose numbers could be reduced while the number of doctors needed to be steadily increased, but this is what has happened. The effects have been complicated by the move towards Project 2000, which aims to change the training of student nurses to a full-time academic course at Queen's University including much more sociology and psychology than at present. They will be seconded to hospital and community work for periods but will no longer play an essential part in the work of the wards.

Male nurses were admitted for training in the hospital as far back as 1948, but it was many years before a man achieved any senior appointment. The first was probably W.J. (Jackie) Carville as Night Charge Nurse in 1972; in 1974 J.A. Ferguson became Principal Administrative Education Officer in the school of nursing for North and West Belfast. In 1975 Horace Reid became the first male nurse to be awarded the gold medal.

In spite of problems and reorganisations, nursing in the hospital has gone from strength to strength since 1948. There were giants of the past such as Sister Mary Galbraith of wards 15 and 16 and later the Outpatient Building, and her sister Kate Galbraith of the main theatres, Sister Lorna Dunn of the recovery ward, Miss Florence Betty of wards 17 and 18 and eventually geriatrics, Sister Benson (Benny) of wards 9 and 10, Sister 'Lofty' Lowry of Ward 22, and Sister E.L.C. Wallace (Wally) of wards 3 and 4. And many others were equally dynamic and, perhaps to their juniors, equally formidable. Whether good nursing is achieved by commonsense or by the 'nursing process', the aim is still the same.

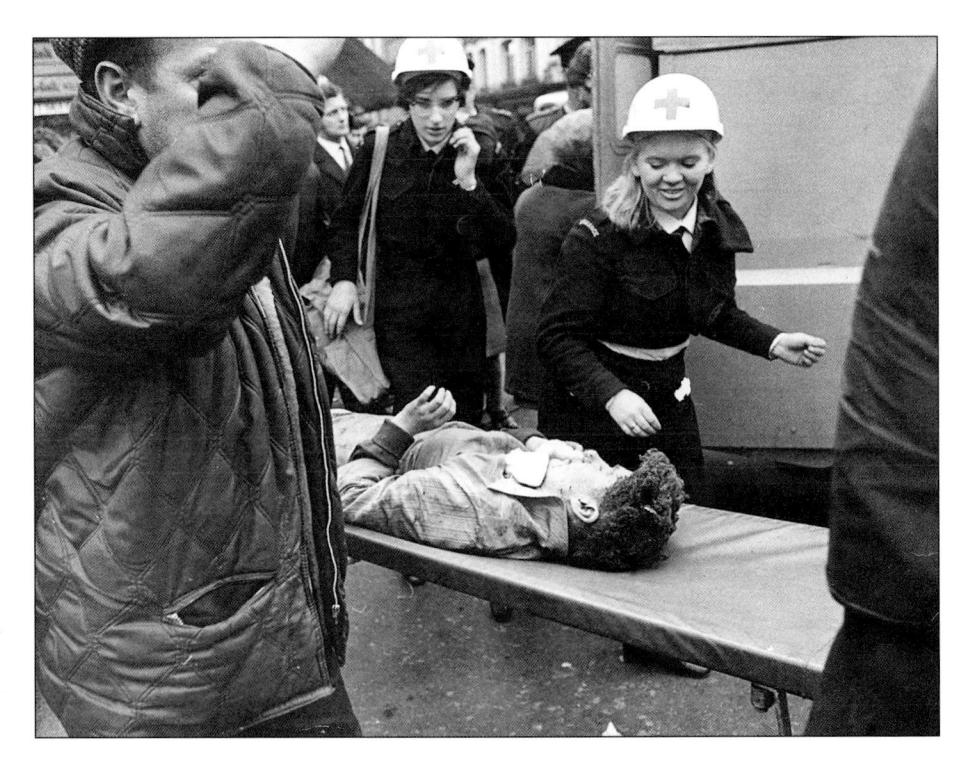

One of the injured being taken away on a stretcher after the Abercorn bombing on 4 March 1972, cheered and comforted by two of the ambulance personnel
BELFAST TELEGRAPH

6

THE SURGICAL SPECIALITIES
AND THE IMPACT OF THE TROUBLES

Surgery in the 1950s was not greatly different from that performed in the 1930s; certainly many radical changes have taken place since then. Certain types of surgery have become rare – such as that for tuberculosis, made unnecessary by drugs such as streptomycin, and peptic ulcer surgery, obviated by the H_2 blocking drugs. There was always some specialisation, but by now prostate and renal surgery have become the domain of the urologist, and the more radical oral surgery has became the responsibility of the maxillo-facial and plastic surgeons.

Moreover, both these fields have largely left the Royal Victoria Hospital. Breast surgery has also changed: the radical mastectomy of the post-1945 era has been replaced by more localised removals, preceded by one or more biopsies. Varicose vein and haemorrhoid operations are less common now, but there is still no answer other than surgery to inguinal and femoral hernia. Arterial vascular surgery really only came in during the 1960s and is already a specialist province with better results in obstruction to lower limb vessels, and aortic aneurysm surgery is now largely a planned procedure rather than a last resort. When all this is said, surgery of the abdominal cavity still forms the mainstay of the surgical lists.

Perhaps the most obvious change in the running of the operating theatre has been the gradual introduction of disposables and the Central Sterile Supplies Department (CSSD). The supply of catgut with or without needles has been expensive but has greatly facilitated fine and accurate suturing. In addition, the introduction of nonirritant fibres such as nylon, Teflon and Dacron has made much of the repair work more reliable. Radio-opaque swabs have been with us since World War Two, but now they are pre-packed, counted and sterile when they come to the hospital. Disposable rubber gloves came in during the 1960s and greatly reduced the work of the theatre nurses who previously had to scrub and sterilise the surgeons' rubber gloves. However, the practice of keeping separate and full sets of instruments for, say, six operations in one day has been adopted only slowly because of the cost. Such an arrangement, while allowing for cleaning centrally rather than in the theatre, and a much more rigorous sterilisation, has not yet become practicable in all operating theatres.

The most conspicuous change affecting all branches of surgery has been the growth of endoscopy. After the early days of Andrew Fullerton and the cystoscope, and the gradual improvements in the bronchoscope and oesophagoscope in the inter-war years, in the 1960s the more sophisticated instruments arrived, such as the choledochoscope and peritoneoscope, accompanied by a general irritation with the technology and ridicule for the surgeon who tried to use them. Manufacturers persisted, however, and quite suddenly in the 1970s abdominal endoscopy (laparoscopy) became a practical and useful technique, particularly for surgery of the Fallopian tubes (usually sterilisation); in the 1980s came laparoscopic cholecystectomy. The advantages were less pain for the patient and a shorter stay in hospital, which benefited everyone. Against this there were surgical problems in the early stages of development of each procedure, and surgery by endoscopy is really only safe for straightforward cases and with experienced operators.

In the USA, the advent of laparoscopic surgery has been accompanied by a move to 'day-stay surgery', but this has been slower to be accepted at the Royal Victoria Hospital. It is easy to believe that this is only due to conservatism on the part of the surgeons, but the main reasons appear to

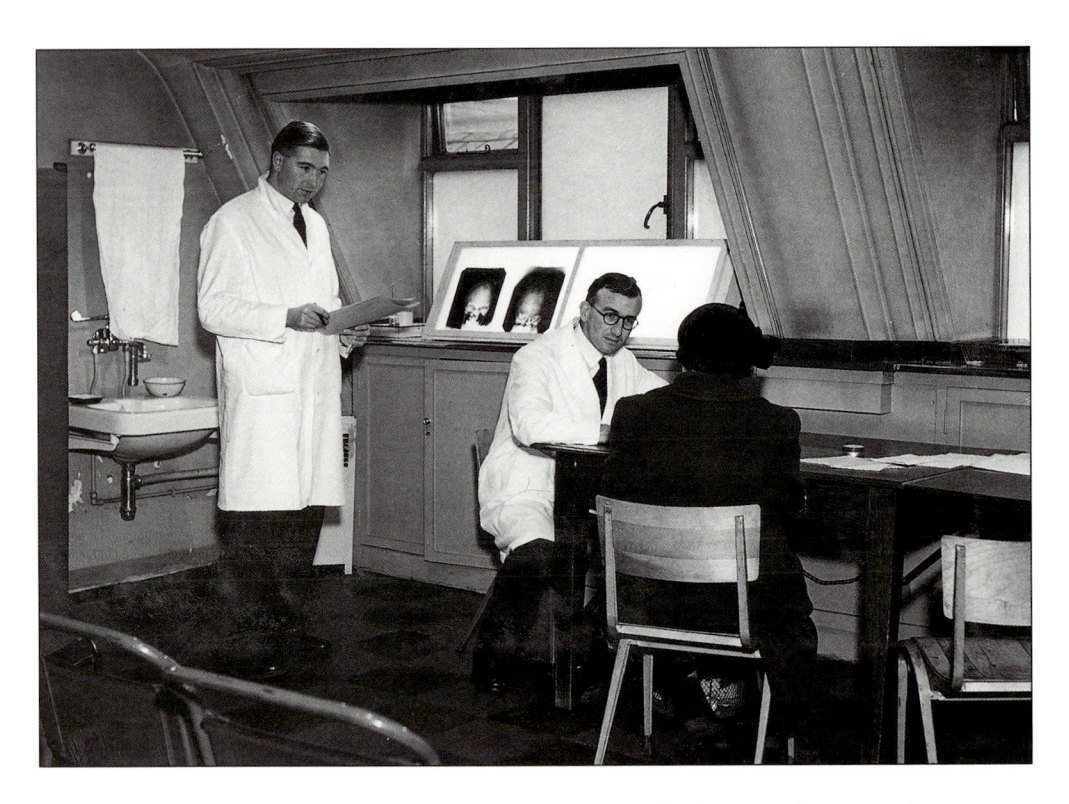

Mr Reggie Livingston (*left*) and Mr Sinclair Irwin in the outpatient consulting rooms on the first floor of the old extern, *c.* 1956
ROYAL VICTORIA HOSPITAL

Harold Rodgers, Professor of Surgery at Queen's University Belfast and Consultant Surgeon to the Royal Victoria Hospital, 1947–73
ROYAL VICTORIA HOSPITAL

be a genuine belief that too early discharge (whether on the same day as the operation or later) is associated with a higher morbidity and the fact that the Royal Victoria Hospital is the final resort in Northern Ireland for difficult cases. This means that the hospital receives a high proportion of complicated cases requiring prolonged investigation, admission and at least high-dependency care post-operatively.

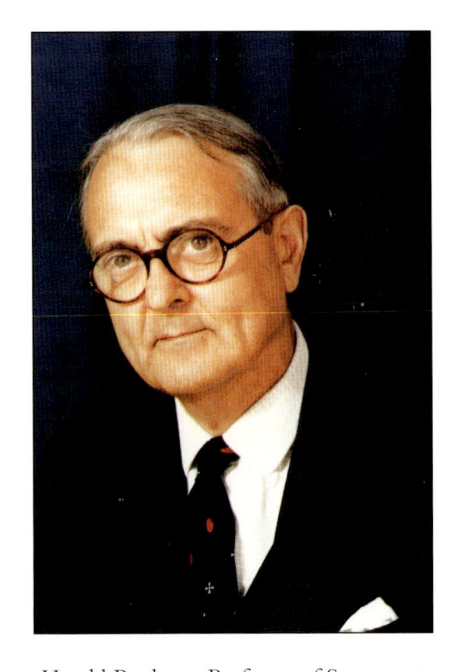

THE GENERAL SURGEONS

Professor Harold Rodgers had been appointed to the chair of Surgery in 1947. The first surgeon to be appointed after the advent of the NHS was Mr J. Sinclair Irwin, who came to the hospital in 1950 to work in wards 13 and 14. He was a son of Sir Samuel Irwin (see page 111) and had served in the RAMC, being captured at Dunkirk in 1940. He had a particular interest in vascular surgery but over the years covered all aspects of general surgery. He gave the annual winter oration in 1965, and eventually retired in 1978. In 1950 also, Mr Ernest Morrison was appointed to wards 19 and 20. He too had served in the RAMC after qualifying; while being a general surgeon, he had a lifelong interest in urology, its advances and innovations, as witnessed by his 1969 annual winter oration. Mr Terence Leslie Kennedy had graduated in 1942 at the London Hospital where his father was a surgeon, before joining the Royal Navy, and then training in London; he too joined the staff of the Royal Victoria Hospital in 1950. He was later president of the Association of Surgeons of Great Britain and Ireland and a member of the Council of the Royal College of Surgeons in London. He was a prolific writer on surgical subjects but particularly on the broad field of gastric surgery, and gave the 1970 annual winter oration on the topic 'Communication in medicine'. He was an incisive debater, an amusing speaker, and a skilled yachtsman.

After the burst of appointments in 1950 there was a lull until 1956 when Mr Reginald (Reggie) Livingston was appointed. He had an early interest in urology but later concentrated on vascular surgery, though a heavy clinical load did not prevent him from performing many extra-curricular tasks in medical administration, the YMCA, the Society of Friends, and the Cripples' Institute. He gave the annual winter oration in 1980 and died in the same year, at the height of his skill and energy at the age of fifty-seven.

In 1957 Mr Willoughby Wilson, a native of Straid, County Antrim, was appointed. One of a notable medical family, he graduated in 1946 and shared with Reggie Livingston a tireless energy for surgery both routine and emergency. His particular interest was in colonic surgery, but inevitably he was heavily involved in the surgery of the Troubles, and he was awarded the OBE for his work in this field in the New Year Honours of 1983. He gave the 1981 annual winter oration. He is married to an anaesthetist, Dr Kaye (née Browne) Wilson.

Mr Richard Welbourn was appointed Consultant Surgeon in the Professorial Unit in 1957; he had been a senior lecturer there from 1952 after graduation at Liverpool in 1942 and service in the RAMC. He was a pupil of Charles Wells's in Liverpool and derived from him a strong interest in gastroenterology, though he later became particularly associated with endocrine aspects of surgery. His major interest was in surgical research, and he was appointed to a personal chair in this field by

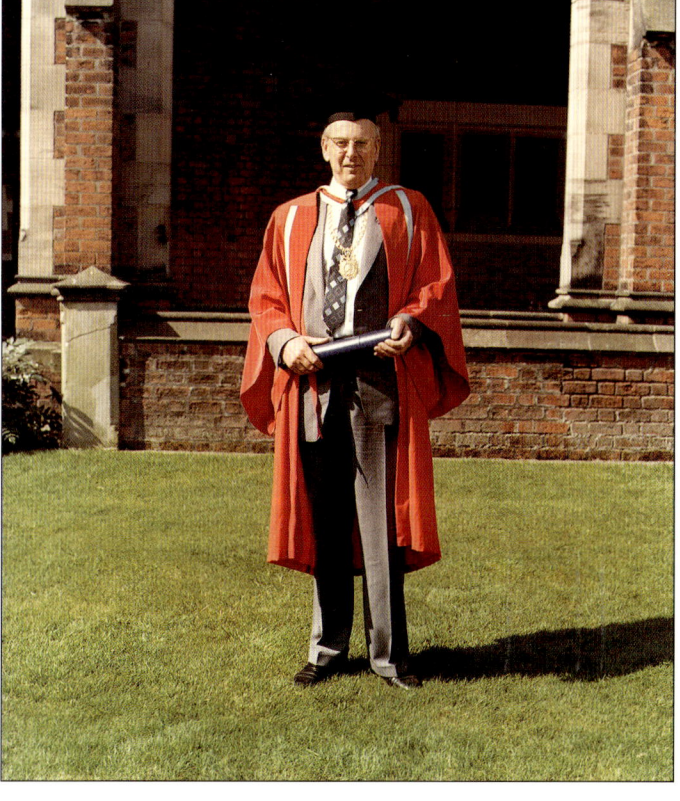

Mr Terence Kennedy, Consultant Surgeon to the Royal Victoria Hospital, 1950–84; he is seen here in 1981 when he was awarded an honorary MD by Queen's University as president of the Association of Surgeons.
ROYAL VICTORIA HOSPITAL

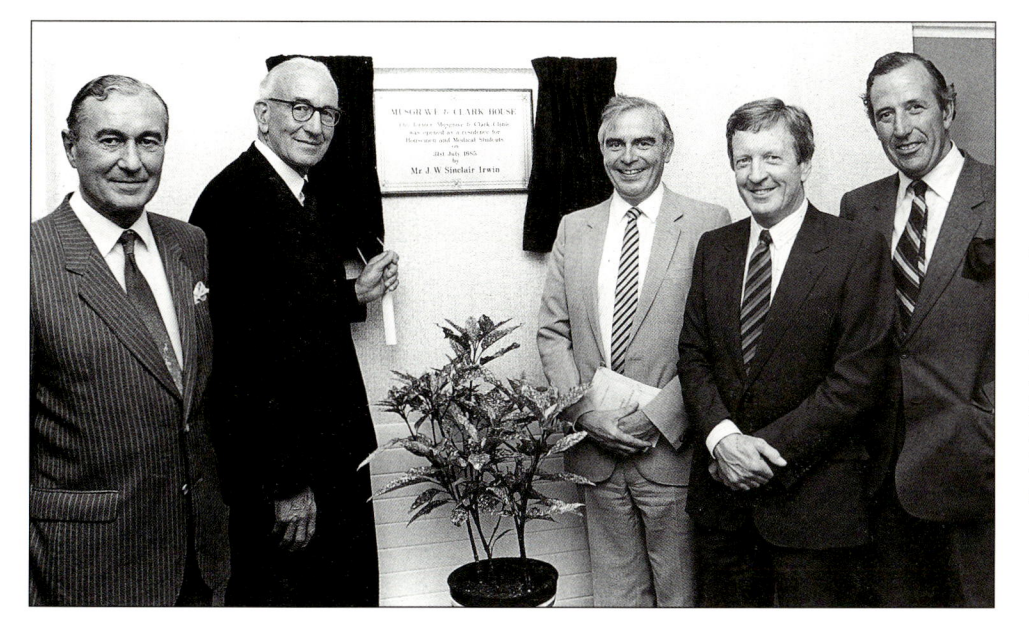

The opening of the refurbished Musgrave and Clark Clinic as accommodation for the resident medical officers in 1985: *left to right*: Mr Willoughby Wilson FRCS Edin, Mr J. Sinclair Irwin FRCS Edin, Mr Patrick Kinder, Dr Desmond Burrows and Dr A.H.G. Love
ROYAL VICTORIA HOSPITAL

Queen's University Belfast in 1958, though he moved on to a chair in the Postgraduate Medical School, Hammersmith Hospital, London, in 1963. He was given a D.Sc. (*honoris causa*) by Queen's in 1985.

In 1966, Mr George Johnston (MB with honours and many medals, QUB, 1956) was appointed. He worked with Mr Terence Kennedy in the field of gastric surgery but his particular interest, passed on by Professor Rodgers (see page 116), was in hepatic surgery and the management of bleeding veins in the oesophagus. He gave the 1990 annual winter oration, entitled 'The enjoyment of life depends on the liver'. He was appointed an honorary Professor of surgery in 1991, was chairman of the Medical Staff, 1993–95, and retired in 1995. Mr Joseph Kennedy, who was also appointed in 1966, was also a Consultant Surgeon in the Belfast City Hospital with a major interest in urology; he joined Mr Morrison's unit, helping to provide a specialist urological service in the Royal Victoria Hospital; he retired in 1996. In 1966 too, Mr Stewart Desmond Clarke was appointed as a General Surgeon, with sessions also in the Belfast City and Musgrave Park hospitals. He was soon to concentrate on starting the renal transplant service for Northern Ireland, based in the Belfast City Hospital; the first renal transplant there was carried out in November 1968. He resigned in 1974 to run the surgical service in Ahmadi, Kuwait, for nine years, before returning to Midhurst, Sussex. Mr Gordon Loughridge, son of Mr James Loughridge FRCSE, was appointed Consultant Urologist to the Royal Victoria Hospital and Belfast City Hospital in 1972, though he worked mainly in the Belfast City Hospital.

On the retirement of Mr Sinclair Irwin in 1978 Mr Aires Barros D'Sa was appointed; like Mr Irwin he too had a special interest in vascular surgery. He had graduated with an MB at Queen's University Belfast in 1965 with many scholarships and with an MD with honours in 1975, and had continued his surgical training in Seattle, USA. He was joined in the vascular unit in 1982 by Mr John Hood, who had essentially the same field of interest. In 1982 also Mr Colin Russell was appointed; his interest was general and endocrine surgery.

When Professor Rodgers retired in 1973 after twenty-six years in university and hospital, he was replaced by Professor Arthur Douglas Roy, a Glasgow graduate, who had been a Consultant Surgeon in the Western Infirmary there and Professor of Surgery in Oman and Nairobi. He retired in 1985 and was followed by Professor Brian James Rowlands. After training at Guy's Hospital, London, and Sheffield, Professor Rowlands had been Associate Professor of Surgery in Texas and brought with him specialist interests in gastrointestinal surgery, nutritional support and intensive care. He resigned in 1997 to take up a chair in gastrointestinal surgery at the University of Nottingham. Mr Thomas George Parks was appointed senior lecturer in 1971 and was given a newly created chair in Surgical Science in 1982. His work has been mainly in colo-rectal surgery, and most of his sessions have taken place in the Belfast City Hospital. Mr George William Odling-Smee joined as senior lecturer in 1974, with a special involvement in breast surgery; with Mr Alan Crockard he was coeditor of *Trauma Care* (1981). Mr Samuel McKelvey was appointed in 1974 but resigned to work exclusively in the Ulster Hospital in 1985. Since then Mr Alan Wilkinson was appointed Consultant in 1985, R.J. (Roy) Maxwell was appointed Consultant in 1987, Mr Keith Gardiner was appointed Consultant and senior lecturer in 1995, and Mr Paul Blair was appointed Consultant and Trauma Director in the same year.

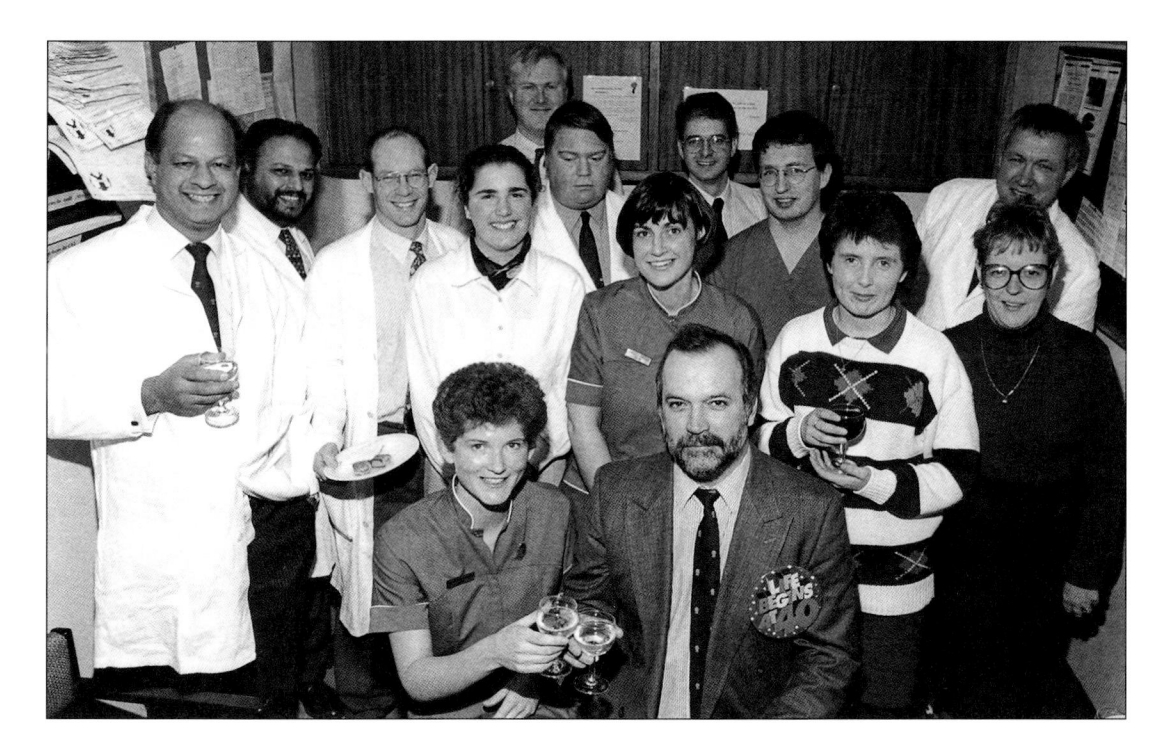

A party in Ward 17/18 to celebrate Paul Blair's fortieth birthday in 1996: *standing, left to right*: Mr Aires Barros D'Sa, Mr D. Kamerkar, Dr Andrew McKinley, Barbara George, Dr Barry Kelly, Mr John Hood, Sister Janet Robson, Mark Jones, Dr Ian Kelly, Maureen McFarland, Enid Burgess, Professor Brian Rowlands, and, in front, Sister Judith McClements and Mr Paul Blair
ROYAL VICTORIA HOSPITAL

ORTHOPAEDICS AND TRAUMA

Orthopaedic surgery has made much progress since 1948 but most of that performed in Belfast has taken place in the Musgrave Park Hospital and need not be reviewed here. The technology of hip surgery has advanced, for treatment both of osteoarthritis and of fractures of the neck of the femur. In addition, external fixation and the use of various kinds of nail have taken away the need for prolonged hospitalisation following many types of lower limb fracture. From time immemorial it has been recognised that the essential treatment of any kind of fracture is to keep the bones together and immobile. This has been achieved traditionally first by splints, then by plaster of Paris, and for femoral fracture by bed rest with traction on the limb. There was always reluctance to undertake any surgery, even in the case of a clean fracture, because of the risk of infection and osteomyelitis. However, the advent of antibiotics encouraged open reduction and the development of nonirritant insertions to hold fractures together.

The first significant advances in the 1940s were the Smith–Petersen pin (to join the fragments of the neck of the femur) and the Steinman's pin through the upper end of the tibia (to apply traction for certain types of fracture). Certainly the simple pin could reduce the period of bed rest for some patients but it was only satisfactory for a few, and a painful hip and prolonged immobilisation in bed, with the risk of bedsores, pneumonia and pulmonary embolus, were still common. An improvement came in the late 1950s with the introduction of the Austin Moore prosthesis for hip replacement, particularly for female patients over seventy years of age; some form of hip replacement soon became standard management. The use of intramedullary nails for simple fractures of long bones from the 1960s onwards was of great benefit in restoring activity in the young.

External fixation has been of particular importance in management of tibial fractures, but it has improved results in upper limb fractures as well. The idea of this type of fixation was developed on the European continent early in the twentieth century and gradually perfected, though it was only really used in the Royal Victoria Hospital from the 1970s, when the Belfast Fixator made by James Mackie and Sons was extensively tried. Modern devices have become lighter and easily obtained, and understanding of the physiology of fracture healing has permitted more movement of the patient generally, and particularly of the neighbouring joints. The other area of orthopaedic surgery practised in the Royal Victoria Hospital was management of injuries, tumours and deformities to the vertebral column, a particular field of Mr Ian Adair.

Mr Norman Martin, who graduated with an MB at Queen's University in 1935 and with an MD in 1939, served in the RAMC in India, Ceylon and Burma (being awarded the MBE), and after further training in Oxford returned to Belfast. In 1948 he was appointed Consultant Surgeon to the Royal Victoria and Musgrave Park hospitals, but he worked mainly in the latter. He was on the Medical Staff Committee of the Royal Victoria Hospital from 1962 until his retirement in 1977. Mr Walter Braidwood also served with the RAMC and after working as Casualty Surgeon in the Royal Victoria Hospital was appointed Consultant Surgeon to the Ards Hospital in 1950. Nevertheless he continued as Visiting Consultant to hold a special clinic for hand injuries in the Royal Victoria Hospital, and he was on the Medical Staff Committee from 1962 until his retirement in 1969.

Robert Irvine Wilson joined the Orthopaedic Department in 1953. He had graduated at Queen's in 1938, served in the RAMC during World War Two in North Africa and Sicily (being awarded the MBE in 1944), and

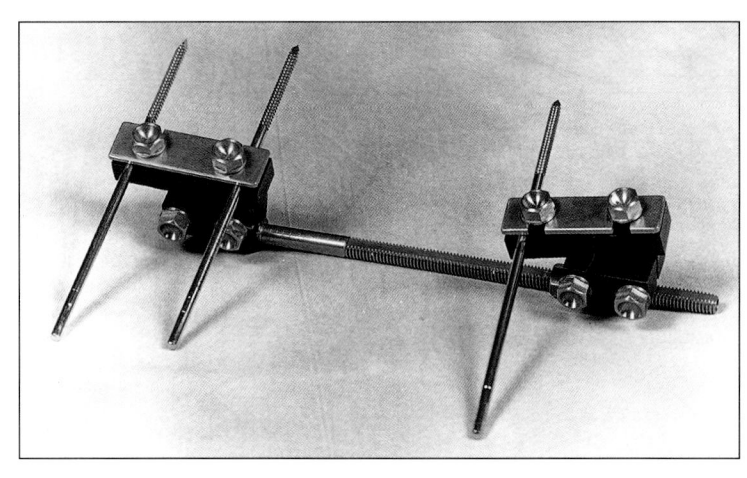

The Belfast Fixator, prototype made in Mackie's foundry: the heavier threaded bar runs parallel with the skin and four pins (three of which are shown) are inserted into the bone, two above and two below the fracture, to maintain the broken surfaces in close contact. The device is surprisingly rigid, can be adjusted to improve alignment, and is more comfortable to wear in hot weather than a heavy plaster.
ROYAL VICTORIA HOSPITAL

married a daughter of R.J.W. Withers (see page 112). At the Royal Victoria Hospital he continued to build up the department, as well as being on the staff of the Musgrave Park and the Ulster hospitals, and giving the annual winter oration in 1976; he was appointed to the first chair in Orthopaedic Surgery at Queen's in 1979. He retired in 1982.

In 1965 Mr Paul Harald Osterberg was appointed, having graduated with an MB at Trinity College Dublin in 1953 and trained as an orthopaedic registrar in London. He gave the annual winter oration in 1989, and retired in the same year. His appointment was followed in 1966 by that of Mr John Henry Lowry who retired in 1988; in 1974 by that of Mr Alan Gurd who resigned in 1976 for a post in the USA; in 1977 by that of Mr Ian Adair; and in 1979 by that of Mr John Templeton who resigned in 1988 to become Professor of Traumatic Orthopaedic Surgery at Keele University. In 1979 also, Mr Raymond Alexander Boyce (Rab) Mollan was appointed, though most of his work was carried out at Musgrave Park Hospital where he made a particular study of congenital dislocation of the hip and bioengineering techniques in orthopaedics. He was appointed Professor of Orthopaedic Surgery in 1982, but eventually retired from the chair and his post in the Royal Victoria Hospital early in 1995 to take a part-time post as deacon in the Church of Ireland. Mr Charles Joseph McClelland was appointed Consultant Orthopaedic Surgeon in 1983, Mr Dennis Mawhinney in 1988, Mr Gerald McCoy in 1990 and Mr Reginald Barr in 1993.

GYNAECOLOGY

In the field of gynaecology and obstetrics it is always obstetrics that makes the headlines, and as the age of viability of the foetus has come down from the old, arbitrary date of twenty-eight weeks it has encroached on its sister speciality. The main change that has taken place in gynaecology since the 1950s have been a decrease in the number of minor surgical procedures such as diagnostic dilation and curettage. On the other hand there has been a great increase in sterilisations; a small number of terminations of pregnancy is also carried out for serious medical or genetic problems, even in Northern Ireland where the procedure is still technically illegal. More positively, a totally new field has developed: the management of infertility. This includes hormonal treatment to stimulate ovulation, extrauterine fertilisation, and the reconstruction of the Fallopian tubes to treat sterility, whether caused by disease or by surgery. As in other surgical fields this has become possible with improvements in the technology of fibre optic laparoscopy; indeed it was the gynaecologists who pioneered the development of laparoscopy, now so widespread in many forms of abdominal surgery.

After the advent of the NHS Mr Gavin Boyd was appointed as

Consultant Gynaecologist to the Royal Victoria Hospital in 1948, but the next appointment of Mr Graham Harley was not until 1962. Then, in 1963, on the retirement of Professor Macafee, Professor John (Jack) Pinkerton succeeded him. Mr Gavin Boyd had graduated with an MB at Glasgow in 1936, and came to the Belfast Department of Midwifery and Gynaecology in 1939, married local doctor Anne Elizabeth Kyle and, apart from his years with the RAMC, settled at the hospital for life. His main interest was always in the field of Obstetrics, particularly in the management of recurrent midterm abortion, in hypnosis for obstetrical pain relief, and in critical assessment of the causes of maternal deaths. He retired in 1978. Dr Graham Harley is also a Scot, but was born in Demerara and graduated at Queen's University Belfast. He married Dr Mona McQuitty, an anaesthetist born in Northern Ireland. His major interest was in the interrelation between the endocrine system and obstetrics and particularly the management of diabetes complicating pregnancy. He was appointed to a personal chair in Obstetrics and Gynaecology in 1978, was chairman of the Medical Staff Committee, 1987–89, gave the annual winter oration in 1991, and retired in 1992, being awarded the CBE.

The new Professor of Midwifery and Gynaecology, Dr Jack Pinkerton, a graduate of Queen's, had served in the Royal Navy during World War Two and held academic posts in Jamaica and Harvard. He then became Professor and Consultant in Obstetrics and Gynaecology in Queen Charlotte's Hospital, London, 1958–63, before taking the chair at Queen's University Belfast. His main interest continued to be medical education, especially in the Third World, and he was vice-president of the Royal College of Obstetrics and Gynaecology. He was awarded the CBE in 1982 and retired in 1985.

In 1966 Dr Charles Whitfield was appointed senior lecturer and Consultant in Midwifery and Gynaecology. He had graduated at Queen's University in 1950 and remained in Belfast as a senior lecturer and later reader in the Department of Midwifery and Gynaecology only from 1966 to 1974. He then went to Manchester as Professor in Obstetrics and Gynaecology and was subsequently Regius Professor of Midwifery at Glasgow.

Mr Reginald (Reggie) Magee graduated with an MB at Queen's University in 1937 and after World War Two was appointed Consultant Obstetrician and Gynaecologist at the Massereene Hospital, Antrim, and the Ards Hospital before being appointed to the Ulster, Royal Victoria and Royal Maternity hospitals in 1948. Although on the staff of the Royal Maternity Hospital, he was not appointed a member of the Royal Victoria Hospital Medical Staff Committee until 1966. Over the years he became increasingly involved in administration, being a member of the Northern Ireland Hospitals Authority and chairman of many NHS committees. In 1972 he became actively involved in politics and in subsequent years was elected a member of the Northern Ireland Assembly as an Official Unionist. About the same time he became a member of the Council of the Royal College of Surgeons in Ireland and was elected president 1986–88, following which he was awarded the CBE. He retired from his Consultant appointment in 1979 but was Group Medical Administrator to the Royal Group of Hospitals, 1979–84.

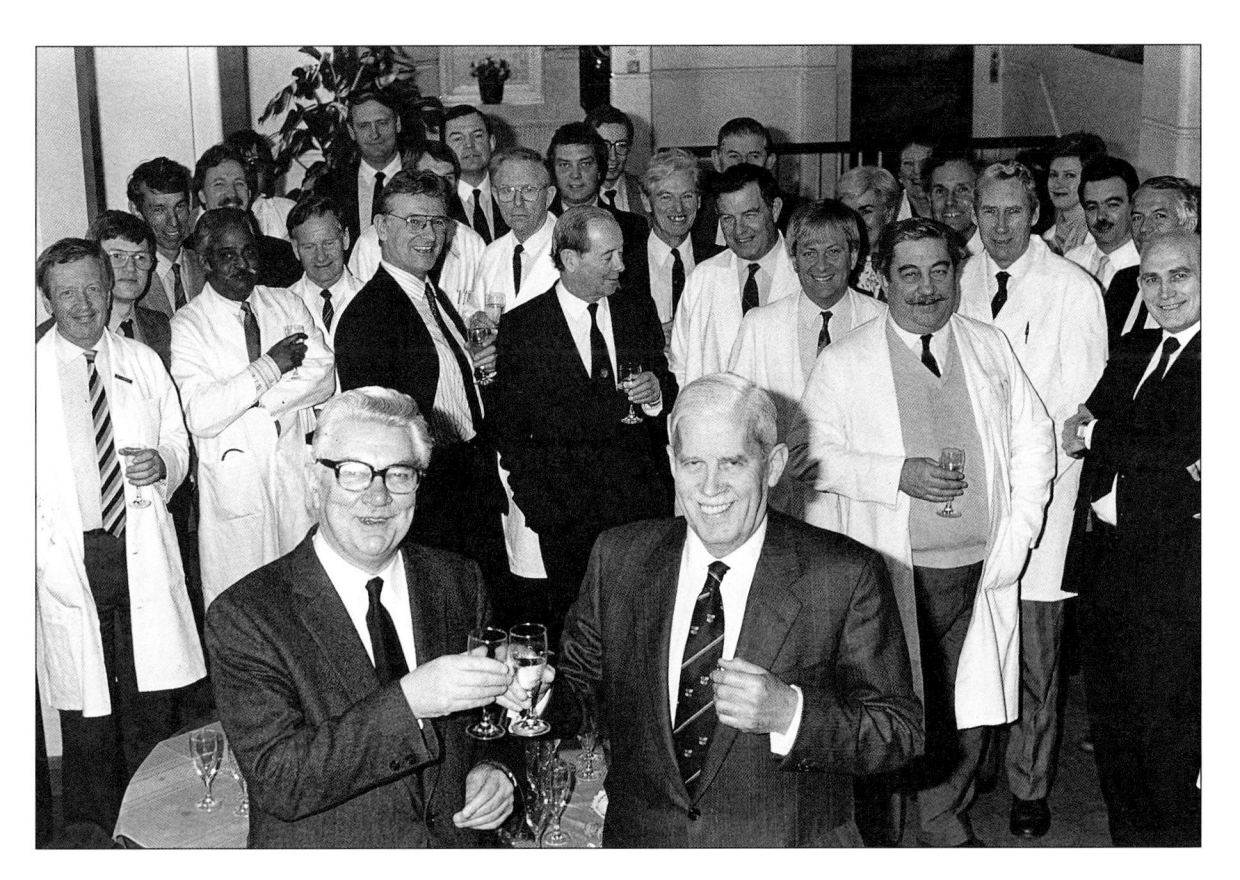

In 1970 Dr William (Billy) Thompson was appointed senior lecturer in Midwifery and Gynaecology and Consultant to the Royal Victoria Hospital. He was appointed Professor of Midwifery (later Obstetrics) and Gynaecology in 1985 to succeed Professor Pinkerton. He has had a career-long interest in the problems of infertility both male and female, and in undergraduate education. Dr Harith Lamki was appointed senior lecturer in Midwifery and Gynaecology and Consultant to the Royal Victoria Hospital in 1972, as was Dr George Murnaghan in 1974. The latter also took on the post of Director of Medical Administration for the Royal Group of Hospitals in 1987. Dr Anthony (Tony) Traub and Dr David Boyle were appointed Consultants to the Royal Victoria and Royal Maternity hospitals in 1980 and 1984, and Dr James (Jim) Dornan was appointed in 1986.

OPHTHALMOLOGY

Although by the pre-1939 era of Mr James Craig and Mr James Wheeler ophthalmology had become almost completely distinct from ear, nose and

New Year 1989: a party to celebrate the awards to Professor John Dundee OBE and Mr Reginald Magee CBE (*front, left and right*). Those visible include Dr Desmond Burrows, Dr Stanley Hawkins, Dr David Wilson, Dr V.K.N. Unni, Dr Howard Fee, Mr George Johnston, Mr Joe McClelland, Mr George Murnaghan, Mr Alan Wilkinson, Dr Dennis Boyle, Mr William Odling-Smee, Dr Jim Dornan, Professor Graham Harley, Dr Rory Corbett, Professor Richard Clarke, Dr Bob Gray, Professor William Thompson, Dr Manton Mills, Miss Liz Duffin, Mr John Gibbons, Professor Ingrid Allen, Professor David Simpson, Mr Derek Gordon, Dr Linda Caughley, Dr Gavin Lavery, Professor Michael Emmerson and Dr Samuel Kielty
ROYAL VICTORIA HOSPITAL

throat surgery, the fields have always been closely associated at the Royal Victoria Hospital. They remained housed together on the corridor of the hospital until their building was demolished in 1960, but had separate floors in the new Eye, Ear, Nose and Throat Hospital, completed in 1965. The first important development in ophthalmology after 1948 was the introduction in the 1950s of the technique of corneal grafting; an extension of the technique of skin grafting, this introduced the public to the idea of transplanting tissues from cadavers into the living.

One of the characteristics of ophthalmic surgery is that it can be carried out safely and effectively under local anaesthesia and this was traditionally always carried out by the surgeon. In the 1940s and 1950s, however, endotracheal techniques were improving steadily and gradually almost all eye surgery came to be carried out under general anaesthesia, with greater comfort for both patient and surgeon. Then, in the late 1980s, the wheel swung back to local block anaesthesia, though this time it was carried out by anaesthetists, whilst better drugs and needles resulted in the patient having conditions quite as comfortable as under general anaesthetic yet with more rapid and safe recovery. The application of microscopical surgical techniques to the eye in 1963 greatly improved the result of intraocular surgery and increased the range of ophthalmic procedures that could be easily and safely undertaken. Similarly the adoption of laser photocoagulation in 1972 for the treatment of retinal disorders was a giant step forward in treating diabetic eye disease and retinal detachments.

The surgical appointments in the field after Mr J.A. Corkey began with Mr Eric Cecil Cowan, who graduated at Queen's in 1952 and was appointed Ophthalmologist to the Ophthalmic Hospital and to the Royal Victoria Hospital in 1960. He retired in 1992. The next appointment was of Mr Victor Alexander Faris Martin in 1964; he had served in the RAF during World War Two and had been a Consultant Surgeon at the Benn and Ophthalmic hospitals since 1950. He retired in 1978. In 1964 Mr Robert Baird was also appointed having been a Consultant at the Benn and Ophthalmic hospitals since 1956 and 1958 respectively. He retired in 1981. Mr Charles Maguire was appointed in 1967 (retiring in 1994); Professor Desmond Archer followed in 1972 and became the first Professor of Ophthalmology in the university. The chair was designated the Sir Charles Blackmore Chair in recognition of the contribution of Sir Charles, a senior civil servant, in raising money for the visually handicapped in Northern Ireland and also of the assistance of the Home for the Blind (of which he was chairman) in helping fund the university department. Mr Stewart Johnston was appointed in 1973 and retired in 1993, Mr William Logan was appointed in 1975, retiring in 1994, Mr John Bryars and Mr Patrick Johnston were appointed in 1978, Mr Trevor Buchanan and Miss Yvonne Canavan were appointed in 1981, Mr David George Frazer was appointed in 1991, Mr Brian Page was appointed in 1989, Mr F.G. ('Frank')

McGinnity was appointed in 1993, and Mr James Sharkey was appointed in 1994.

EAR, NOSE AND THROAT SURGERY

The antibiotic era probably made more changes in this field than in any other branch of surgery, and much acute and chronic ear disease has virtually disappeared. This in turn has enabled surgeons to concentrate on the field of tumours of the whole region and on the surgical treatment of deafness. Tumours of the pharynx and larynx pose some of the most difficult management problems in surgery. The actual surgery inevitably interferes with respiration and swallowing, and a safe outcome has only been possible with technical advances in anaesthesia. In addition, the long-term social and psychological management of patients after laryngectomy and other mutilating surgery has shown that patients can cope with such problems and that radical surgery is well worthwhile.

Acoustic neurinoma is a benign tumour but important as a cause of deafness and potentially lethal when it expands into the brain. Its management is of interest because of the co-operation required between several departments in diagnosis and surgery. Surgical treatment of other causes of deafness and of the broader problems of Ménière's disease (including tinnitus and vertigo) have also expanded steadily. In all these fields improvements in the operating microscope have played a large part.

Otosclerosis, in which the mechanism of the ear 'seizes up', is an inherited condition; surgical treatment by fenestration really only began in the early 1950s. The other cause of deafness was, of course, infection of the middle ear and mastoid cavity and it is only in recent years that surgery for this problem has ceased to be required.

At the beginning of the NHS, ear, nose and throat surgery in the Royal Victoria Hospital was still in the hands of Mr J.R. Wheeler, Mr Frank MacLaughlin and Mr Kennedy Hunter, and Mr Henry Aitken was appointed as a new Consultant. Mr Henry Aitken graduated at Aberdeen in 1928 and trained as an ear, nose and throat surgeon in Sheffield and Birmingham before joining the RAMC during World War Two. He was appointed as Consultant Surgeon at the Benn and Royal Victoria hospitals in 1948. He retired in 1972 to live in Bridlington, Yorkshire.

The speciality was in great difficulties until 1965 when the new block was opened. However, several consultant appointments were made in preparation for this: of Mr Robert McCrea in 1959, followed by Mr David Craig and Mr Gordon Smyth in 1964. Mr 'Bob' McCrea, who was born in Fintona, County Tyrone, trained as an ear, nose and throat surgeon at Belfast and Newcastle upon Tyne. Throughout most of his life his main interest was in the field of malignant disease, but when poor health caused him to reduce his heavy surgical load, he did pioneering work for deaf children in the field of audiometry. He retired in 1982 and upgraded his Open University BA to an Honours BA before he died in the following year. A hospital lecture in Otolaryngology was established in his honour in 1986. Queen's graduate Mr David Hanna Craig was appointed ear, nose and throat surgeon to the Belfast Hospital for Sick Children in 1938 before joining the RAMC during World War Two. After the war he was Consultant at the Royal Belfast Hospital for Sick Children and the Belfast City and Benn hospitals, before being appointed to the Royal Victoria Hospital in 1964; he was particularly noted for his skill in handling fractious and distressed children. He retired in 1974 and subsequently published *Belfast and its Infirmary*, a history of the Belfast City Hospital (1985).

Mr Gordon Smyth was the son of Dr Jack Smyth, Physician and Biochemist of the Royal Victoria Hospital (see page 132). Gordon Smyth trained as an otologist in Memphis, Tennessee, and Belfast, and from his appointment in 1964 he devoted himself to all aspects of ear surgery; his large series of tympanoplasty operations was unique in the world both in its size and in the detail of his critical assessment of results. He was not only a brilliant surgeon but a dynamic organiser and enthusiastic communicator. He published nearly two hundred papers on his work, taught all who came, in both operating theatre and in courses, and lectured at meetings all over the world. With all his activities he managed to see his patients seven days a week, to follow up almost indefinitely, and to give a considered plan of treatment for every patient. His distinctions included a D.Sc. from Queen's University Belfast, an invitation to give the Toynbee Lecture of the Royal College of Surgeons of England (which had to be given for him after his death) and the obituary tribute of a colleague that he was the leading British middle-ear surgeon of the 1970s and 1980s.

Mr Harold Shepperd graduated at Queen's in 1947 and trained as an ear, nose and throat surgeon in London and Belfast. His first appointment was to the Lagan Valley Hospital, Lisburn, County Antrim, in 1959; he was appointed a Consultant at the Royal Victoria Hospital in 1966, retiring two decades later in 1986. He had a broad range of interests in his speciality and also managed to continue an attachment with the Royal Naval Reserve for nearly thirty years. The next appointment to the department was Mr Alan Kerr, who graduated in 1958 and trained at Belfast and the Harvard Medical School before taking up his Consultant post in 1968. He was the first Professor of Otorhinolaryngology at Queen's University, from 1979 to 1981. His appointment was followed in 1972 by that of Mr Robert (Roy) Gibson who had trained in Belfast and St Louis, Missouri. Mr Michael Cinnamond trained in Belfast and the Toronto Children's Hospital before being appointed Consultant in 1976. He was appointed Professor of Otorhinolaryngology at Queen's in 1981 and held the chair for fifteen years, before resigning from it and his post at the Royal Victoria Hospital in 1996. More recent appointments have been those of Mr Francis D'Arcy

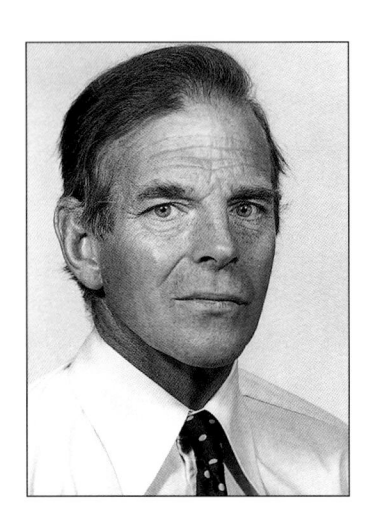

Mr Gordon Smyth, Consultant Otolaryngologist to the Royal Victoria Hospital from 1964 until his death in 1992
ROYAL VICTORIA HOSPITAL

in 1979, Mr A. Peter Walby in 1983, Mr David Adams in 1984, and Mr William Primrose in 1986.

NEUROSURGERY

Probably the earliest planned neurosurgical operations in the Royal Victoria Hospital were carried out by Professor Fullerton in the 1920s, followed more actively in the 1930s by Mr Barney Purce, but the results from these operations were fairly disastrous. Inevitably, of course, only quite advanced problems were submitted to neurosurgery, mainly cerebral tumours and abscesses, and with the knowledge of the period, a mortality of 50 per cent is hardly surprising. Mr Cecil Calvert operated with Mr Purce before World War Two but it was his return from service in 1945 that led to the setting up of a neurosurgical unit in the following year, encouraged by Dr Sydney Allison. In 1945 Mr Calvert had a few beds in wards 9 and 10, and in 1946 he was given twelve beds in wards 11 and 12, operating in the fracture clinic theatre (off the extern hall). Mr Calvert gave the opening address for the winter session of the hospital in 1946; reviewing the history of neurosurgery, he showed that even in World War One good management of penetrating head wounds by British surgeons, using experience from the Boer War, had brought the mortality down from 60 per cent to about 30 per cent. The use of sulphonamides and penicillin and better surgical and anaesthetic technique during World War Two, especially in Sir Hugh Cairns's unit in Oxford, meant that in that conflict the corresponding mortality fell to about 10 per cent.

The Neurosurgical Department was well established by 1947, though it did not have its own dedicated operating theatre until the end of the year. During 1947 there were 109 neurosurgical operations, including 28 for brain tumour, 28 ventriculograms, 12 head injuries, 11 spinal problems, 10 brain abscesses and 10 myelograms. The technique of arteriography was starting and the first of these procedures in Belfast was carried out; altogether it is evident that investigation, particularly by x-ray contrast, was already playing a large part in diagnosis. Dr Sydney Allison's neurology unit was set up in 1948 but the complete building of Quin House for the partnership of neurology and neurosurgery, with its x-ray and EEG facilities, was not opened until 1953.

Neurosurgeons at this stage were well aware of the problems of raised intracranial pressure, and the advantages of using external ventricular drainage to remove excess cerebrospinal fluid, and of dehydration therapy, were established. With these considerations went the special problems of bleeding within the cranial cavity; diathermy, silver clips and fibrin foam had come into use. The role of ensuring adequate ventilation or active hyperventilation to minimise bleeding and lower pressure came in the 1960s.

The 1950s saw the introduction of the operation of prefrontal leucotomy, now rarely performed, for certain forms of schizophrenia; there was also early work on the surgical treatment of Parkinsonism. In the same period, collaboration with the endocrinologists made removal of the pituitary (either for tumour or for management of breast cancer) a possibility; this work developed into effective treatment of acromegaly. Interestingly, in all these fields new drugs have removed the need for surgery; with drugs, benefits and side effects can be balanced in the course of treatment. The collaboration with otolaryngologists in the surgery of acoustic neurinoma has been mentioned earlier. In the whole range of planned neurosurgery the introduction of the operating microscope in the early 1970s was probably the biggest technical advance of the twentieth century.

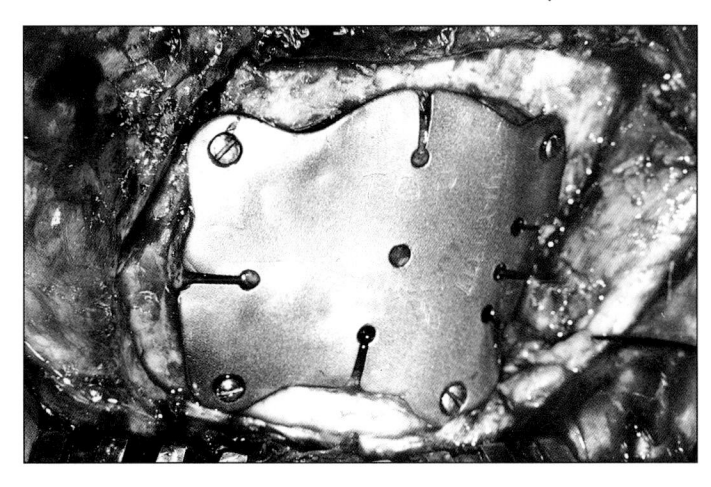

But it is the management of head injuries caused by both road traffic accidents and civil disturbance that has taken up much of the time of the neurosurgical unit. Mr Alan Crockard was involved in research on raised intracranial pressure at the height of the Troubles and described it in his Calvert Lecture of 1973. Mr Derek Gordon, in a review of head injuries fourteen years later, stressed the interdependence of accident and emergency unit, intensive care unit, neurosurgical ward and neuroradiology, the last now strengthened by the introduction of CT scanning. Another interesting collaboration came with the development of titanium plates in the School of Dentistry to cover defects in the skull following trauma.

Titanium plate specially made to cover a defect in a patient's skull, screwed in position (technique first described in an article by D.S. Gordon and G.A.S. Blair in 1974)
MR D. GORDON AND ROYAL VICTORIA HOSPITAL

The first neurosurgeon to be appointed after Mr Calvert was Mr Rainier Campbell Connolly (MRCS, LRCP St Bartholomew's, London, 1941) who was appointed Consultant Neurosurgeon in 1950 but resigned in 1952 to take up a post in a Birmingham hospital and later returned to St Bartholomew's. He was followed by Mr Alex Taylor, who had graduated in Aberdeen in 1941, served in the RNVR and trained as a neurosurgeon in Edinburgh. He was appointed Consultant in 1952 and had a particular interest in spinal cord surgery; he resigned because of ill health in 1974. Mr Colin Gleadhill was appointed Consultant in 1957, having graduated with an MB in Edinburgh in 1939 and an MD in 1941. He was especially interested in cerebral vascular problems and in the pituitary; he retired in 1979. His daughter Dr Valerie Gleadhill was married to the accident and emergency consultant Dr Peter Nelson (see page 220).

The fourth neurosurgeon of this early group was Mr Derek Gordon, who graduated at Queen's in 1948 and trained in Belfast and at the Massachusetts General Hospital, Boston. He was appointed Consultant

Neurosurgeon in 1960 and published many papers on the work of the department, being awarded the OBE in 1976 for his work with trauma during the Troubles (and the CBE in 1988). He gave the winter oration in 1984 and retired in 1989.

There were no further appointments until 1974 when Mr Ian Bailey was appointed Consultant Neurosurgeon. He had trained in King's College Hospital, London, and had set up the neurosurgical unit in Makere College, University of East Africa, Kampala, before settling in to an active life of surgery and research in Belfast. He retired in 1995. Mr Alan Crockard also was appointed Consultant Neurosurgeon in 1974, but he resigned in 1978 to take up a post in the National Hospital for Nervous Diseases, Queen Square, London. Subsequent Consultant appointments have been Mr Dermot Byrnes who trained in Dublin and Edinburgh before being appointed Consultant in 1979; and Mr Thomas Fannin, who was appointed in the same year. Mr John Gray was appointed Consultant Neurosurgeon in 1989 and Mr Stephen Cooke was appointed in 1996.

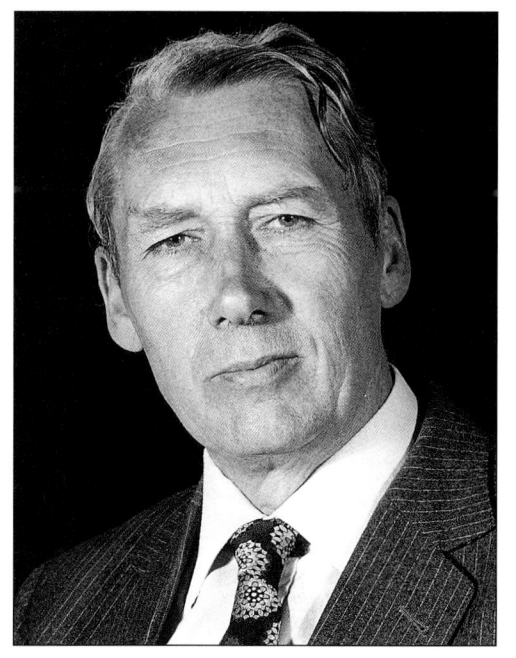

THORACIC AND CARDIAC SURGERY

The early history of thoracic surgery is reviewed in the 1947 presidential address to the Ulster Medical Society by Mr Barney Purce (see pages 114–15), one of the Royal Victoria Hospital's most distinguished general surgeons, who was also, remarkably, a pioneer in both neurosurgery and thoracic surgery. In his address Mr Purce reviews thoracic problems with which we are still familiar, including missile injuries resulting from war or car accidents. The particular problems of the open chest had already been understood and overcome by the anaesthetists, though artificial respiration was still only possible for short periods, during surgery, rather than for long-term life support. However, empyema was still common, presumably because efficient exploration of chest wounds was not practised and effective antibiotics were not freely available. (Certainly isolated chest wounds were still dreaded during World War Two, whereas by the period of the Troubles full recovery would be the expected result.) Mr Purce had performed the first lobectomy for bronchiectasis (a chronic chest disease of children) in 1939 and the disease was still fairly common at the time of Mr Purce's survey and into the 1950s, though now it is rare. The surgery of tuberculosis was well established by 1947, but was still largely collapse therapy to rest the diseased area of the lung. This had started with artificial pneumothorax or paralysis of the phrenic nerve but thoracoplasty, an extensive operation on the chest wall, was also well established. On the other hand surgical excision of the diseased lobe or lung would not become practicable until streptomycin became widely available in the

Mr Derek Gordon, Consultant Neurosurgeon to the Royal Victoria Hospital, 1960–89
ROYAL VICTORIA HOSPITAL

1950s. The other factor that would increase the safety of chest surgery was blood transfusion: the Northern Ireland Blood Transfusion Service was just being set up at the time of Mr Purce's address.

Surgery for lung cancer was practised in the 1940s but the disease was not as well recognised at that time and the few patients who reached the surgeon appeared too late to be surgically treatable. It was only in the early 1950s that Richard Doll's papers began to appear linking the disease with smoking. Only then did people become aware of its early symptoms such as cough, 'flu-like feelings', shortness of breath, chest pain and coughing up blood. The situation had changed radically by 1956, when Mr T.B. Smiley could review 91 operations. Similarly oesophageal cancer was usually only seen when severe obstruction was present and palliative treatment with radium was the best that could be offered. At this time only 2–5 per cent of patients with either type of cancer were surviving for five years.

In 1947, surgery for tuberculosis was carried out principally at the Whiteabbey and Musgrave Park hospitals; this work was later concentrated in a new unit at Forster Green Hospital. In the Royal Victoria Hospital surgery for lung and oesophageal cancers developed steadily, and such operations soon dominated thoracic theatre lists. In subsequent years, thoracic surgery has increased its scope alongside great advances in anaesthesia, and with the benefit of improved diagnostic facilities. Surgery for benign oesophageal problems developed, as did the management of various benign and malignant mediastinal tumours, including also removal of the thymus gland for certain cases of myasthenia gravis (a rare disease associated with severe muscular weakness).

Since 1969, the thoracic surgical unit has been much involved in the acute management of penetrating chest injuries. Many old lessons in this field have had to be relearnt, and new protocols have had to be developed. Success in alleviating acute chest pain over this period has been the result of close co-operation with the anaesthetists, both in the operating theatre and in pre- and post-operative intensive care. Distinctive techniques such as high-frequency jet ventilation have allowed oxygenation without true breathing, and total intravenous anaesthesia has allowed unconsciousness to be maintained without the taking in of anaesthetic gases through the lungs.

In 1947 two new thoracic surgeons had already returned from the war and were working in the hospital under the government's rehabilitation scheme. Mr T.B. (Tom) Smiley had graduated with an MB at Queen's in 1939 and almost at once joined the RAMC. He was posted to the Far East and was in Singapore when it fell, only escaping death when a Japanese bayonet was deflected by his cigarette case. He survived the war years as a prisoner and was later awarded the Military Cross; he had also made contacts that induced him to become a thoracic surgeon. For this he trained at the Brompton Hospital, London, and then returned to Belfast, where he was appointed Consultant in 1951. He carried out the first mitral valvotomy in Ireland in 1950 while still a registrar, and he started open-heart surgery in 1960, but he always carried out the full range of adult thoracic surgery. He was an enthusiastic extrovert, often singing while he was operating ('The Lord's My Shepherd'); outside medicine he was a keen huntsman. He gave the annual oration in 1974 on 'Medical students and their education' and retired early, in 1977, to spend a year as Visiting Professor of Surgery in Kuala Lumpur before settling in Norfolk where he died in 1981. His brother James, his wife Elizabeth and two of his sons became doctors.

Mr John A.W. Bingham, another Queen's graduate, had already completed his surgical training before World War Two, in Windsor and Roehampton. He served throughout the war in India and the Far East. After the war he too worked in the Brompton Hospital. On returning to Belfast he was appointed Thoracic Surgeon to the Royal Belfast Hospital for Sick Children in 1947 before joining the Consultant staff of the Royal Victoria Hospital in 1951. He continued throughout his life to operate in the thoracic and closed cardiac field, on both adults and children. In personality he was in marked contrast to his colleague Tom Smiley, with few words on any occasion, and he resisted all attempts by his colleagues to get him married. His operations were quick and quietly uneventful and even if a rare mishap did occur, it seemed to be repaired before the anaesthetist a few feet away was aware of it. He was devoted to golf and retired in 1976, but after several heart attacks he died in 1983. He was first cousin of Dr William Bingham, anaesthetist, who is father of Dr Ann Bingham, dermatologist, both of the Royal Victoria Hospital.

The third member of the thoracic team, and until 1977 the only other member, was Mr H. Morris Stevenson, son of the surgeon Mr Howard Stevenson (see page 108). He qualified at Queen's with honours and many prizes in 1943 and served in the RNVR before training in thoracic surgery at the Brompton Hospital. He was appointed Consultant Thoracic Surgeon at the Royal Victoria Hospital in 1953 and was active in all types of thoracic and closed cardiac surgery, as well as in the early stages of open-heart surgery in Belfast. He gave the annual winter oration in 1982 and retired in 1986.

A more recent appointment in thoracic surgery was Mr John Gibbons (MB Leeds, 1954) who trained at the National Heart Hospital, London, and was Accident & Emergency Consultant at the Royal Free Hospital, London, before being appointed Consultant Thoracic Surgeon at the Royal Victoria Hospital in 1977. He retired in 1993, having maintained close links with the RAMC throughout his career. Mr James (Jim) McGuigan was appointed Consultant Thoracic Surgeon in 1988 and Mr Kieran McManus likewise was appointed Consultant Thoracic Surgeon in 1993.

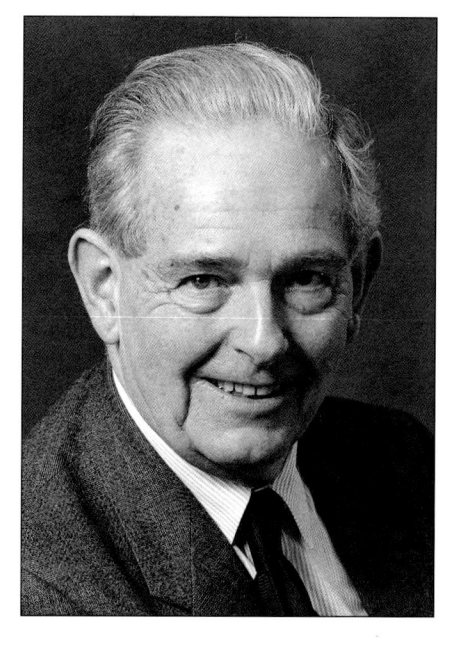

Mr Morris Stevenson,
Consultant Thoracic Surgeon to the
Royal Victoria Hospital, 1957–86
ROYAL VICTORIA HOSPITAL

Surgery of the heart and great vessels began only after World War Two. Mr Purce performed the first ligation of a patent ductus arteriosus (a common but important congenital shunt) in 1947. The mitral valvotomy, carried out in the Royal Victoria Hospital by Mr Smiley in 1950, with Dr Maurice Brown giving the anaesthetic, was the first actual operation on the heart in Northern Ireland. The procedure involved stretching the partly closed mitral valve with the finger while at the same time taking care not to make the valve incompetent. The first operation was successful; the extent of the need is indicated by a report three years later of 121 cases treated by surgery, including three pregnant patients. By 1957 there had been four hundred such operations altogether, carried out in the Royal Victoria Hospital by Mr Smiley, Mr Bingham and Mr Stevenson. The operative mortality by this time had fallen to 1.4 per cent, and it continued to fall, whilst some improvement was noted in 80 per cent of patients. The operation remained the mainstay of thoracic surgical lists throughout the 1950s, 1960s and 1970s, only becoming less common when open-heart surgery could permit repair with better results and an acceptably low mortality.

The next surgical procedure on the heart to become established in the late 1950s was closure of a simple atrial septal defect (the simplest kind of hole in the heart). For this procedure the patient was cooled to 30–32° centigrade in a galvanised bath of iced water, then laid on the operating table on a water-circulating blanket, and the operation was started. The circulation to the heart could then be cut off and the defect closed with stitches in four to eight minutes. This worked well so long as the diagnosis by the physicians was absolutely correct – which was not always the case with the radiological techniques then available. The other hazard was ventricular fibrillation (a form of cardiac arrest) which occasionally resulted from excessive cooling. Pulmonary valvotomies were also carried out in this period using the same techniques; all these operations for congenital defects of the heart were carried out by the three cardio-thoracic surgeons.

The techniques then available could be used for only a small minority of cardiac problems, and disaster was likely if physician, surgeon or anaesthetist made any mistake in diagnosis or treatment. Open-heart surgery offered more flexibility if there were any difficulties, but it involved the revolutionary concept of replacing the heart, during an operation, by two pumps in series and replacing the lungs by some type of oxygenator. The first open-heart operation in the UK was performed at Hammersmith Hospital in 1958. Over the subsequent decades, there has been a steady improvement in the oxygenators from the early Melrose disc oxygenator, which required a priming volume of four litres of fresh blood, took about half a day to set up and a day to clean afterwards, and damaged the blood more and more during every hour in which the patient was exposed to it.

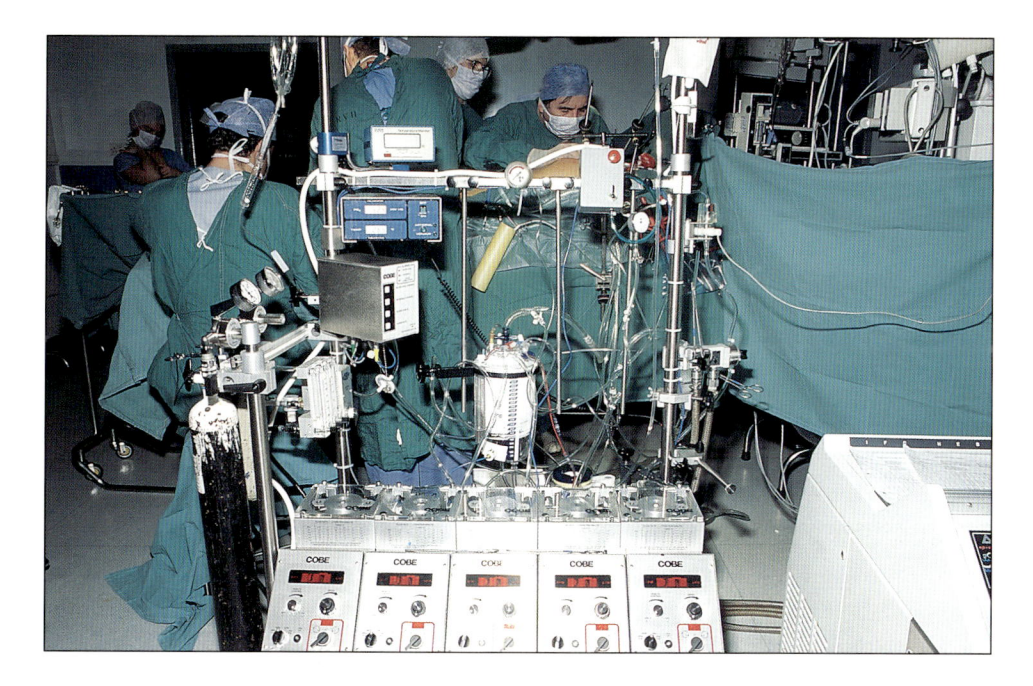

Now we have disposable plastic equipment which can be set up in a few minutes, which requires no blood except to replace blood lost, and which can be run for several hours (though still restricted to a finite surgical procedure).

It was in 1960, in the Royal Victoria Hospital, that the first patient underwent open-heart surgery in Belfast. Again the pioneer was Mr Smiley, with Dr Maurice Brown as anaesthetist. In the following year Mr Stevenson took over, working in the Royal Belfast Hospital for Sick Children, with Dr Harold Love and Dr Gerry Black as anaesthetists. Dr Richard Clarke, Dr Manus O'Donnell and Dr Connor Mulholland were Registrar pump operators and cardiologists.

One difficulty of the earlier days of open-heart surgery in Belfast was that the easier conditions had been treated by closed techniques, leaving the more difficult and chronic problems as a challenge for the new procedure. The selection of patients was made entirely by the cardiologists, and in the early years the flow of cases was too slow to allow a sufficient expertise to be built up by the team. At all events, for a variety of reasons the unit moved back to the Royal Victoria Hospital, and stuttered to a halt in 1965. In the following year Professor Alphonsus D'Abreu from Birmingham was asked to report with plans for a new approach; these proposals, plus a large injection of funding, enabled the hospital to make a fresh start.

This was made in June 1968 with Mr Patrick (Pat) Molloy as leader of the team and Dr Morrell Lyons, fresh from a year in Houston, Texas, as the full-time Anaesthetist. Dr Richard Clarke was part-time Anaesthetist with the team, Sister Liz Lattimore was the senior theatre sister, and Mr Jim McIlroy and Mr Ernie Stewart were the pump technicians. Mr Molloy was energetic and optimistic, prepared to work all the hours in the day, and the team soon built up to five cases weekly, taking on the full pre- and

Pumps (*foreground*), oxygen cylinder and flowmeters (*left*) and membrane oxygenator (*centre*), forming the 'heart–lung machine' and showing the compact disposable plastic equipment now available
ROYAL VICTORIA HOSPITAL

post-operative selection and management of patients.

Mr Patrick John Molloy had graduated with an MB at Otago University, New Zealand, in 1952 and trained in thoracic and cardiac surgery in Guy's Hospital, London, and Broad Green Hospital, Liverpool, where he was Consultant Thoracic Surgeon before being appointed Consultant Cardiac Surgeon at the Royal Victoria Hospital in 1968. Whilst still relatively young, he was an excellent organiser and a good leader; he had the great ability to carry the team with him however hard he expected them to work. He and his wife Jewel were very hospitable and the parties given in their large house on the Malone Road were memorable. Equally memorable was the fact of his nine daughters followed eventually by an Irish son; it was the worry of bringing up a large family in strife-torn Belfast that induced him to return to his native New Zealand in 1973.

Mr John (Jack) Cleland, a Queen's graduate who trained in cardiac and thoracic surgery in Belfast and at the Mayo Clinic in Rochester, Minnesota, before returning from the USA to the Royal Victoria Hospital as Senior Registrar, was appointed Consultant Cardiac Surgeon in 1971. He was joined on Mr Molloy's resignation by Mr Hugh O'Kane, a Queen's graduate who had trained in St Louis and the Mayo Clinic. In spite of increasing pressure for more operations to be performed, there were no further appointments until that of Mr A.E. 'Freddie' Wood, who was appointed in 1982 to have a major responsibility for the surgery of congenital heart disease. He resigned in 1983 and Mr Dennis Gladstone was appointed in 1987. More recent appointments have been Mr Mazen Sarsam and Mr Gianfranco Campalani, both of whom were appointed Consultant Cardiac Surgeons in 1993, and Mr Simon MacGowan, appointed in 1996. Mr Jack Cleland retired in 1995.

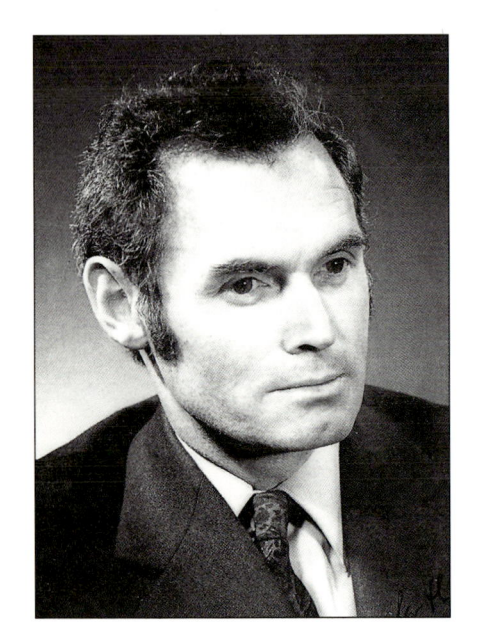

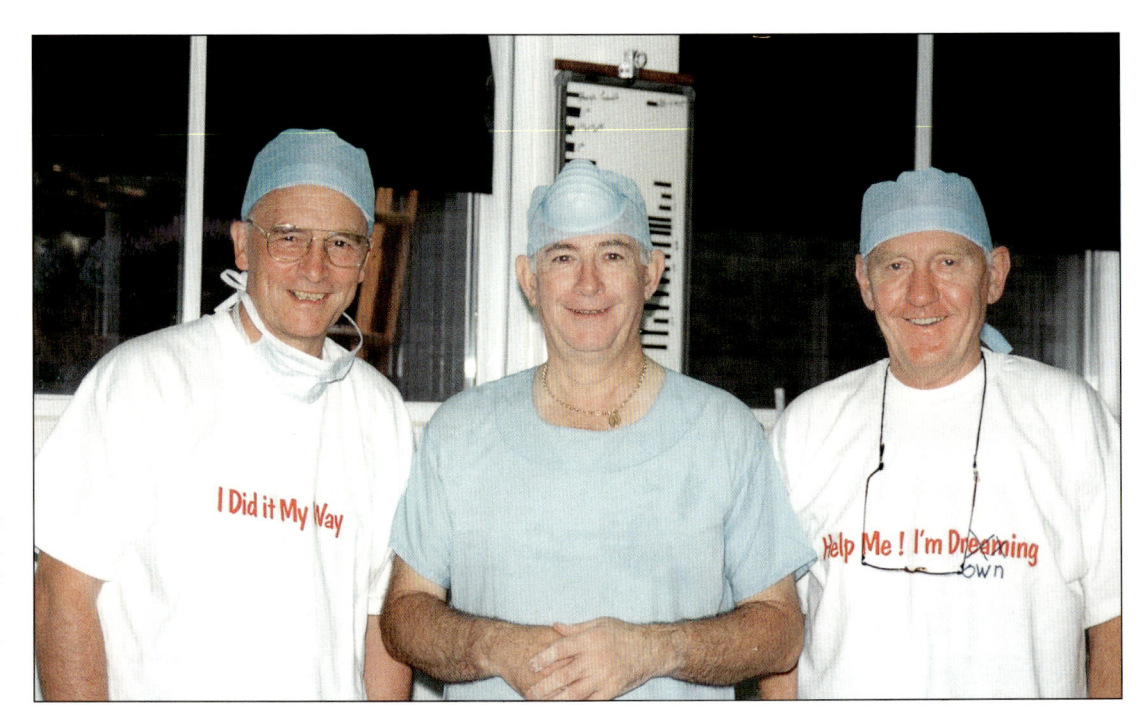

Mr Patrick Molloy, Consultant Cardiac Surgeon to the Royal Victoria Hospital, 1968–73, the major force in restarting open-heart surgery in the hospital
ROYAL VICTORIA HOSPITAL

Left to right: Dr Morrell Lyons, Cardiac Anaesthetist, Mr Jack Cleland, Cardiac Surgeon, and Ernie Stewart, pump technician, on Mr Cleland's last day in the operating theatre in 1995; all had worked in open-heart surgery since 1958.
ROYAL VICTORIA HOSPITAL

After its inception the new team carefully gained experience with the repair of simpler congenital defects and single valve replacements. The initial results were excellent, and very quickly they moved to the more difficult valve operations and to younger and younger 'blue' babies with Fallot's tetralogy and transposition of the great vessels. The arrival of Mr O'Kane coincided with the proven beneficial effects of coronary arterial surgery and this quickly became the dominant type of operation (70 per cent, with valve surgery at 16 per cent and congenital at 14 per cent of the total).

From the outset one of the strengths of the newly established unit was its ability for total patient care in the cardiac recovery ward, later named the Cardiac Surgical Intensive Care ward. The first sister was Lorna Irwin; she was followed by Hazel Harper and then by Sara Gray. Initially the patient stay averaged four or five days, but the 1980s brought a period of marked improvement in the post-operative status of all patients and this, allied to a pressure for greater throughput as workloads increased, saw the stay drop to two to three days. The Cardiac Surgical Intensive Care ward became a bottleneck restricting further expansion, and in 1992 an extension to the unit of a further five beds was opened by Mr J.W.S. Irwin. Soon afterwards a High Dependency Unit was opened in Ward 12 as a step-down facility before return to the general ward. This expansion of the unit, and the shortening of the time spent under intensive care in particular, meant that the number of surgeons could be increased from three in 1987 to five in 1993, with the workload now limited only by the available funding.

The Consultant Anaesthetists working in cardiac surgery have in general been solely committed to the unit and it is appropriate to list them here. Dr Morrell Lyons, a Queen's graduate, undertook training in cardiac anaesthesia in Houston, before being appointed as the first full-time Consultant Cardiac Anaesthetist in 1968. He was elected president of the Association of Anaesthetists of Great Britain and Ireland from 1994 to 1996 and was awarded the OBE in 1996. Another Queen's graduate, Dr J.D. (Jim) Morrison, was appointed in 1971 but resigned in 1974 to take up a post at the Izaak Walton Killian Hospital in Halifax, Nova Scotia. Dr Ian Carson was appointed in 1975 but reduced his commitment in 1993 to become Medical Director of the Royal Hospitals Trust. Dr Ian Orr held an appointment from 1983 to 1986, resigning for a post at Craigavon Area Hospital. Dr Peter Elliott, son of Dr Jim Elliott (see page 209), had already been a Consultant Anaesthetist since 1985 when he took on sessions in the unit in 1987 and became full-time in 1992. Dr Terry McMurray, after a year in the Groote Schurr Hospital, Cape Town, and Dr Fiona Gibson (Mrs McNulty) were appointed in 1987. Dr Moyna Bill was appointed in 1991 and after a year in Leyden took up a post in the unit in 1992. Dr A.S. (Sally Anne) Phillips was appointed in 1994, and Dr William McBride was appointed in 1996, both the latter having spent a year in Durham, North Carolina.

PLASTIC SURGERY AND BURNS

The impetus to start a plastic surgery unit is thought to have been provided by the *Reina del Pacifico* engine room explosion in 1947, when many burn casualties were brought from the ship to the hospital. These were treated first with sodium hypochloric and salt (Milton) solution, using equipment specially flown over from London, but the patients later had to be transferred to East Grinstead, Surrey, for plastic surgery. The Throne Hospital was an obvious venue for a plastic surgery unit since it had sufficient space and an operating theatre, where repair of hernias and other routine procedures were regularly being carried out.

The first plastic surgical operation recorded at the Throne Hospital was in September 1950 when a fractured malar (cheek bone) and facial scars were operated on by Mr Norman Hughes. Dental operations began in 1953 and over the next few years the combined speciality built up until in 1967 about two thousand plastic and dental procedures were performed; general surgical procedures had dropped to 10 per cent of the total operations at the Throne. The types of plastic procedures carried out in the hospital ranged from treatment of extensive burns with cross-leg flaps to treatment of advanced sepsis in a mandible. Occasionally emergencies were brought in requiring major plastic surgery, but in the absence of a twenty-four-hour x-ray and laboratory service at the hospital for crossmatching blood, the hospital was unsatisfactory for emergency work.

Surgery in the Throne Hospital for the first half of the twentieth century had been carried out in a little theatre sited on a half-landing midway between the two floors of the building. There was no lift and patients were taken to and from it on stretchers (or walking if possible). In 1954, however, a gift of £15,000 from the Royal Victoria Hospital Ex-patients' Guild made it possible to build a new twin-theatre suite with modern preparation and changing rooms. The Northern Ireland Hospitals Authority contributed a further £10,000 to complete the project, but it was not until 1964 that a bed lift was installed. The beds situation was improved in that year by the reallocation of the convalescent beds that still remained to plastic and general surgery. In the same year a portable lift for transferring severely burned patients from bed to bath was purchased. A dental laboratory had already been opened in 1962 to support maxillo-facial surgery, and in 1966 a very expensive operating microscope was purchased.

The decision had already been made, however, to transfer plastic surgery to a purpose-built unit in the Ulster Hospital, and in November 1968 the speciality moved to its new home (taking the operating microscope). The

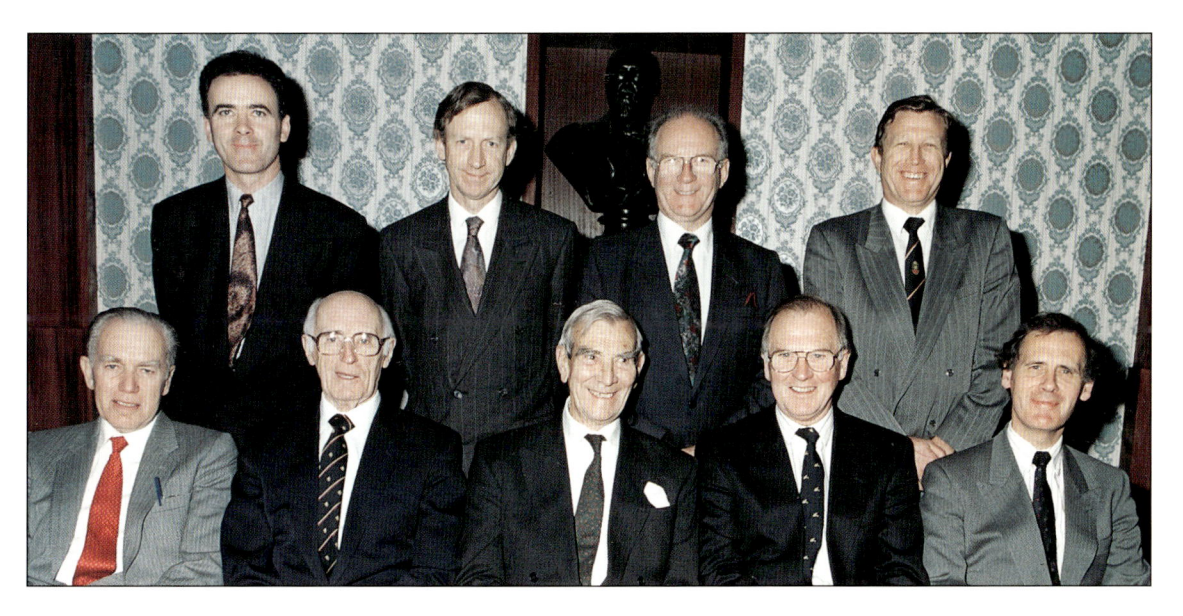

Throne Hospital continued taking routine oral surgery until 1975 and then reverted to its nonacute role, mainly for geriatrics. It was closed in 1992.

The first Plastic Surgeon appointed was Mr Norman Campbell Hughes, in 1950. He had graduated at Queen's University in 1937, and served with the RAMC during World War Two, with a commando unit in Norway and in the Middle East. He then trained at East Grinstead, Surrey, and in 1950 was appointed Consultant Plastic Surgeon at the Royal Victoria Hospital and Royal Belfast Hospital for Sick Children. He gave the annual winter oration to the Royal Victoria Hospital in 1968 on 'A short history of plastic surgery' and led the unit through its move to the Ulster Hospital in that year. He was a leading member of the planning team of the Royal Victoria Hospital and served on the Northern Ireland Hospitals Authority, being awarded the OBE in 1979. He retired in 1979 and in 1992 he unveiled a plaque naming the burns unit in the Royal Victoria Hospital the Norman C. Hughes Regional Burns Unit.

Mr W.R. (Wilbert) Dickie graduated at Queen's in 1940 and subsequently worked with the British Red Cross in China; he trained in plastic surgery in the Manchester Royal Infirmary and the Throne Hospital. He was appointed Consultant Plastic Surgeon at the Royal Belfast Hospital for Sick Children in 1954 and the Royal Victoria Hospital in 1958; he moved with the unit at the Throne to the Ulster Hospital in 1968 and retired in 1980.

Mr John Colville graduated at Queen's in 1955, trained in Belfast and Pittsburgh, and was appointed Consultant Plastic Surgeon to the Royal Victoria Hospital and Royal Belfast Hospital for Sick Children in 1968. He had a particular interest in hand surgery and was president of the British Society for Surgery of the Hand in 1988 and of the British Association of Plastic Surgeons in 1990. He retired in 1990.

Mr R.M. (Ronnie) Slater was Consultant Plastic Surgeon 1971–91; Mr Robert (Roy) Millar was appointed in 1978; Mr Michael Brennen and Mr

At the opening of the Norman C. Hughes Regional Burns Unit, 1979, plastic and maxillo-facial surgeons at the Royal Victoria Hospital: *standing, left to right:* Mr James Small, Mr Alan Leonard, Professor Michael Emmerson and Dr Richard Kendrick; *seated, left to right:* Mr John Colville, Mr William Dickie, Mr Norman Hughes, Mr Ronald Slater and Mr Roy Millar
ROYAL VICTORIA HOSPITAL

Alan Leonard were appointed in 1979.

Throughout the period when the plastic surgery unit was in the Throne Hospital, the outpatient clinics were held in the Royal Victoria Hospital, and there they have continued to the present time, attended by the various plastic surgeons on the staff of the hospital. With the departure of the plastic surgery unit from the Throne to the Ulster Hospital, however, it was soon felt that a unit specially for burns was needed in conjunction with the emergency facilities of the Royal Victoria Hospital. A burns unit (Ward 38), with 14 beds and an operating theatre, was therefore set up in 1979 with Mr Roy Millar as the Surgeon in Charge and Dr Hilary Johnston as the Anaesthetist. It has continued to treat mainly burns, with a small number of plastic procedures and more recently breast reconstruction being carried out.

DENTISTRY

The Dental School of Queen's University Belfast and the Dental Hospital have essentially functioned together and with considerable overlap. Before 1946 all the dental staff were part-time; the first full-time appointment in Dentistry was of Dr James Henderson Scott MD, D.Sc. as lecturer in Anatomy for Dental Students. After his death in 1976, Dr P.D. Adrian Owens was appointed lecturer (1971–77), senior lecturer (1977–82) and then reader (1982–). It was recognised as a great step forward when, in 1947, Professor Philip J. Stoy was appointed as the first Professor of Dentistry, a full-time appointment like those of the post-war medical professors. He was born in Wolverhampton and graduated with a BDS with first-class honours from Birmingham University in 1932. He then held lectureships in Dental Mechanics and Dental Surgery in Bristol, and served in the Royal Navy before being appointed to the chair in Belfast. Here he introduced the five-year degree course (BDS) in 1950, with the same entrance requirements as for medicine. He was founder fellow of the new Faculty of Dentistry of the Royal College of Surgeons in England and of its sister faculty in Ireland, and he remained the senior professor and leader of the School of Dentistry until he retired in 1973. He is commemorated by a bronze bust in the School of Dentistry and was given an honorary MD by Queen's University Belfast in 1987. The present dental building represents the fruits of his energy: although it was not opened until 1965 and he had worked for nearly twenty years in the cramped quarters of the King Edward Building, it had been discussed almost from his appointment.

The School of Dentistry was established within the Faculty of Medicine in 1920 and after Professor Stoy was appointed to the chair of Dentistry he was elected to the new post of Dental Assistant Dean within the Faculty of Medicine. Subsequent Dental Assistant Deans have been Mr C.P. Adams

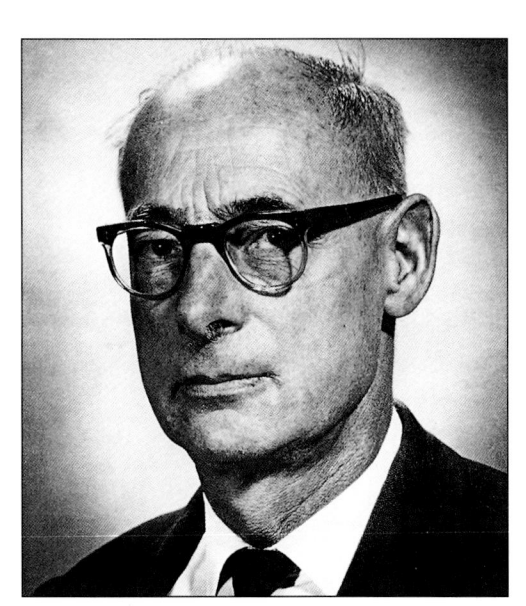

Professor Philip Stoy, first Professor of Dentistry at Queen's University Belfast, 1947–73
ROYAL VICTORIA HOSPITAL

(1974–77), Professor W.A.S. Alldritt (1977–80), and Professor F.V. O'Brien (1980–83). Since a reorganisation in 1983, Dr P.D.A. Owens (1983–84), Professor F.V. O'Brien (1984–88), and Professor I.C. Bennington (1988–) have been designated directors of the School of Clinical Dentistry.

The advent of the National Health Service with its promise of free dental treatment gave people a more positive attitude to their dental health. Gradually the number of applicants for places in the School of Dentistry rose, and altogether dentistry seemed a more intellectually rewarding career. There is more scope now for root fillings, for replacing the visible part of the tooth with a crown, for cast inlays of gold or less conspicuous materials. As a result the majority of the population can hope to retain most of their teeth into middle age, and certainly it is very rare now for a doctor to recommend total clearance of all the teeth, as was often done in the past on dubious grounds. The positive attitude of both dentists and public has been greatly helped by improvements in local anaesthetic drugs and technique. This view has persisted in spite of the reduction in government financial support, and the teeth of the public are better than in the 1940s, although the high consumption of sweets and sweetened drinks and reluctance to accept fluoridation point in the opposite direction. The position of Dental Surgeons in the hospital, however, was slow to change and it was not until 1983 that they (21 in total) were invited to join the Medical Staff Committee. The other change affecting the public image of dental surgeons came in 1996 when the General Dental Council allowed them to use the title 'Dr' if they wished.

The Department of Dental Surgery described in Chapter 4 was the original nucleus of the Dental Hospital and School of Dentistry, and a surprising number of the early staff (mostly part-time) were still in post when Professor Stoy was appointed. The most senior were Mr Herbert Elwood LDS, lecturer (1921–51); Mr W. Muirhead Hunter LDS, lecturer (1921–50); Mr J.S. O'Neill LDS, lecturer (1920–54); and Mr W. Marshall Swan LDS, lecturer (1920–50). Mr James Lyons LDS, in post 1927–52 (lecturer in Dental Materia Medica from 1935), and Mr David Rankin LDS, in post 1927–48, were of nearly as long standing; their appointments were followed by those of Dr James C. (Jim) Smyth LDS, LRCPI, LRCSI, dental surgeon (1937–58), and Mr Robert S.L. Sloan DDS, lecturer (1946–49). Dr Smyth was unusual for the time in having the double qualification, both medical and dental. He was president of the Ulster Medical Society in 1959, and was a president of the British Dental Association.

Since 1948, Dental Surgeons (later Oral Surgeons) have included Mr J.K.H. Benson, lecturer (1953–54); Mr Arthur S. Prophet DDS, lecturer (1954–56); Mr Ian A. Finlay BDS, lecturer (1961–64, who left when he was appointed Professor of Oral Surgery at Trinity College Dublin); Dr Owen Tuohy MB, MDS, lecturer (1964–67, who left when he was appointed Professor of Oral Medicine at the Dublin Dental Hospital); Dr 'Frank' V.

O'Brien, MB, BDS, lecturer (1969–73), Professor (1973–91, with responsibility for Dental Pathology); Mr John McGimpsey B.Sc. (Hons.), BDS (Hons.), MDS, FDS, FFD, lecturer (1972–73), senior lecturer (1973–96), Professor from 1996; Mr 'Gerry' C. Cowan BDS, FDS, FFD, lecturer (1978–85), senior lecturer from 1985; and Dr John Marley B.Sc. BDS, FDS, Ph.D., lecturer from 1993. Professor Philip J. Lamey B.Sc., DDS, MB, FDS, FSD was appointed to a new chair in Oral Medicine in 1994.

The field of oral and maxillo-facial surgery (surgery of the mouth and bones of the face) was introduced into Northern Ireland by Mr Roy Whitlock MDS, FDS. He had been a squadron-leader in the Royal Air Force and then trained at East Grinstead before being appointed Consultant Oral Surgeon to the Royal Victoria Hospital in 1953. Until this time major surgery of the mouth had been the province of the general surgeon, often with very poor results. Mr Whitlock joined Mr Norman Hughes, who had founded the plastic surgery unit at the Throne Hospital in 1949, and a new era of collaboration between plastic and maxillo-facial surgeons began. Now, even the most radical operation – removal of half the tongue and lower jaw, for example – could be undertaken with the prospect of a good functional and cosmetic result. The Plastic and Maxillo-Facial Unit remained at the Throne Hospital until 1968 when it moved to new wards and new theatres in the Ulster Hospital. Routine oral surgery was continued at the Throne Hospital until 1975, when the number of beds for such surgery at the Royal Victoria Hospital was increased and a theatre in the former neurosurgical unit in Quin House was provided.

Mr Whitlock retired in 1983 and was awarded the OBE. Mr John Gorman MDS, FDS was Consultant Oral Surgeon at both the Royal Victoria and the Ulster hospitals from 1960 to 1991, and Dr Charles McKay MDS, Ph.D., FFD was Consultant Oral Surgeon at the Royal Victoria and the Belfast City hospitals from 1962 to 1980. Dr Richard Kendrick MB, FDS, a graduate in Dentistry from Guy's Hospital, London, and in Medicine from Queen's University Belfast, succeeded Mr Whitlock as Consultant Oral Surgeon at the Royal Victoria and Ulster hospitals in 1983. Dr McKay was succeeded in 1980 by Mr Terry Swinson BDS, FDS and Mr Gorman was followed in 1991 by Mr Peter Ramsay-Baggs MB, BDS, FRCS Edin, FDS.

Orthodontics, or the study of the correct alignment of the teeth, was established by Mr H.T.A. (Theo) McKeag BDS, who was a lecturer from 1920 and orthodontist to the hospital from 1924. He built up the prestige of this speciality, becoming a reader in 1952 and retiring in 1959. He was joined by Mr C. Philip Adams BDS, lecturer (1954–64), reader (1964–74) and Professor from 1974 until his retirement in 1984. Mr William A.B. Brown BDS was lecturer (1959–64). Mr Andrew Richardson BDS, M.Sc., FFD was lecturer (1964–68), senior lecturer (1968–73), reader (1973–85) and Professor from 1985. Mr Donald Burden B.Sc., BDS, FDS, FFD, Ph.D. was lecturer (1990–94) and senior lecturer from 1994.

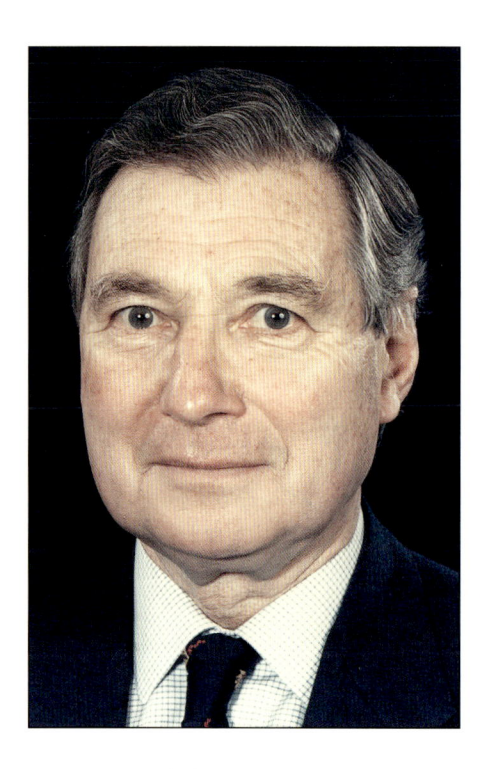

Mr Roy Whitlock, Consultant Oral and Maxillo-facial Surgeon, 1953–83, working at the Royal Victoria, the Throne and the Ulster hospitals
ROYAL VICTORIA HOSPITAL

Dental mechanics, later known as prosthetics and essentially the making of plates and crowns, et cetera, was established in 1927 with the appointment of Mr John (Jack) A. Clarke as lecturer; he remained in post until 1965. Part of the department moved to Queen's in 1929 because of lack of space, but the department was reunited in the new building in 1965. Mr Clarke was succeeded by Mr George Blair MDS, lecturer (1965–71), senior lecturer (1971–87), who was involved in closing defects in the skull (arising largely from bomb, bullet and other missile injuries) with plates of titanium. These plates could cover up to 20 square inches in area and were cast from impressions specially made during a preliminary cleaning-up operation. The plate was then fixed in position with screws at the definitive neurosurgical procedure (see page 192). Mr Philip Saunsbury M.Sc. LDS was lecturer (1953–66) and senior lecturer (1966–78). Mrs Anne Dimmer BDS, FFD, FDS was lecturer first in Dental Surgery (1968–71), and then transferred to Prosthetics in 1973. Mr Eric Scher MB, M.Sc., BDS, FFD was senior lecturer (1977–81). Mr Ian Bennington BDS, FDS, FFD was senior lecturer from 1978 to 1982 and professor from 1982. Mr Thomas Clifford BDS, FDS was lecturer from 1982 to 1985 and senior lecturer from 1985, and Mr C.A. 'Andy' Burnett BDS, FDS was lecturer from 1990.

The Department of Conservative Dentistry was established after World War Two by Mr Ralph Smith BDS who was lecturer in Dental Surgery in 1953–68, lecturer in Restorative Dentistry in 1968–75 and senior lecturer and head of the department from 1975 until 1978, when he retired. Mr John Desmond Eccles was lecturer in Conservative Dentistry from 1959 to 1964, but resigned for a post as senior lecturer and later Professor of Conservative Dentistry in Cardiff. Mr Neil Swallow MDS was appointed Professor in 1978; he resigned in 1983. Professor J.D. Eccles then returned to Belfast and held the chair from 1984 to 1988. After 1988 the chair was left unfilled and Prosthetics, Periodontics (the study of gums and gum disease) and Conservative Dentistry were grouped together as Restorative Dentistry. Dr J.F. Mageean LDS, Ph.D. was lecturer in Dental Surgery (1968–71), and in Periodontics (1971–72); he was senior lecturer in Periodontics (1972-74). Dr John Kennedy B.Sc., MDS, Ph.D., FDS was lecturer in Conservative Dentistry (1973–78) and senior lecturer from 1978, Mr David Russell BDS, M.Sc., FDS was senior lecturer from 1986, Mr Sean Sheridan BDS was Consultant from 1989, Mr David Hussey BDS, FDS was lecturer (1983–89) and senior lecturer from 1989, and Miss Christina Mitchell BDS, FDS, Ph.D., was lecturer from 1990.

Periodontics was established as a separate department in 1965 with Mr Stanley Alldritt (formerly lecturer in Oral Surgery, 1959–65) as Professor until his retirement in 1987, after which the chair was left unfilled. Mr S. Blackwood MDS was lecturer in Dental Surgery (1967–71), in Periodontics (1971–75) and senior lecturer in Periodontics (1975–83). Mr G.J. (Gerry) Linden B.Sc., BDS, FDS was lecturer (1984–85) and senior lecturer from

1985; currently he is Assistant Director (research). In 1990 Dr Christopher Irwin B.Sc., Ph.D., BDS was appointed lecturer, and in 1994 Mr Brian Mullally BDS, MDS, FDS was appointed senior lecturer in Periodontics.

Children's and Preventive Dentistry was established in the 1930s by J. Cuthbert McNeill, who was already on the staff of the Belfast Hospital for Sick Children and was on the staff of the Dental Hospital from 1931 to 1967. Thereafter work in this field was carried out in both the Royal Belfast Hospital for Sick Children and the Dental Hospital. Mr Robert (Bob) H. Elliott LDS (brother of Dr 'Jim' Elliott, anaesthetist) was lecturer (1933–74). Mr David Stewart MDS was lecturer (1959–66), senior lecturer (1966–69), reader (1969–79), and Professor (1979–87); he retired in 1987. Mr D.C. Kernohan MDS was lecturer (1966–69) and senior lecturer (1969–76). Mr William Desmond Pielou B.Sc., MDS was Consultant from 1967 until he retired in 1987. Mr Ian Saunders BA, MDS, FDS, FFD was Consultant and honorary lecturer from 1974. Mr A.D. (Tony) Valentine, formerly senior lecturer in Children's Dentistry in Sheffield, was senior lecturer (1979–82) and Professor from 1982. Mr Martin Kinirons BDS, Ph.D., FDS, FFD was lecturer (1983–85) and senior lecturer from 1985. Dr Ruth Freeman M.Sc., BDS, Ph.D. was lecturer (1990–94) and senior lecturer from 1994.

There have been six part-time lectureships over the years, usually held by consultants at the hospital. The lecturers in Dental Anaesthetics were Dr Maurice Brown, Dr Sylvia Browne and Dr Susan Atkinson. Those in Dental Radiology were Mr Harry Morrow, Dr J.O.Y. Cole, Dr Denis Gough and Dr Clive Majury. Dental Pathology is covered on pages 168–69. Those in Dental Medicine were Dr William Strain, Dr Seamus Coyle, Professor 'Gary' Love and Dr 'Mike' Callender, and those in Dental Surgery were Mr John Megaw, Mr Millar Bell, Mr Rodney Curry and Mr Colin Russell. The lecturers in Law and Ethics in the School of Dentistry were Professor T.K. (Tom) Marshall and Professor Jack Crane.

ANAESTHESIA

The most obvious changes in anaesthesia over the past fifty years have been in the way patients are anaesthetised. In 1948 the majority of patients went to sleep breathing an anaesthetic mixture; this process was more or less smooth according to the skill of the anaesthetist. The anaesthetic was inevitably given by a face mask and, whilst most adults were prepared to accept this, a high proportion of children found it frightening and unpleasant.

The introduction of intravenous anaesthetics enabled anaesthesia to be induced via a small needle, almost without the patient being aware of it. The rapid-acting barbiturate thiopentone had come in during the 1930s but it had a relatively long action and caused residual drowsiness lasting six to twelve hours; work over the next half-century has established propofol as an improvement for most situations, leaving the patient more awake afterwards and even feeling hungry! In the 1950s, the intravenous anaesthetic was given with a glass syringe and needle (often blunt), these being either taken out or strapped to the arm. Now we have excellent disposable plastic cannulae which can remain in position for days.

There has also been some progress with the inhalational anaesthetics, in the move from chloroform (which is toxic to both heart and liver) and ether (which is explosive), to chemically related compounds with minimal toxicity. The safety margin with these substances is small, however, and they are expensive, so new apparatus has been developed to regulate and measure precisely the concentration inhaled and to ensure an adequate supply of oxygen at the same time. So the Boyle's machine of the mid-century with its coloured cylinders of oxygen, cyclopropane and nitrous oxide, and glass bottles to vaporise the liquid anaesthetics, has been replaced by piped gases and heavy, temperature-controlled vaporisers. Research in the Royal Victoria Hospital has contributed significantly to the understanding of both these groups of anaesthetics as well as of the newer muscle relaxants. For instance, it was the early work on thiopentone which demonstrated that as a barbiturate it could not have analgesic properties but instead heightened the sensitivity to pain. Similarly it was work in the Department of Anaesthetics that demonstrated the dangers associated with intravenous anaesthetics using a solvent known as Cremophor EL.

The 1920s and 1930s saw the introduction of Sir Ivan Magill's endotracheal tube to make thoracic surgery possible by allowing ventilation of the lungs to be controlled; it also made head and neck surgery easier by taking the anaesthetist and his equipment well away from the patient. The post-1945 era has seen almost all patients having tubes inserted; this procedure requires the widespread use of muscle relaxants but ensures adequate ventilation of the lungs, without any risk of contamination with irritant stomach contents. Since about 1985, the laryngeal mask has taken over from both tracheal tube and face mask, but its uses and limitations are still uncertain.

The use of muscle relaxants necessitates controlled ventilation of the lungs, and whilst mechanical ventilators were only being introduced in the 1950s, now ventilation is a universal accompaniment of all but the most minor anaesthetic. In 1960 the only ventilator in regular use in the hospital was the Blease Pulmoflator in the theatre of wards 15 and 16 (for thoracic surgery); the neurosurgical theatre had one for occasional use. Like the equipment for administering the anaesthetic, ventilators have become increasingly complicated, with controls, safety valves and devices for measuring gas concentrations and volumes.

The third type of equipment needed by the anaesthetist in the operating theatre is required to monitor the patient's bodily functions. We have moved from simple measurement of blood pressure by hand in the 1950s, to automated visual displays of blood pressure, ECG, temperature, oxygen saturation, carbon dioxide levels, et cetera. How these measurements are made depends on the length and complexity of the operation, but they usually mean much safer anaesthesia and minimal risk to the patient, although there is considerably increased cost in capital equipment and disposables.

As already noted in the case of ophthalmic surgery, the use of local anaesthetic techniques has fluctuated over the twentieth century. They avoid the risks associated with unconsciousness, but introduce others deriving from the drugs used and the possibility of infection close to the spinal cord; they often require more technical expertise than is required to administer a general anaesthetic. They therefore have a definite place where early and full recovery is wanted and particularly for operations on the lower part of the body and for localised areas such as the hand or the eye. As with every type of anaesthetic, safety with local techniques can never be guaranteed but is most likely with well-trained practitioners and constant vigilance.

The other feature of all modern anaesthetics is the intravenous infusion of fluid, which was almost nonexistent fifty years ago, except when patients were visibly dehydrated. Now patients receive a range of fluids before, during and after their anaesthetic, tailored to their needs, including a wide range of blood products and nutrients, and all through clear plastic tubing rather than the irritant and potentially contaminated red rubber tubes of previous times.

The recovery room is certainly one of the greatest advances in anaesthetic management, since the risks of anaesthesia and surgery persist long after the operation has ended. Until the main theatre block was opened in 1964, patients were taken back to the ward, turned on their side and left to wake up with more or less observation by nurses according to pressure of other work. The addition of recovery wards to the main theatres and others since then have meant that (provided nursing numbers can be maintained) there is one-to-one nursing until the patient can safely be left. At the same time more careful attention to pain relief can be applied; over the last ten years this has progressed to patient controlled analgesia (PCA), in which the patient really does administer his or her own pain relief, with preset safeguards and under trained nursing supervision.

Anaesthetic rooms were also felt to be a great advance when they were introduced with the main theatre block. Their principal advantage is that in them the anaesthetist with nurse or technician can anaesthetise the patient in quiet surroundings away from the intimidating atmosphere of the operating theatre. In addition, a second anaesthetist can start anaesthesia on a new patient while the first anaesthetist is finishing the anaesthetic for the earlier patient. However, now that there are fewer anaesthetists and theatre nurses, and if the second patient is very ill, there are fewer advantages in starting the anaesthetic in a separate room and subsequently having to move the anaesthetised patient into the operating theatre.

THE ANAESTHETISTS

The large number of anaesthetists in any general hospital is striking, but even in 1948 there were no less than eight trained anaesthetists working in the Royal Victoria Hospital. Seven of these were not graded as Consultants because they were also engaged in general practice and had no royal college to grant them a recognised qualification. However, they were certainly specialists and those who remember Dr John Boyd, for instance, will testify to his masterly skill with the anaesthetic technique he used in cases involving children. The actual number of anaesthetists was considerably smaller than that of surgeons, but of course surgeons spend much of their time in wards and outpatient clinics. On the whole the two specialities have grown side by side and this, together with the time now spent by anaesthetists in intensive care and post-operative care, probably accounts for the fact that in 1997 there are approximately thirty Consultant Anaesthetists working in the Royal Victoria Hospital.

The first consultant anaesthetist to be appointed after World War Two was Dr Wilfred Maurice Brown, a Queen's graduate, who had served with the Royal Navy during the war and had suffered from severe facial burns after being torpedoed in the Mediterranean. After the war he trained in anaesthesia at the Westminster Hospital, under Dr Ivan Magill, and returned to Belfast to a Visiting appointment at the Royal Victoria Hospital in 1946. He worked mainly in thoracic anaesthesia but also was Consultant Anaesthetist in the Samaritan Hospital and lecturer in Dental Anaesthesia. He gave the annual winter oration in 1959 on 'The conquest of pain', retired in 1976 and published his autobiography in 1988.

In 1950 another Queen's graduate, Dr J.F. (Minty) Bereen, who had served with the RAMC and been an anaesthetist in Stockport, was appointed Consultant Anaesthetist to the neurosurgical unit at the Royal Victoria Hospital. He remained in the unit throughout his career, responsible not only for the operating theatre but also for the neuroradiological procedures. He gave the annual winter oration in 1964 and retired in 1977, being awarded the OBE.

Queen's graduate Dr James (Jim) Elliott trained as an anaesthetist in Belfast and was appointed a Consultant at the Royal Victoria Hospital in 1954, having a special interest in thoracic anaesthesia. He gave the annual winter oration in 1978 and retired in 1980 to live in his native Portaferry in County Down. His wife, Dr Peggy Hamilton, and two of his sons are

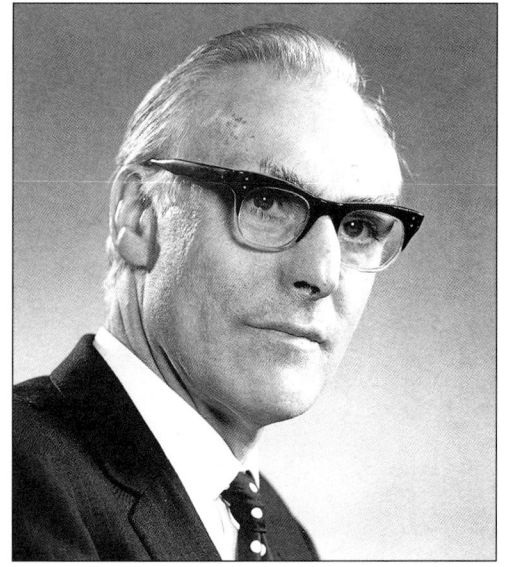

Dr Maurice Brown, Consultant Anaesthetist to the Royal Victoria Hospital, 1946–76
ROYAL VICTORIA HOSPITAL

doctors. Dr James (Jim) Reid, who had been Consultant Anaesthetist at Banbridge Hospital, was appointed Consultant at the Royal Victoria Hospital, also in 1954. Like most of the earlier anaesthetists, he had a special interest in thoracic anaesthesia, and was also on the staff of Whiteabbey Hospital and the Forster Green Hospital. He retired in 1986.

In 1958 a joint Consultant and Senior Lecturer post in Anaesthetics was created and Dr John W. Dundee was appointed, though he was not elected to the Medical Staff Committee until 1961. He had graduated at Queen's University in 1946 and studied further at Liverpool, where he became a Consultant and senior lecturer. He had also been research fellow for a year at the University of Pennsylvania. He came to Belfast with an exceptional basis of research mainly on the intravenous anaesthetic thiopentone, but also on the technique of hypothermia. He was given four rooms on the first floor of the recently opened Institute of Clinical Science, and these served as a base both for the hospital Department of Anaesthetics and for the university research and teaching side. Although Dr Maurice Brown was the Senior Anaesthetist, Dr Dundee quickly became the driving force for teaching, starting practical classes with anaesthetic gases and drugs (nonaddictive) held in or near the Department of Anaesthetics for medical students, a complete course of lectures and tutorials for the trainee anaesthetists, and 'interesting case' meetings for Consultants and trainees. In particular, training was organised for the benefit of the trainees both to help them pass exams and to give them a broad academic base, long before the Northern Ireland Council for Postgraduate Medical Education or the various educational bodies for Anaesthetics in London and Dublin were formed.

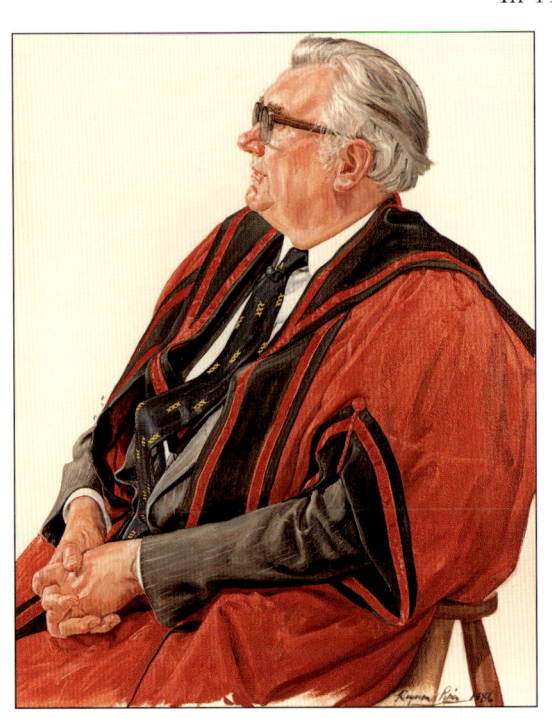

Professor John W. Dundee, first Professor of Anaesthetics at Queen's University Belfast, 1964–86, in his Liverpool Ph.D. gown; portrait by Raymond Piper
QUEEN'S UNIVERSITY BELFAST

Dr Dundee was appointed Professor in 1964 and the staff of the department slowly expanded, so when it became clear that there would be no further space available on the Royal Victoria Hospital site, he took up the suggestion to move – to the new Whitla Medical Building – in 1976. He had also been on the staff of Musgrave Park Hospital for some years but continued to have his main clinical sessions with Mr Morris Stevenson (thoracic surgery) and in intensive care until he retired in 1986. He was an international figure in research into Anaesthetic Pharmacology and a phenomenal writer of books and particularly of scientific papers. He was a founder fellow of the Faculty of Anaesthetists of the Royal College of Surgeons in Ireland in 1959, was Dean from 1969 to 1973, and was awarded the OBE in 1989. He gave the annual winter oration in 1985.

Dr Richard Samuel Jessop Clarke – son of Dr B.R. Clarke (see page 152) and brother of Mr S.D. Clarke (see page 182)– studied medicine at Queen's University graduating in 1954. He had a research post in Oxford and then trained in anaesthetics in Belfast and St Bartholomew's, London, before being appointed Consultant in the Royal Victoria Hospital and lecturer at Queen's University Belfast in 1965. He was given a personal chair in 1980 and was Professor of Anaesthetics from 1988 to 1994. His clinical work was mainly in cardiac anaesthesia and in intensive care. He was Dean of the Faculty of Anaesthetics of the RCSI (1991–94), gave the annual winter oration on 'A corridor to the past' in 1993, and was appointed honorary archivist of the hospital in the same year.

Later Consultant staff in the university department have been Dr J.P. Howard Fee, who after being Consultant Anaesthetist in the Mid Ulster Hospital was appointed Consultant and senior lecturer in 1982 in the Royal Victoria Hospital. His clinical work was with orthopaedic surgery and intensive care. He was appointed Professor of Anaesthetics in 1996. Dr Rajinder Mirakhur (MB Jammu and Kashmir 1967) was appointed Consultant Anaesthetist to the Royal Victoria Hospital in 1980 with a major clinical commitment to ophthalmic anaesthesia and an increasing involvement in research into muscle relaxants. He was appointed senior lecturer in 1990 and given a personal chair in 1996.

As described in Chapter 5, many anaesthetists, despite having Consultant or Senior Hospital Medical Officer status, were only admitted to the Medical Staff Committee in a block in 1962. They are listed here in alphabetical order: Dr G.W. (Gerry) Black who trained in Belfast and Pennsylvania, and was also Consultant Anaesthetist to the Royal Belfast Hospital for Sick Children where he later concentrated his work. He was Dean of the Faculty of Anaesthetists of the RCSI (1982–85), and retired in 1990. Dr Sylvia Browne was appointed Senior Hospital Medical Officer in 1962 and Consultant in 1974, and was also a lecturer in Dental Anaesthesia; she retired in 1990. Dr J.C. (Mac) Clarke was also Consultant to the Ulster Hospital where he later concentrated his work until he retired. Dr W.R. (Bob) Gilmore was also Consultant to the Forster Green and Whiteabbey hospitals and later to the Ulster Hospital, where he eventually concentrated his work; he retired in 1987.

Dr R.C. (Bob) Gray, a graduate of Trinity College Dublin, trained at Lurgan and Portadown and the Royal Victoria hospitals with a research fellowship at the latter to investigate the scope for intensive care. He was appointed Consultant in charge of the new intensive care unit in 1962; he retired in 1987.

Dr John Houston was a Senior Hospital Medical Officer and also a general practitioner in Bangor, County Down; he retired in 1964. Dr Vida Lemon (who qualified in New Zealand) was also Consultant to the Ulster Hospital; she retired in 1964. Dr Harold Love was also Consultant to the Royal Belfast Hospital for Sick Children where he later concentrated his work, as well as being Dean of the Faculty of Anaesthetists of the RCSI, 1976–79; he retired in 1984 to take up the post of part-time Medical

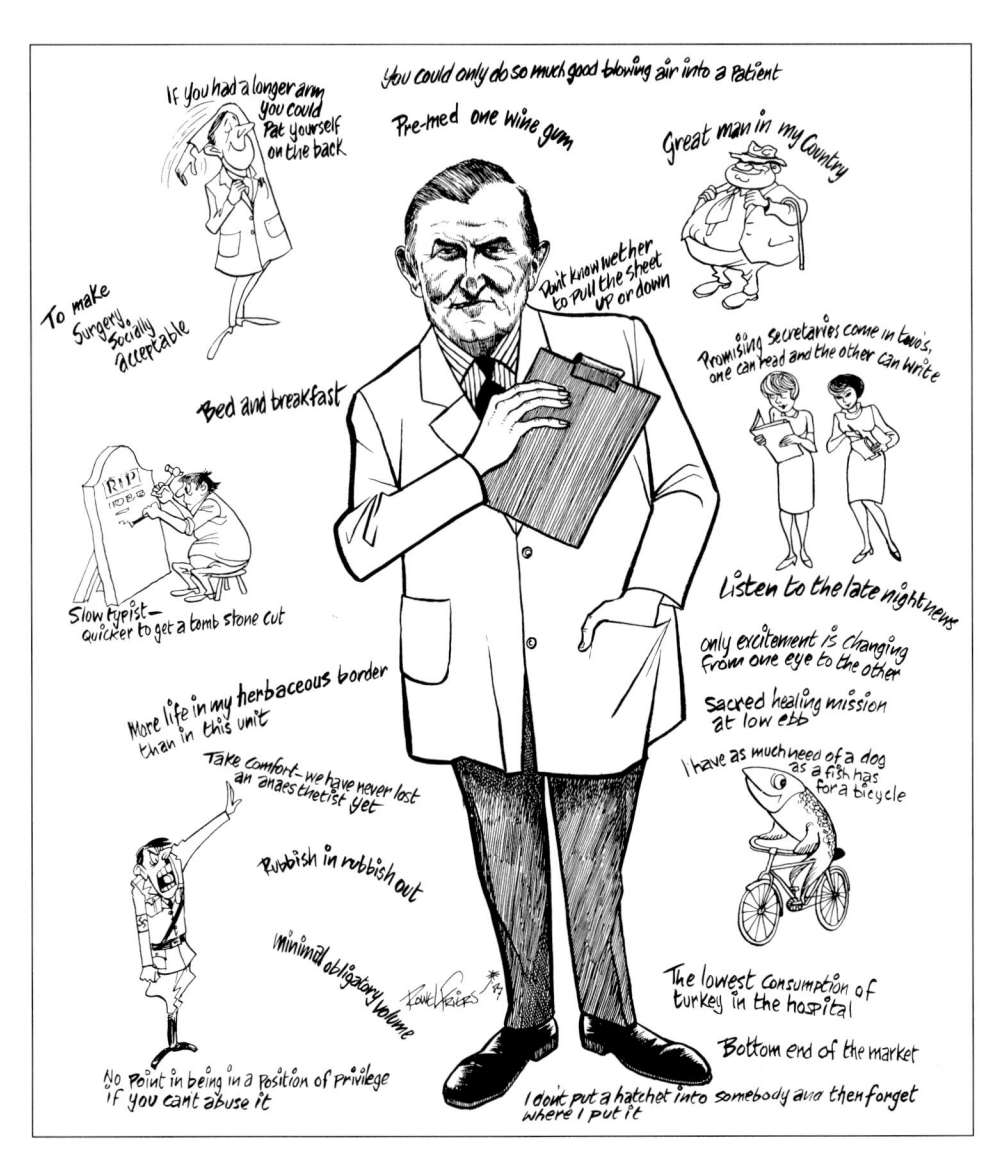

Dr Bob Gray, drawn on his retirement in 1987 by Rowel Friers, with some of his maxims
ROYAL VICTORIA HOSPITAL

Superintendent, 1984–87. Dr Florence McClelland, like Dr Love a graduate of Queen's, was also Consultant to the Royal Maternity Hospital; she retired in 1967. Dr Charles Reid had been specialist anaesthetist in the RAF and was also Consultant at the Musgrave Park Hospital; he resigned in 1977. Dr Eric Scott was appointed Consultant in 1959 and resigned in 1963.

The following Consultant Anaesthetists have retired or died. Dr Sheila Bell (née Wilson, wife of Mr Millar Bell FRCS) was appointed in 1964 and was also Consultant Anaesthetist to the Samaritan and Belfast City hospitals where she concentrated most of her work until she retired. Dr John Dorman was appointed in 1964 and was also Consultant Anaesthetist to the Belfast City and Musgrave Park hospitals where he later concentrated his work until he retired in 1977. Dr David Barron was appointed in 1965 having previously been Consultant to the South Tyrone Hospital. He was also Consultant to the South Belfast Group where he later concentrated his work; he retired in 1988. Dr R.M. (Robbie) Nicholl was appointed in

1966, having previously been Consultant to the South Down Group. He retired in 1992.

Dr William (Billy) Bingham, first cousin of Mr John Bingham, the thoracic surgeon, was appointed in 1967 having previously been a surgeon in the RNVR and Consultant in the Lurgan and Portadown Hospital; he retired in 1981. Dr W.F. Keith (Tub) Morrow was appointed in 1969 having previously been Consultant to the Banbridge, Dromore and South Armagh hospitals. He worked partly in the intensive care unit and after his death the Morrow Memorial Lecture on a topic related to intensive care was established in his memory. Dr Edmund (Ed) Richey was appointed in 1970 but resigned in 1977 for a post in Whiteabbey Hospital. Dr Shaun Young was appointed in 1977; he died in 1990 at the age of forty-six.

The anaesthetists involved in cardiac surgery are listed in the section on cardiac surgery above since their work is largely confined to this unit. All other anaesthetists still in active practice in the Royal Victoria Hospital are listed below in order of appointment. Dr M.A. (Mike) Lewis, a Trinity College Dublin graduate, was appointed in 1967 and has always had a major involvement in the Royal Maternity Hospital. Queen's graduate Dr Dennis Coppel was appointed in 1970 and has also worked in Dallas and in Jerusalem. He has had a long involvement in thoracic anaesthesia, was chairman of the Medical Executive Council, and became the Senior Anaesthetist in the intensive care unit on the retirement of Dr R.C. Gray. Dr V.K.N. Unni (MB Kerala 1961) was appointed in 1977 having previously been Consultant to the Mater Infirmorum Hospital, Belfast. He has a major interest in neurosurgical anaesthesia. Dr Richard McBride was appointed in 1978 and has a major interest in anaesthesia for vascular surgery. Dr Hilary Johnston, like Richard McBride a Queen's graduate, was appointed in 1979 as the Anaesthetist responsible for the burns unit. Dr Henry Craig was appointed in 1980 having previously been a Consultant in the Mid Ulster Hospital. Dr David Wilson was appointed in 1981 and has a major interest in obstetric anaesthesia. Dr Emer McAteer was appointed in 1983 and resigned in 1986 for a Consultant post in Leeds General Infirmary. Dr Julian Johnston was also appointed in 1983 and has a major involvement in the intensive care unit. Dr Kenneth Harper was appointed in 1987. Dr Gavin Lavery was appointed in 1987 with a major involvement in intensive care. Dr Kenneth Lowry, a Manchester graduate, was also appointed in 1987 with a major involvement in intensive care. Dr Emmett Sharpe was appointed in 1988. Dr Clive Stanley and Dr J.H. (Joe) Gaston were appointed in 1990, the latter having previously been consultant in Fredericton, New Brunswick, and in Riyadh, Saudi Arabia. Dr Peter Farling was appointed in 1991 with a major interest in neurosurgical anaesthesia. Dr Susan Atkinson was appointed in 1992 and became a lecturer in Dental Anaesthesia in 1995. Dr Una Carabine and Dr Kevin McGrath were appointed in 1993, Dr Ciaran Rafferty in 1994, and

Dr Declan Fogarty and Dr Eamon McCoy in 1995, Dr McCoy having already invented a new type of laryngoscope which won many prizes and is commercially marketed.

INTENSIVE CARE

The concept of intensive care probably derived from the work of doctors Lassen and Ibsen in Copenhagen who had to manage a massive epidemic of poliomyelitis in 1952 with a high proportion of patients requiring artificial ventilation. Up to this time, artificial ventilation was usually done with the iron lung, a box enclosing the whole body (apart from the head), which permitted air to be sucked into the lungs during inspiration in the normal way. Unfortunately many of the patients also had difficulty in swallowing and coughing, and as a result saliva and even vomitus could also be sucked into the lungs. These problems, together with a shortage of iron lungs, led to the idea of 'positive pressure' ventilation of the lungs via a endotracheal tube or tracheostomy. In this way the lungs could be kept clear of secretions by suction and the ventilation could be provided by 'bag-squeezers' in the form of medical students.

In Belfast in the early 1950s, patients with severe poliomyelitis were treated in Purdysburn Fever Hospital under Dr Fred Kane; the mortality was as high as 90 per cent. Patients with severe respiratory difficulties in the Royal Victoria Hospital were occasionally managed in an iron lung in scattered locations round the hospital and with similar results.

When Dr John Dundee arrived in Belfast as lecturer in Anaesthetics in 1958, however, the new and challenging Copenhagen work was fresh in his mind. Dr Bob Gray was a Senior Registrar in the hospital at the time and a research fellowship for two years (1959–61) was obtained for him to investigate how anaesthetists could play a part in improving the management of patients with respiratory failure. The results were encouraging and Dr Gray gave the Calvert Lecture in 1961. In addition there was support from other anaesthetists, from professors Owen Wade and Peter Elmes, who had interests in chest disease, and from doctors Hilton Stewart and Sydney Allison, neurologists. Eventually in 1961 the neurologists and venereologists agreed to give up two beds in Ward 22 to start a Respiratory Failure Unit (RFU) which later became the Respiratory or Regional Intensive Care Unit (RICU). A room was also formed by closing in a balcony, which was common room, tea room and bedroom for doctors, when the frequent visitors could be driven out! As demand rose, the number of patient beds rose to four and occasionally to six. Dr Gray was appointed the Consultant in Charge of the unit in 1962 on a half-time basis, with Professor John Dundee and Dr Richard Clarke contributing two sessions each (though, in practice during the entire week, Dr Gray was seldom out of the unit).

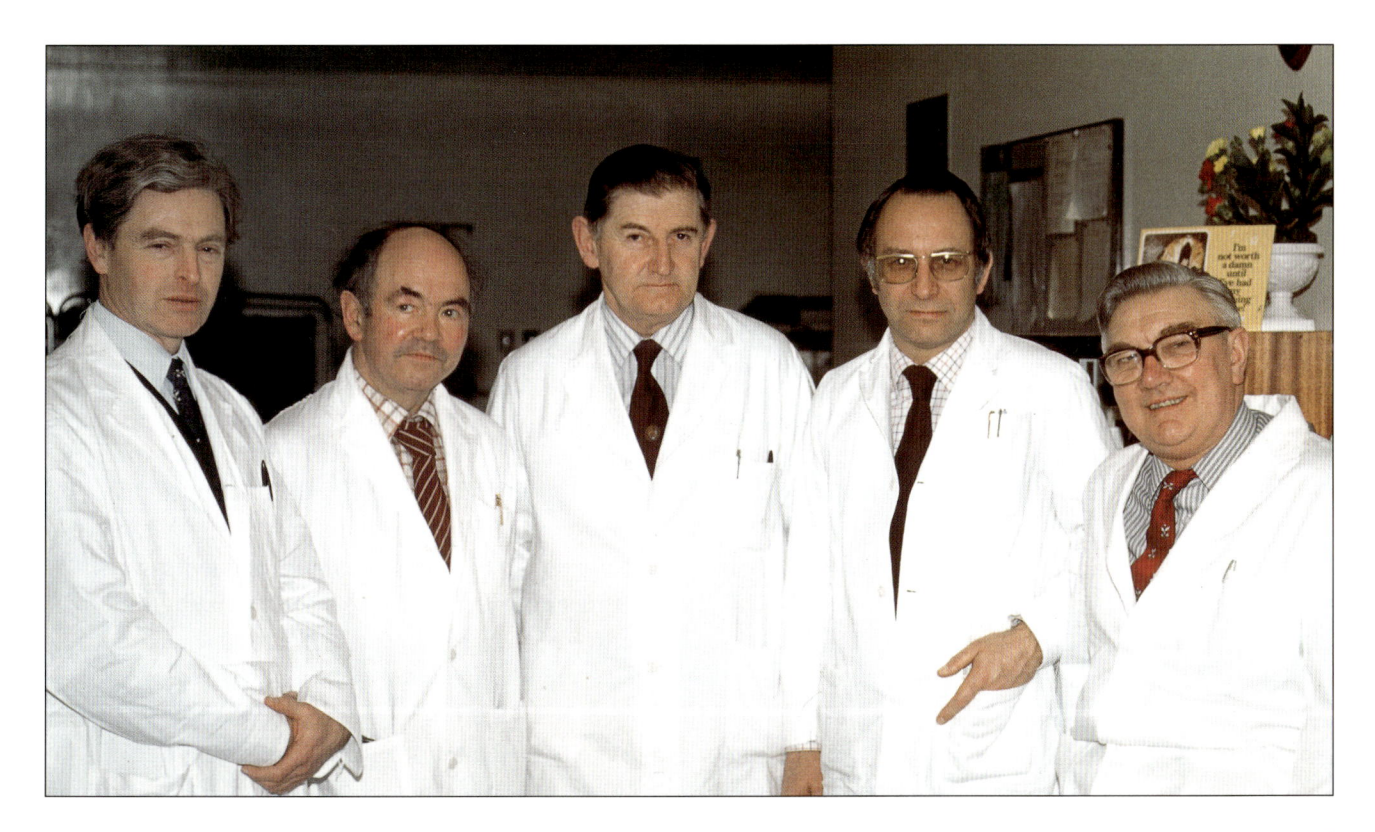

The Consultant Anaesthetists of the Intensive Care Unit in 1980: *left to right:* Professor Richard Clarke, Dr Keith Morrow, Dr Robert Gray, Dr Dennis Coppel and Professor John Dundee
ROYAL VICTORIA HOSPITAL

The demand for intensive care provision escalated rapidly with the advent of highly sophisticated and technologically advanced modern medicine. Surgeons, physicians and the public recognised the need for one-to-one nursing and medical care devoted to the critically ill. The number of patients admitted to intensive care clearly reflected this, with a rise from eighty-four patients in 1965 to almost six hundred in 1995.

Medical staffing was increased in 1970 when Dr 'Tub' Morrow and Dr Dennis Coppel were appointed. They were later joined by Dr Julian Johnston in 1983 and Dr Gavin Lavery, Dr Ken Lowry and Dr Howard Fee in 1987, when Dr Gray and Professor Dundee retired.

The patients admitted to the intensive care unit over the years have changed; certainly lessons have been learnt as to who would benefit most from management in the unit. When the unit first opened, large numbers of patients with cerebro-vascular accidents (strokes) were admitted but it was found that when such patients need assistance with their respiration, the prognosis is already very poor. The same is probably true of many patients with chronic bronchitis. Other conditions such as poliomyelitis have virtually disappeared, thanks to immunisation, though neuromuscular disorders in general have good prospects of recovery.

Tetanus was particularly prevalent in the 1950s and 1960s and had proved difficult to treat because of pain; the distressing nature of the disease often caused death from the severity of the muscle spasms or the efforts to treat with sedation alone. Nowadays with the introduction of a vigorous regime of muscle paralysis, artificial ventilation, physiotherapy, feeding and generally energetic nursing, carried out over one to two months, full recovery is to be expected. Indeed during the 1960s the Northern Ireland Hospitals Authority let it be known that all patients with tetanus in Northern Ireland should be transferred to the Royal Victoria Hospital intensive care unit to ensure their best chance of recovery. Fortunately tetanus, like poliomyelitis, can now be prevented by immunisation.

Self-poisoning used to form about 15 per cent of admissions to the intensive care unit around 1960 but, as is well known but inadequately explained, this problem has diminished with the Troubles. On the other hand, admissions from trauma have increased with the Troubles, the unit has received many patients with bullet wounds, and multiple injuries from bombings and some of the more severe punishment beatings. Nevertheless, all these put together do not match the steady volume of admissions from road traffic accidents. Soon after the intensive care unit opened it was realised that all head injuries and some other forms of brain damage could benefit from artificial ventilation for a limited period, and it has been the regular practice to provide it ever since. Some of the longest-stay patients are suffering from multiple organ failure following major trauma, sepsis and massive haemorrhage. These, like the patients with head injuries, show that an intensive care unit, although for continuity it is managed by the anaesthetists, is really an area of the hospital where the skills of surgeons, physicians, nephrologists, bacteriologists and haematologists are all pooled for the benefit of the patient.

It was soon apparent that having an intensive care unit – with its own sister (Noelle Gibson, 1962–75), medical staff at all levels, physiotherapists coming several times a day, and one nurse per patient – inside a neurological ward was unsatisfactory. Sister 'Lofty' Lowry was sister in charge of Ward 22 (neurology) and was not always happy to see the turmoil created by just two intensive care patients. By 1969 a committee was planning a new eleven-bed unit and it opened in 1970 in the link block across the corridor from the casualty department. It had six beds in cubicles and six on an open plan, plus storage space, a workshop, sister's office and resident doctor's suite. At the height of the Troubles, however, a policeman guarding a patient was shot dead in the unit on a Sunday afternoon. After this the entrance was moved away from the rather public Casualty Department and provided with an elaborate security presence including bulletproof glass.

In 1992 a major refurbishment of the unit was completed at a cost of £350,000. The money was raised by Revive, a charity solely devoted to supporting financially the intensive care unit. A waiting room, sleeping accommodation and a counselling room were provided for patients' relatives. A large seminar room was made available for medical and nursing staff, which doubles as a recreation area. For ease of nursing, the cubicles were converted to an open area, one being left for isolation purposes. The need to expand the unit to accommodate more patients was accepted by the Hospital Council and in 1996 three more beds were provided, bringing the bed complement to fourteen, thus making the intensive care unit in the Royal Victoria Hospital one of the biggest in the UK. Consultant staff had office accommodation provided in an adjoining Portacabin. A new twenty-bed intensive care unit is included in the plans for the new block to be opened in the year 2000.

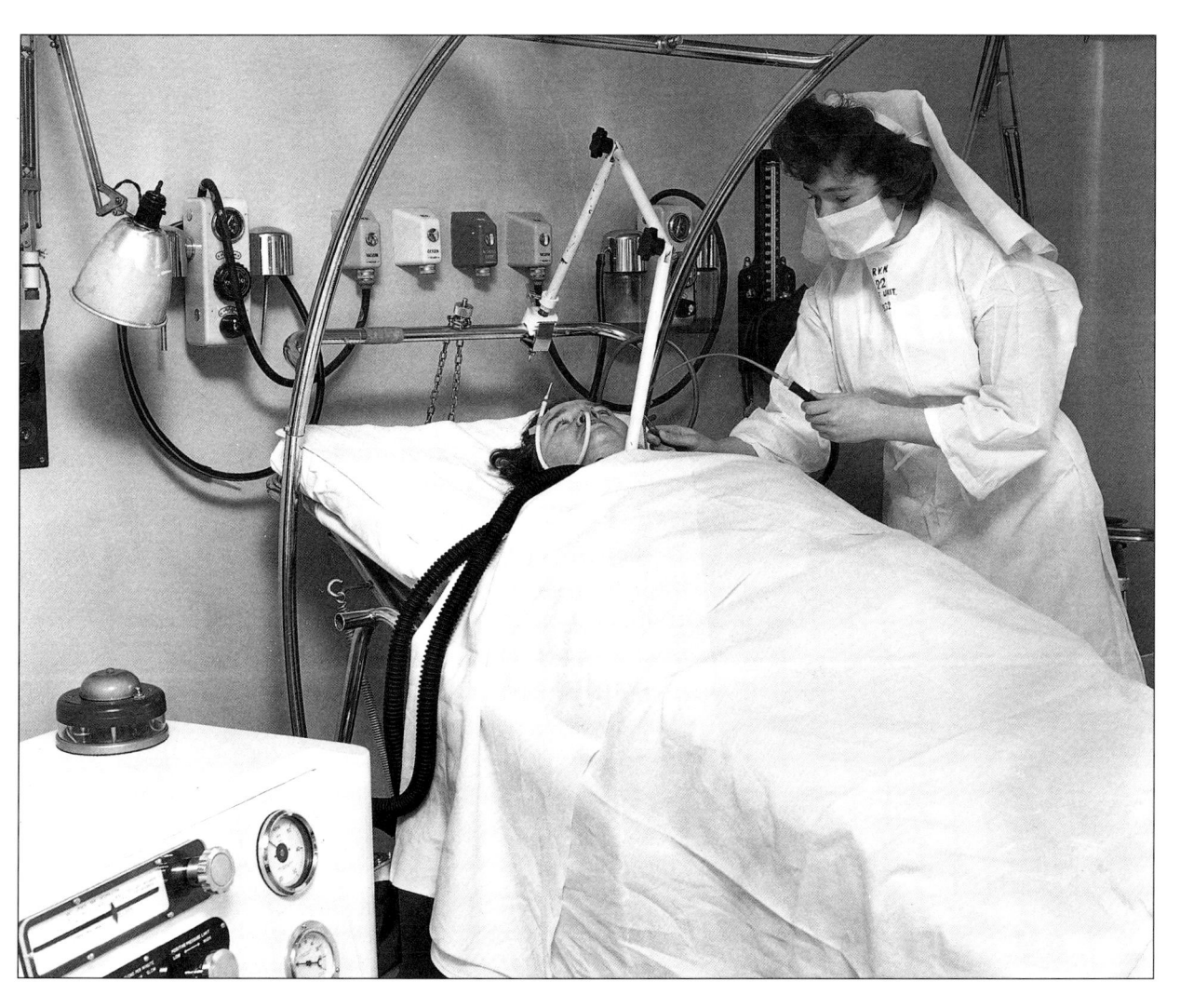

When Sister Noelle Gibson resigned in 1975, Sister Elizabeth McAlister followed, 1975–78, then Sister Margaret Fenton, 1978–80, and Sister Eleanor Blair, 1980–94. The present sister is Joanna McCormack. James (Jim) Wilson was appointed technician in charge of the unit's equipment in 1970 and was helped by many others at different times. He now has a wider brief within the Anaesthesia, Theatre and Intensive Care (ATICS) Directorate.

Sister Noelle Gibson with a patient in a circo-electric bed in the Respiratory Failure Unit (Ward 22) in 1963; note the simple but robust Cape-Wayne ventilator
ROYAL VICTORIA HOSPITAL

THE IMPACT OF THE TROUBLES AND THE A & E DEPARTMENT

The Royal Victoria Hospital and its predecessors have survived two hundred years of 'Troubles' in Northern Ireland. As noted in Chapter 1, the first of these episodes, in 1798, actually led to the hospital closing completely for several months. The riots of 1864 were well described in Surgeon Murney's report, which collected information on 316 injuries from 73 doctors within the city.

Of course the term 'Troubles' itself reflects this history. This name was given to the conflict that followed the partition of Ireland in 1921, and in case our generation should think ourselves unique the following verses about Dr Thomas Houston (then in his thirties) may be quoted:

> The gunmen lurked round the Dunville Park
> The lamps were out and the streets were dark
> On the Grosvenor Road a corpse lay stark
> And the 'Specials' walked in dread.
>
> But Tom in the lab ignored the thugs
> And nightly tended his much loved bugs
> And coaxed the juice from the rabbits' lugs
> Then – calmly drove home to bed.

However, the present violence, which dates essentially from the civil rights marches of 1969, has had a different kind of impact on the hospital. For one thing, a high proportion of those injured were brought to the Royal Victoria Hospital, which has had nearly thirty years of nightly violence, punctuated by episodes with large numbers of casualties. Very many patients with severe injuries have been brought in by a dedicated ambulance service, patients who could and did recover with skilful treatment. Finally, there has been the proximity of the hospital, situated as it is in the heart of republican west Belfast, to much of the conflict and the fact that many of the hospital staff had some personal knowledge of the injured on one or other side. This last fact in no way influenced the treatment or attention given to the injured, but it heightened tension. It also meant that patients' relatives were often in and out of the hospital, meeting relatives of other patients with whom they were in conflict. This frequently led to abrasive remarks, but with tact on the part of the nurses, real violence within the unit has been avoided.

Injuries have occurred as a result of civil disturbance intermittently during the twenty-eight years, since 1969, but over most of this period the number of severe injuries in any particular month resulting from road accidents has been higher. It is the road traffic accidents, many of them alcohol-related, that have provided a steady stream of work for the Accident and Emergency Department at night and justified a sufficiently senior 'on call' rota of surgeons and anaesthetists. The victims of civil violence are an additional sporadic load on the hospital and may be divided into four categories:

1 Riot victims – common in 1969–71 with largely minor injuries, but with a few more serious gunshot or plastic bullet injuries.

2 Isolated shootings, usually with high-velocity bullets, and often instantly fatal. A minority have been brought rapidly to hospital and have recovered after heroic efforts by both patient and staff.

3 Punishment shootings and beatings. These were rare in the 1970s but have become more common and were unaffected by the 1994 cease-fires by the IRA and loyalist paramilitaries.

4 Bomb explosions, which have never been as common as shooting incidents, though in the early 1970s as many as eleven occurred in a single day. The numbers killed from this cause have been fewer than those from gunshot wounds, but because of the generally greater number of casualties occurring at one time and the whole emotive effect, such incidents live more in the public memory.

Those living outside Northern Ireland frequently comment, 'You must have a very wide experience of severe injuries in the Royal Victoria Hospital', but this is only partly true. Road traffic accidents are seen all over the developed world, and gunshot injuries are seen much more frequently in the major US cities, or indeed in Johannesburg, than in Belfast. It is the number of injuries from bomb explosions that have occurred here added to the much higher number of gunshot injuries than in other cities of the UK that makes the Belfast experience different. Certainly it has resulted in at least thirty scientific papers and an involvement in at least ten major conferences on trauma over the years. For the reader who wants not only the facts about the injured but the full emotional overlay, the best publication to come out of the early Troubles is Alf McCreary's *Survivors* (1976).

In the forefront of the hospital's involvement in the Troubles has been the accident and emergency department (A & E, more commonly known as Casualty). It has received the whole spectrum of casualties, from the people at the edge of an explosion who needed mainly comfort and support, to the CID ('carried in dead'). Most patients only required to have their wounds cleaned and stitched, but the real satisfaction in such a department is in the rapid treatment of life-threatening situations – the ABC (Airway, Breathing, Circulation) management of any emergency which comes into action as the patient enters the door. The other important role of such a department in a large disaster is triage, that is, the sorting of patients into those who need urgent resuscitation, those who need prolonged and complicated surgery, and those who can be put somewhere comfortable to have their minor injuries treated when staff become available. Perhaps one of the most unpleasant jobs that confronted the A & E staff in the early Troubles was cleaning those who had been tarred and feathered – a traditional Irish punishment for those suspected of being informers or at least of fraternising with the enemy. This was more recently replaced by 'kneecapping', beating up with clubs or shooting dead.

It happened that in 1967 a returned medical missionary from India, Mr William Rutherford FRCS Edin, was appointed as Casualty Surgeon. He had graduated at Trinity College Dublin in 1944 and worked as medical officer at Limadwala Missionary Hospital in Gujarat, India, from 1947 to 1966. What might have been simply a stepping stone turned out to be a fulfilling task well suited to his careful and caring temperament. He published much on the problems of casualty management (with Dr Peter Nelson and others) including a textbook of *Accident & Emergency Medicine* (1980), and at the height of the Troubles he was awarded the OBE for his work, from which he retired in 1986.

A succession of other doctors have worked in the A & E Department over these years. Dr Peter Gerald Nelson, son of Professor Gerry Nelson (see page 192), graduated at Queen's University in 1966. He then worked in research in cardiology in the Royal Victoria Hospital and in King's College Hospital, London, before returning in 1975 to a post as Accident and Emergency Consultant in the Royal Victoria Hospital. He was a kind and generous doctor as well as a flamboyant sportsman and after his early death was commemorated in the Peter Nelson Prize for A & E Medicine.

Dr Christine Dearden was appointed an Accident and Emergency Consultant in 1986 on the retirement of Mr Rutherford, and Dr Peter Nelson was followed in 1992 by Mr Laurence Rocke, who had been Consultant in the A & E Department of the Mater Infirmorum Hospital. Dr Brian McNicholl was appointed in 1996.

No picture of the A & E Department would be complete without mention of Sister Kate O'Hanlon, who by her personality and her good humour held the unit together at the height of the Troubles and was awarded the MBE on her retirement. As Mr Rutherford once remarked, 'Running Casualty is really very simple: you have to love everybody, you have to listen to everybody; and when in doubt you do just what Sister O'Hanlon tells you!'

THE BOMB AND THE BULLET

Anyone writing about disasters and the Royal Victoria Hospital must inevitably write of the incidents that affected him or her personally, and in my lifetime at the hospital there have been many, starting with the casualties seen after the *Reina del Pacifico* engine room explosion in 1947. Then there was the crash at Nutt's Corner airport in 1953, in which some medical student colleagues died, though others happily escaped unharmed. In the same year bodies were brought in from the sea after the wreck of the

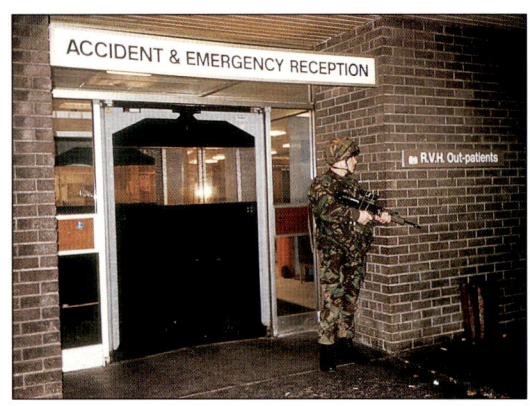

An armed soldier keeping guard outside the Accident and Emergency Department, when military personnel were being treated inside
ROYAL VICTORIA HOSPITAL

Left to right: Sister Gwen Ross, Mr William Rutherford and Sister Kate O'Hanlon in the Accident and Emergency Department
ROYAL VICTORIA HOSPITAL

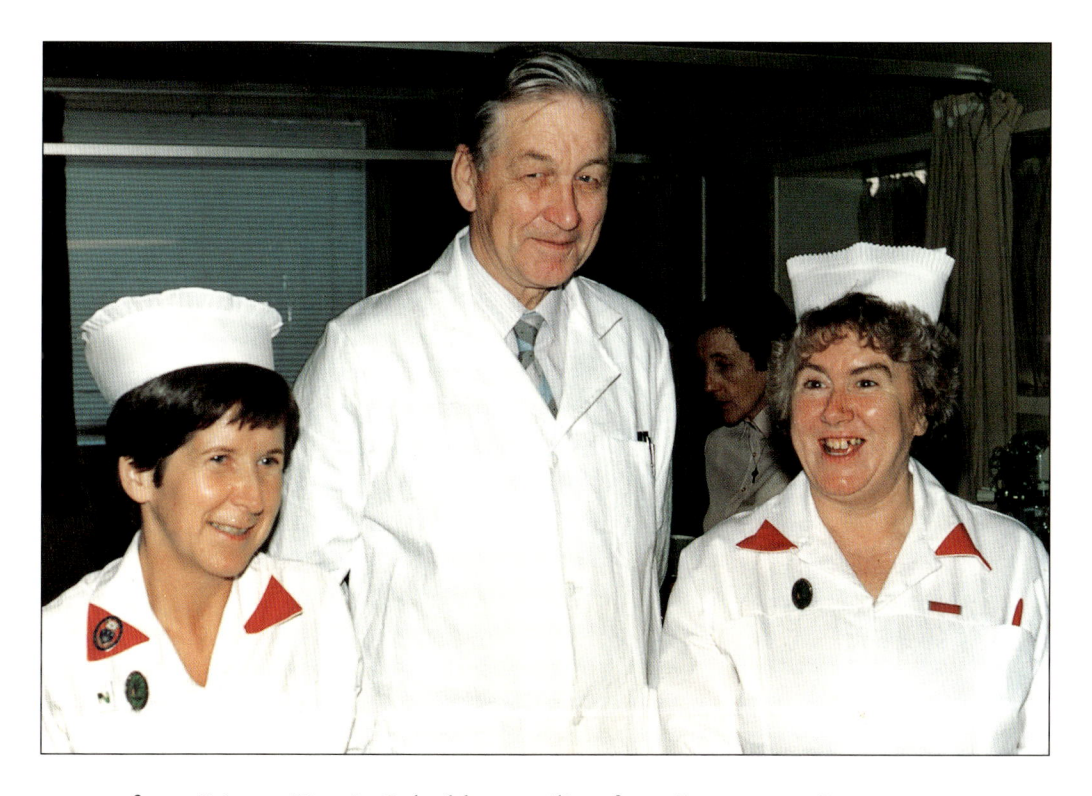

car ferry *Princess Victoria*. It had been sailing from Stranraer to Larne on a particularly wild day and after tossing about for hours finally sank off Donaghadee with the loss of 133 lives. But these were accidental disasters, whereas, after the Red Lion pub bombing, to see a young physical education teacher in the intensive care unit who lost one of her legs was a different type of horror. She was only one of thirty-five patients brought to the Royal Victoria Hospital on the same day from two bombings. After the explosion in McGurk's bar in December 1971, twenty-three people who had been dug out of the rubble were taken to the hospital. Then came March 1972 when there were four explosions including that in the Abercorn restaurant, resulting in 335 patients needing treatment in the Royal Victoria Hospital.

The Abercorn bombing was memorable for several reasons. It was a small bomb, 5–10 lb, but exploded in a confined space. There was no warning. It was indiscriminate, killing and injuring ordinary shoppers, mainly young women, and the injuries were horrendous by any standard. The most famous victims were two sisters, Jennifer McNern aged twenty-one and Rosaleen aged twenty-two, who were shopping on that Saturday afternoon and stopped to rest for a cup of coffee in the Abercorn. After the bomb went off, both were taken unconscious to the Casualty Department of the hospital; Jennifer lost both legs while Rosaleen lost both legs and an arm. They had other injuries, particularly to their lungs, requiring treatment in the intensive care unit, but in the end they recovered and two months later they were able to move to Musgrave Park Hospital for fitting with artificial limbs. Five months later Rosaleen was married to her longstanding fiancé; Jennifer was one of the bridesmaids. Another victim,

Jimmy Stewart, who was a sheet metal worker, lost both legs; yet another, Irene Arnold, a waitress in the restaurant, lost both legs and an eye. There were very many injuries, of all types, and no less than sixty perforated eardrums. Two girls died: Anne Owens and Janet Bereen, the latter a daughter of Dr Minty Bereen, the Neurosurgical Anaesthetist. He was in the hospital anaesthetising some of the victims that evening, and it was midnight before he heard that his daughter was one of the two who had been killed instantly. No one claimed responsibility for the Abercorn bombing and there were many rumours, the most widely held being that one of the victims had brought the bomb into the restaurant and left it under a table while they had coffee.

The effects of explosions on the body have been studied during and since World War Two; in practice they depend on the size of the explosion and the proximity of the victim to the source of the blast. They can also be grouped into (1) the effects of the explosion itself, (2) the effects of the explosion throwing the body against nearby surfaces, and (3) the effects of missiles thrown out by the explosion hitting the body. The most severe effects include amputation of limbs and disruption by the blast of air-containing spaces in the body: lungs, eardrums and intestine. Close proximity can also produce flash burns to uncovered skin. However, the one lesson that emerges from studying the effects of explosions is their unpredictability. Much depends on the direction the victim is facing and the presence of walls and other objects to take the force of the blast or to reflect it.

Major disasters result in the mobilisation of all the different experts within the hospital. The most severely injured victims may go at once to the intensive care unit where they are prepared for surgery. Others (usually those with damage to a major blood vessel) go at once to the theatre. The biochemical and haematology laboratories are also mobilised at an early stage. The demand for blood is considerable, and it is to the credit of the blood transfusion service that all requests have been met. Many types of expertise can be involved in treatment, sometimes on the same patient, surgeons taking their turn to operate according to anatomical relationship and urgency. Those involved in emergency management include neuro-surgeons, thoracic, orthopaedic, plastic, vascular, general, ophthalmic, ENT, and maxillo-facial surgeons.

Special problems in the intensive care unit include management of head injuries to ensure that the brain has the best chance of recovery. There is also management of pain, of generalised bleeding tendencies, and of infection. A particular problem of bomb explosions that has generated attention is blast damage to the lungs. This, in fact, is rare and may not be present even in those with major loss of limbs. It results from the blast damaging the alveoli, or small chambers in the lungs, and forcing fluid into them. It is therefore very difficult to treat, but can be managed along similar lines to fluid overload or damage by poisonous fumes.

Damage to the lungs alone in any injury often has a good prognosis because it is usually clean, whereas intestinal injuries are infected from the outset and may result in a stormy convalescence after surgery. It is clear, however, that all injuries in bombings are likely to be infected by foreign material driven into the wound, whereas bullet injuries are unlikely to be grossly contaminated.

There is, however, a world of difference between the effects of a bullet from a low-velocity pistol even at close range and those of a marksman's bullet from an Armalite or AK47 Kalashnikov rifle. The former pushes tissues out of the way, only damaging what it penetrates. The latter has a track several centimetres wide with shockwave damage to neighbouring structures, which is often disastrous if they are brain or spinal cord. At the lower end of the scale also is the plastic bullet which is low-velocity but which can kill because of its weight alone.

The Troubles have tested the Royal Victoria Hospital as never before, but it has come out with a record to be proud of. The staff have all turned up for work, often unasked, and have pulled together not just once in a lifetime, but day after day in the 1970s. At the medical level we have learned that when all the experts are brought together, near miracles can be achieved; this lesson could be applied to the management of road traffic injuries in a trauma centre. We have learned (or relearned) that dirty wounds cannot be simply cleaned and stitched up – a process of 'debridement' with 'delayed primary suture' is needed. Finally we have learned lessons of general application – that we can do without blood in the emergency management of injuries, that time (minutes) is important in resuscitation and especially in repair of vascular injuries if full recovery is to occur, and that people (particularly young people) can overcome horrendous injuries and go on to get married or take a higher degree, apparently spurred on rather than crushed by their experiences.

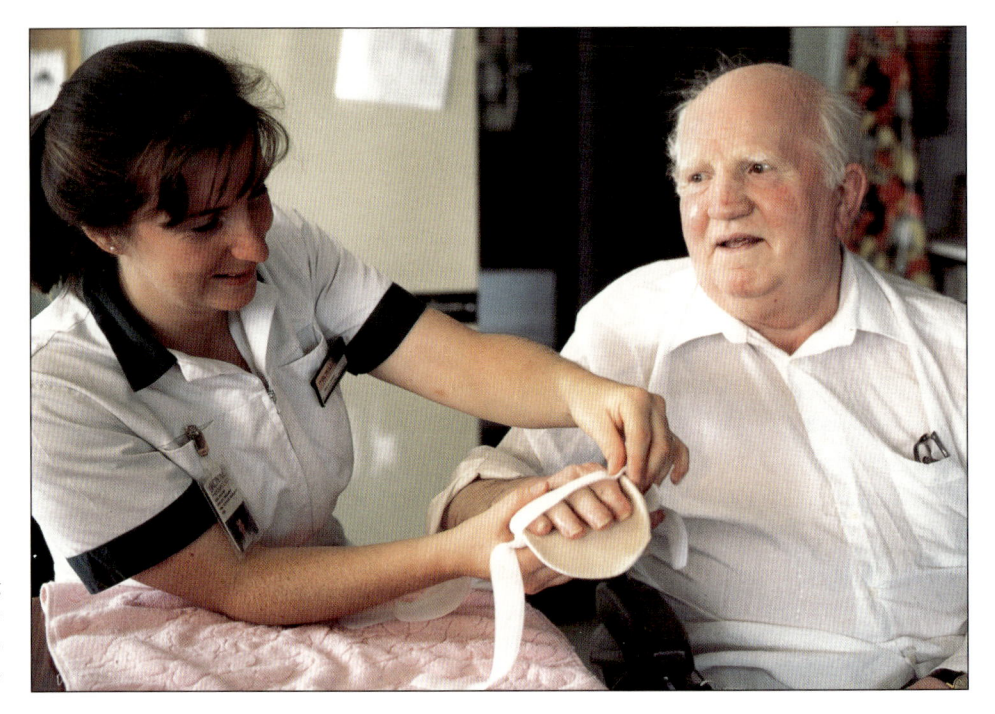

Helen Caves,
Occupational Therapist, fitting
a splint for a patient in the
geriatric wards, 1996
ROYAL VICTORIA HOSPITAL

7

OTHER CARING PROFESSIONS AND
FUNDRAISING COMMITTEES

THE STORY OF THE ROYAL VICTORIA HOSPITAL is not just the story of its medical and nursing staff. Many other groups of people work in the hospital, and they too are essential to the welfare of the patients. Some groups, like the dispensary/pharmacy staff, have existed since the beginning of the hospital; others, such as clinical psychology, have only a short history and involve a few part-time staff. The fundraising groups kept the hospital alive in its voluntary days before 1948 and still play a valuable part when money for particular objects is scarce. They help to integrate hospital and community in a way that, if more obvious in the hospital of a small town, is equally necessary in a specialist area hospital that also serves as the general hospital for a community. The Working Men's Committee is the oldest of these fundraising groups and has been described on pages 85–87.

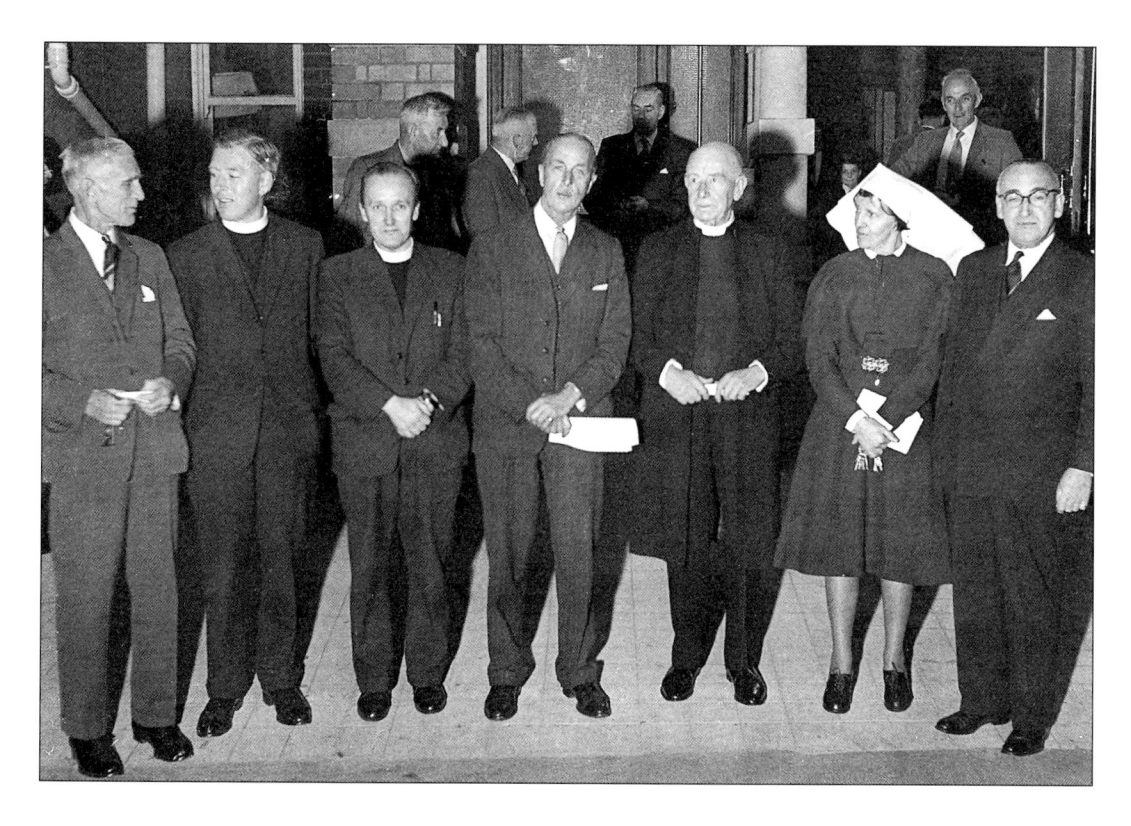

THE CHAPLAINS

The role of the clergy of Belfast in connection with the hospital in its early years seems to have been largely to preach charity sermons and to help in fundraising. There is no record of their providing pastoral care, though presumably they did so on request. We first read of official chaplains in 1875, but even then there was only a suggestion to appoint, on a salaried basis, chaplains belonging to the various recognised religious bodies. This aroused considerable controversy, however, and public discussion occupied a whole page of the *Belfast News-Letter*. The idea of salaried chaplains was thereafter rejected, and there was at best lukewarm support for a proposal put to the Committee of Management that patients should be asked if they wished to have a visit from their clergymen.

During the twentieth century specific clergy have represented the main Christian denominations and the Jewish community, though they were unsalaried until the advent of the NHS. In general those involved have been from the neighbouring churches: from the Drew Memorial Church of Ireland church on the Grosvenor Road, from Broadway Presbyterian church on the Falls Road, from the Grosvenor Hall Methodist mission on

At the opening of the shelter in the quadrangle provided by the Working Men's Committee in 1962: *left to right:* a member of the Working Men's Committee, the Reverend Eric Gallagher, the Reverend James Arbuthnot, Brigadier Thomas Davidson, the Reverend Dr Hugh Scott, Miss Nora Earls and Sir Ian McKinney.
ROYAL VICTORIA HOSPITAL

the Grosvenor Road, and from St Paul's parish on the Falls Road.

With the advent of the NHS it became official policy for the Northern Ireland hospitals to appoint and pay chaplains on the nomination of the appropriate authorities in the Church of Ireland, Methodist, Presbyterian, and Catholic churches. In the case of the Royal Group of Hospitals, it was the custom initially for the Churches concerned to continue the nominations as outlined above. The contractual obligation of the chaplains was to do a weekly round of visiting patients of his (or later her) denomination, to offer spiritual comfort, and, very important, to notify by post the minister of the patient concerned. There was no obligation to have any responsibility for staff members or to arrange or participate in religious or other hospital community activities.

Former patients of the early 1950s and long-serving members of staff will recall the genial and gentlemanly Reverend Hugh Scott, the Presbyterian minister who for many years was the doyen of the chaplains' group, the remarkable and knowledgeable Canon Charles Sansom, and that six foot six or thereabouts giant of a man, the Reverend Robert Cunningham from the Grosvenor Hall. There were more frequent changes of personnel in the case of the Catholic priests, with the result that in those years the Catholic chaplain rarely had the opportunity to establish himself in the same way, though in a later period Father Peter Ford was chaplain for many years.

Over the decades there have been inevitable changes in personnel. One recalls chaplains such as Wilbur Gillespie (Presbyterian), Canon Sansom's successor James Arbuthnot, the Reverend Eric Gallagher (Methodist chaplain, 1957–79) and many others. As time went by each chaplain tended to share his work and his emolument with a colleague, some of whom were to make their mark; the names of Deaconess Mary Angus (Presbyterian), Henry Pedlow (Church of Ireland) and Joseph McCrory (Methodist) are among those still remembered.

Throughout the years there was a camaraderie among them; as often as not they dined together on Mondays. They never considered themselves restricted to the terms of their contract. There was participation in the annual nurses' carol service in Bostock House, the introduction of Sunday morning services for both Catholic and Protestant patients, an afternoon service for all patients in the geriatric wing. More unusual still was the introduction of a nightly epilogue on Radio Royal. (The business of gaining access to the transmitting machine had its problems. The author recalls the frequent struggle with the lift and the night on which, with him inside, it refused to stop at the ground floor and finished up with a bump on the floor of the lift well.)

Each group within the hospital has its own tradition of great moments and memorable events. Unquestionably the months and years of the heavy and indiscriminate bombing of places like the Abercorn and La Mon saw the chaplains at their best. Like their medical colleagues they did not require to be called in. They went as soon as they learned of a major incident. Denominational barriers were ignored. The victims of whatever faith were the first priority and the necessary communication process was initiated as soon as convenient. Those who shared in the harrowing task of providing comfort to victims and relatives will never forget the trauma and despair tinged with hope of those terrible days. In retrospect, whilst every duty and every patient is unique, that period was their finest hour.

In the late eighties the chaplains saw the fulfilment of a long-cherished dream, the opening of a chapel beside the entrance to the main corridor. Many people were involved in this project, but Sydney Callaghan deserves credit for seeing the task through to its completion. The chapel is now open daily for anyone to use, and the chaplains conduct prayers in it on Monday mornings as well as Sunday services and other acts of worship.

The present chaplains with their colleagues are as follows: Church of Ireland, Reverend Gary R. Shaw; Presbyterian, Reverend Derek J. Boden; Methodist, Reverend David J. Kerr; Catholic, Father Paul Byrne; and other denominations, Reverend James A. Lemon.

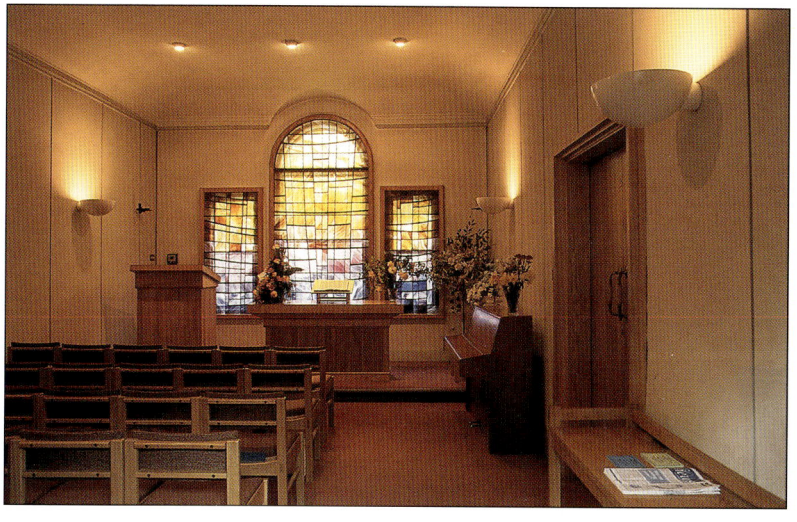

The chapel, constructed in the old board room beside the main entrance to the hospital and opened on 21 September 1988
ROYAL VICTORIA HOSPITAL

THE ALMONERS AND SOCIAL WORKERS

References to the need for an almoner appear in the Royal Victoria Hospital archives from about 1931, and a decision to appoint one was made in 1936. It was the Medical Staff Committee who, frustrated by the delay, made direct contact with the Association of Hospital Almoners to clarify the almoner's role and seek advice about finding a suitable candidate.

Elinor Gough, a trained social worker from St Thomas's Hospital, London, became the first almoner appointed to the hospital in October 1938. By December that year she had submitted a report analysing the work she had done already and outlining her suggestions for how she might best organise her department in future. Her main task was to ensure that patients receiving treatment free were not prevented by home circumstances from benefiting to the full from that treatment. So impressed were the Management Committee that her report was circulated and by the next month she had received permission to employ an assistant almoner and to accept professional course student almoners for placements. Within

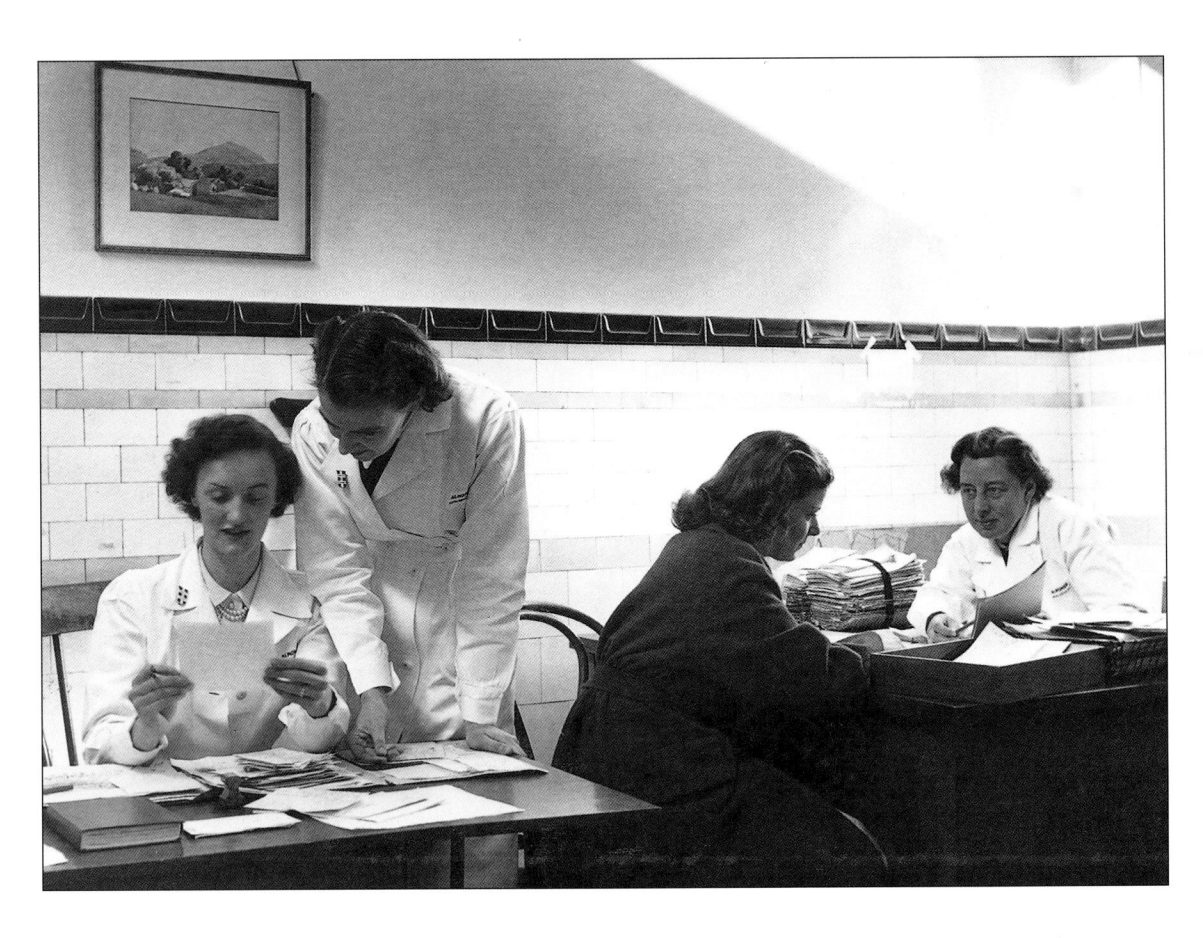

The almoners' office in 1953, with Betty Hall on the right
ROYAL VICTORIA HOSPITAL

three months, therefore, she had secured additional staff to increase the service to patients and had taken steps to establish the teaching tradition of the department in line with the hospital's own high educational profile.

The scope of the almoner's work and that of the medical social worker has always been broad and requires a knowledge of the legislation and of the Churches and public bodies available to provide help. One of their main tasks is to arrange for accommodation and help for patients leaving hospital; without this, discharge arrangements would be slowed down with much worry for patients and ward staff. Almoners also help with domestic problems while the patient is in hospital, and advise victims of domestic and civil violence. Finally, they provide counselling for patients with cancers or other conditions that may be life-threatening or may radically disrupt their life (for example, amputations).

The outbreak of war in 1939 added to the almoner's tasks. With the then limited administrative structures, Elinor Gough was involved in the hospital's emergency planning group and had special responsibility for the welfare and co-ordination of records of service personnel, refugees and survivors of the bombing who passed through the hospital. The hospital annual report for 1941 mentions the almoners as among other staff on duty during air raids. Elinor Gough's report for the same year refers to rehabilitation work with the injured and their families.

At this time (and for many years to come) money had to be raised from

Friendly Societies and voluntary organisations to help patients who could not afford the cost of, for example, surgical appliances, extra nourishment or treatment in a specialist unit in another area. The Poor Law system was still the only community provision, and the hospital itself was supported entirely by public contributions.

Elinor Gough returned to London in 1943, but left a staff of four at a time when no other local hospital had yet appointed social workers. She had established regular meetings between the almoners and Consultant staff, and clear communication through her regular reports.

Betty Hall, who succeeded her, was to serve the hospital for thirty years as departmental head, having already been a student and spent three years working for Elinor Gough. With the reorganisation in 1973 she became Principal Social Worker (Health Care) in the North and West Belfast area, but she still had the Royal Victoria Hospital department among her responsibilities until her retirement in 1977. She was greatly respected for the high standards of care she insisted upon from her staff and the good staff relations she fostered. Throughout her life she kept in touch with former staff and students, and the department was known for its friendliness. Betty Hall was known for her commitment to providing professional training in co-operation with the increasing number of university courses seeking good-quality teaching and experience for their students. She took a leading part in the professional development of social work in Northern Ireland and was on the NI Advisory Committee on the Training of Social Workers and its sister Committee for the Training of Health Visitors. She was awarded the MBE for services to social work in 1955.

As the department expanded to offer additional service to new areas of the hospital, both on site and at the Throne, at the Northern Ireland Fever Hospital and Radiotherapy Centre and at Haypark Hospital (for geriatric and convalescent patients, until it closed in 1986), many senior staff taught students. Betty Hall's deputy, René Boyd, became the main fieldwork teacher, taking units of three or four students concurrently. Rene Boyd became Assistant Principal in Charge of the department in 1973 and in 1977 became Principal Social Worker in North and West Belfast on Miss Hall's retirement. She had worked in the Royal Victoria Hospital for twenty-seven years.

The department had many homes as it grew. What Matron Elliot called 'the crutch cupboard' (for that is what it had been) was the first move after Elinor Gough gently declined the pleasant office allocated to her in favour of a table in outpatients where she was more readily accessible to patients, staff and relatives. Then the department went to the tiled office at the bottom of the old extern, which was reminiscent of a public convenience but was close to the outpatient clinics and the ward corridor. When the old extern was given an upstairs in 1947, part of this was clinic space and part was shared by the Central Registry and some almoner staff. The old room was floored at frieze level, and the series of little heads of Queen Victoria were bisected; it seemed disrespectful to be resting one's feet on the Queen's nose. Some staff at one period were officed in unused bedrooms in the East Wing and were dependent on a very eccentric lift. Interviews with relatives or patients had to take place in borrowed space elsewhere, as these offices were too distant. Finally in 1968, thanks to advice from the King's Fund (an independent committee advising on NHS matters) about the siting of social work services, the present excellent accommodation on Level 5 of the outpatient block was made available with its specially planned student accommodation and adequate privacy for interviewing.

When the department celebrated its twenty-first birthday in 1959, it was well established within the hospital. While the inception of the NHS in 1948 had removed many of the practical problems such as funding appliances or special treatments elsewhere, the complexities of new medical treatments, the greater emphasis on stress-related illnesses, and the particular importance of social work in the developing field of geriatric medicine ensured a continuing and increasing need for social workers.

In 1973 the major reorganisation of Northern Ireland's health and social services placed all hospital-based social workers on the budget and under the management of the social services structure in their unit of management. Although this technically meant that such staff in the Royal Group were now seconded into the hospitals, the presence of the District Social Services Officer on the district executive team gave some input at the higher hospital management level and some continuity.

At the onset of civil disturbances in 1969 some of the hospital social workers volunteered to help in the community for a period when the movements of population caused great strain on existing social services. Within the hospital, social workers, like other staff, were faced with many emotional and ethical dilemmas. Home visiting was difficult and often dangerous, and patients and their families were under great stress. Staff in the hospital were on night emergency call in north and west Belfast – social workers were often the only professionals to go into some areas at night. There was also a duty hospital social worker for the Royal Victoria Hospital.

In major disasters the social workers were on call for the hospital; much of what they learnt through this work has contributed to the establishment of 'trauma teams' of social workers within the area boards.

In 1988 the department celebrated its fiftieth birthday. Margaret Bamford (Assistant Principal Social Worker 1985–89) inspired her social workers to write a series of practice articles which appeared in ten successive issues of *Social Work Today* nationally; the first of these issues had a picture of the hospital on the cover. A dinner in the hospital, a study day and a reunion of former staff were all attended by Elinor Gough and Betty Hall as special guests.

Further reorganisations within the Northern Ireland Health Service have given cause for concern about funding and management issues in the changing structures. Social workers, whose work is vital in bridging the gap between hospital and community, can often fall between the two; some satisfactory arrangement – perhaps joint funding – is needed to ensure that this hospital-based service remains responsive to patient need and continues to ensure the appropriate use of both hospital and community resources.

THE PHARMACY

The history of the hospital's pharmacy service actually goes back further than the history of the hospital itself, since the original pharmacy dates from 1792, five years before the house in Factory Row was rented. A 1765 Act of the Irish Parliament had enabled funds to be made available for building infirmaries and for the purchase of medicines, but the act made no provision for the employment of dispensers in these infirmaries, this being apparently carried out by the physicians or surgeons. The planning committee of 1792 for the new hospital was not restricted by the 1765 Act, however, and one of its first actions was to appoint a resident apothecary, whose duties were not only the compounding and dispensing of all medicines prescribed by the Attending Physicians, but also to keep the accounts and a register of patients. The first apothecary was a Mr Hull, engaged at the relatively generous salary of £40 per year. He resigned in 1795 and Richard Devlin was elected in his place. We have most of the names of his successors throughout the nineteenth century, the most notable being James Murray, mentioned on page 7.

In 1814 the funding situation changed as a result of an act that empowered the governors of any infirmary in Ireland 'to procure the medicines from the Apothecaries' Hall in Dublin or from any wholesale dealer in medicines' and to 'pay to any apothecary who shall have duly served an apprenticeship to the art and mystery of an apothecary a sum by the year not exceeding thirty pounds as a salary for the compounding, making up, preparing and administering medicines to and for the use of patients of such infirmary'. In the early part of the century the cost of drugs used is not included in the annual hospital balance sheet. Presumably it was very low or was included in the apothecary's salary, which by 1832 (with residence allowance) had gone up to £56 13s. 4d. per year.

After 1854, there appears to have been no apothecary for some years; at about this time the Council of the Pharmaceutical Society issued a circular drawing the attention of hospital boards to the importance of having duly qualified pharmaceutical chemists or licentiates of the Apothecaries' Hall to do the dispensing, rather than students, nurses or other unqualified persons. The message was really only heeded two decades later: a dispenser was appointed in 1880 and a pharmaceutical chemist from 1881 onwards.

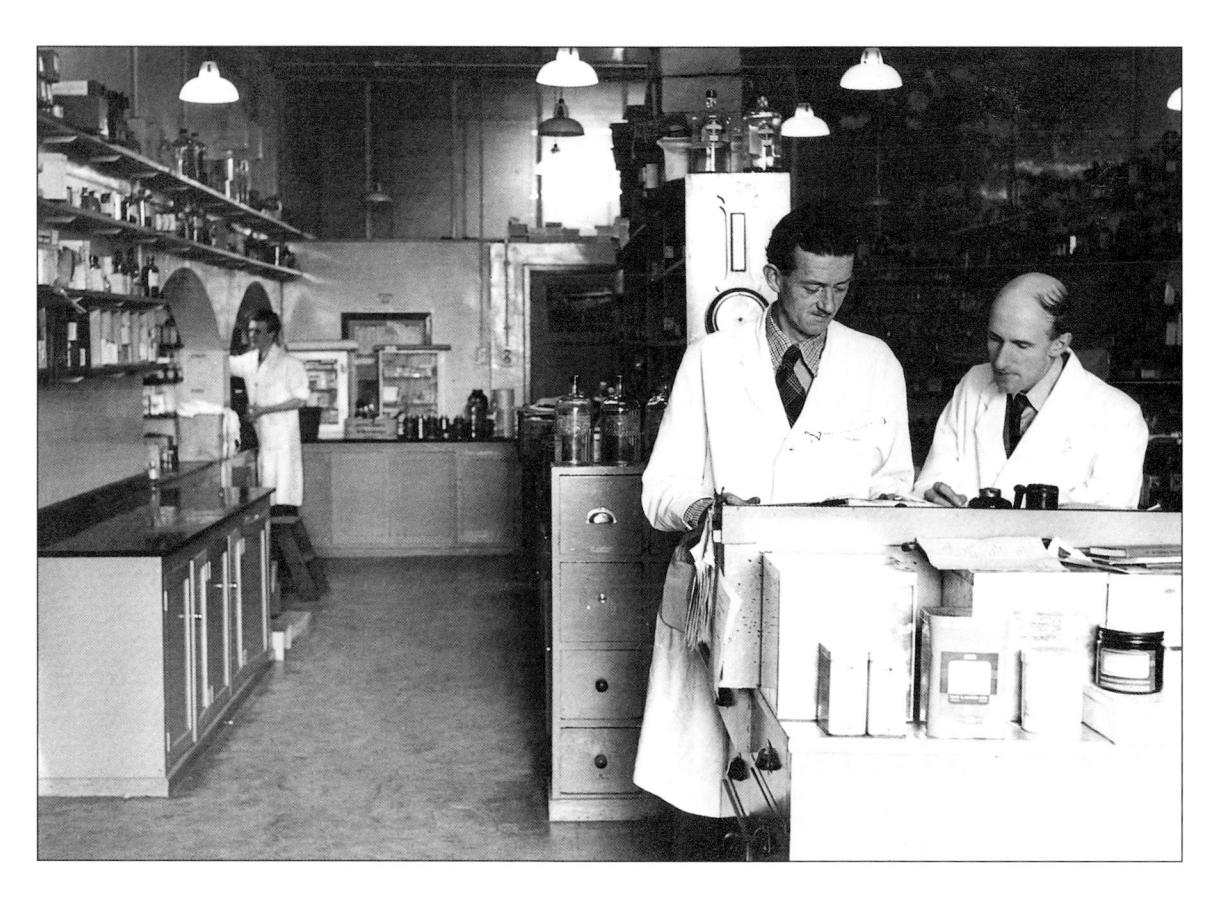

The pharmacy in 1953: *foreground:* John Restrick (*left*) and George McIlhagger
ROYAL VICTORIA HOSPITAL

The pharmaceutical chemists over the next twenty years were Alexander Chapman, George Young, W.J. McDade, David Elliott and James Cole, all of whom had the licentiate or membership of the Pharmaceutical Society of Ireland.

The whereabouts of the dispensary in the Belfast General Hospital is now uncertain; it is not marked on the plan. Certainly if the dispenser/chemist compounded the range of mixtures, pills, pessaries, et cetera, described in Whitla's *Pharmacy, Materia Medica and Therapeutics*, he would have been a busy man requiring several assistants and more than one room.

Mr James 'Matt' Cole LPSI, having come to the Royal Victoria Hospital in 1900, served the hospital as Chief Pharmacist right through until 1944 and was reported to be 'one of the most valued officials of the hospital and very popular with generations of housemen and nurses'. He was replaced by Mr John Restrick Ph.C. and by 1953 six pharmacists were employed, including also George McIlhagger, Alex Strahan and Norma Pielou. John Restrick was followed in the position of Chief Pharmacist by George McIlhagger (1963–74), Wilfie Black (acting, 1974–75), Roy Markwell (1975–89), and Sean O'Hare (1989–).

Another well-known worker in the dispensary from the 1920s was Hugh Patterson, the porter. Hugh started work in the hospital as a boy and spent all his working life there, living in hospital accommodation during many of his working years. His work in the dispensary involved the

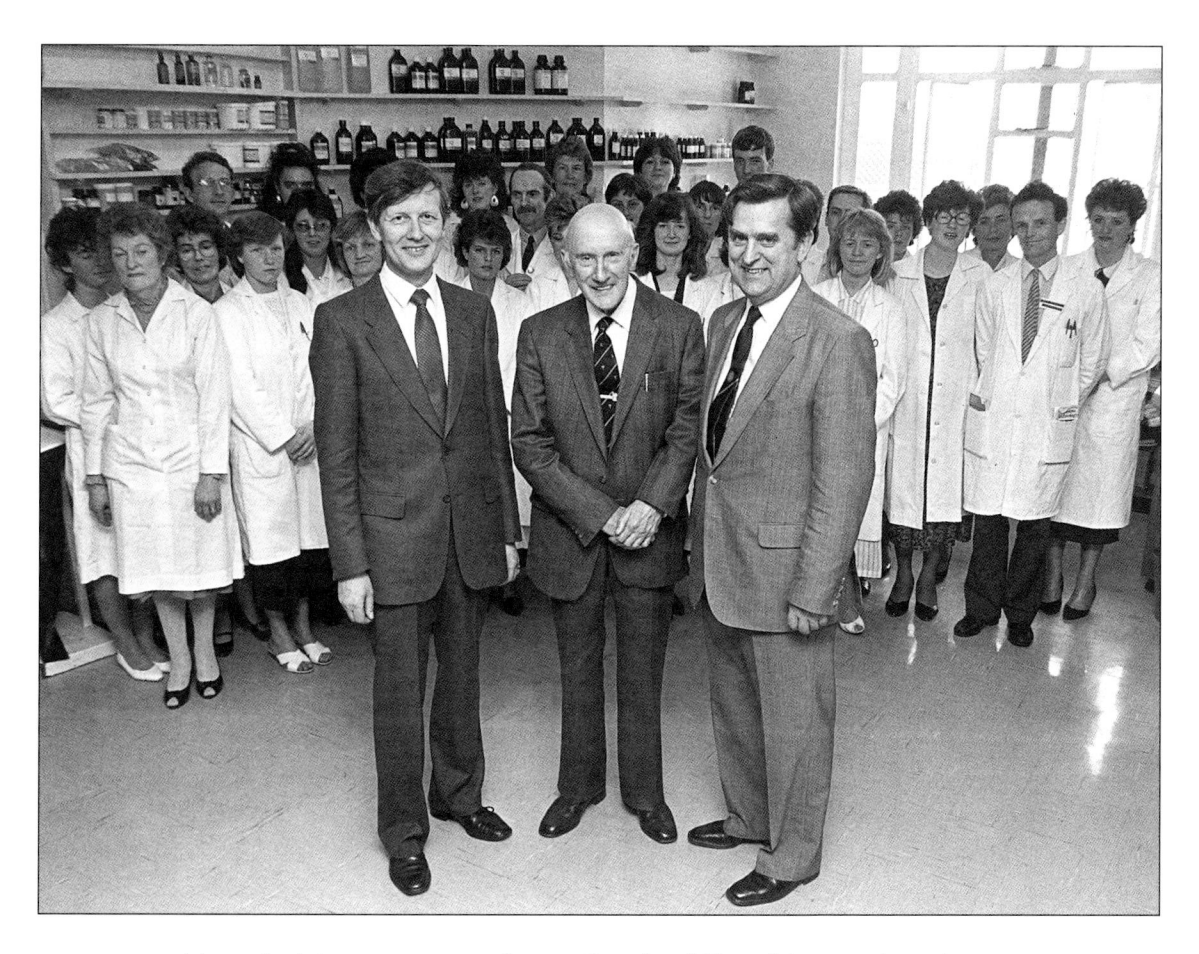

The pharmacy staff in 1985: *foreground, left to right:* Roy Markwell, Chief Pharmacist, George McIlhagger, retired Chief Pharmacist, and John Simpson, chairman of the Eastern Health and Social Services Board
ROYAL VICTORIA HOSPITAL

repacking of spirit soap, green soft soap, Lysol and Dettol in container sizes suitable for the wards; when this was finished he did other specific tasks such as bedpan washing.

In the years since 1953 the number of pharmacists and the range of work performed by them have expanded, and the pharmacist's role has changed from being medicine preparation and dispensing alone. Probably the biggest change occurred in the early 1970s when Noel Hall recommended in a report that such specialist tasks as drug information, quality control, production, and ward and clinical services should be taken on, and pharmacy technicians and assistants were introduced. Pharmacists could now undertake wider-ranging roles, while technicians and assistants could perform the tasks of preparation and provision of medicines, under supervision.

The hospital dispensary of the Royal Victoria Hospital was sited for many years on the main corridor opposite Ward 4; it moved to the archways below Ward 5 in 1951 and became known as 'the pharmacy'. An Intravenous Fluid Sterile Production Unit was already established in these archways and all intravenous fluids were prepared in this unit under the supervision of Alex Strahan. The unit had arisen from the need to prepare individual doses of the very scarce penicillin in a special Penicillin Room. The main work of preparing intravenous fluids continued in this area under the archways until the move in 1971 to a purpose-built manufacturing unit near the Works and Maintenance Department – the new Sterile Fluids Unit. Another facet of its work was the preparation of parenteral nutrition solutions, particularly for children; one pharmacist, Susie Rosbotham, was delegated to start a nutrition service in the Sterile Fluids Unit.

Further expansion in the main dispensary could not occur until the early 1960s, when the old Medical Records Department was acquired for more storage space and development of the production area for regularly demanded medicines, antiseptics, et cetera. A particular need was for space for a drug information service; this was developed in 1975, but for years it shared telephones and other equipment with the main pharmacy – an irritating situation but one that certainly kept it in close contact with what was going on in the rest of the hospital. A fire in the production area in July 1987 forced yet another redevelopment and more intensive use of the space available, which will continue until the department finds a new home in the hospital in the year 2000.

The cost of medicines and dressings has risen dramatically over the last ninety years. A typical month's invoices for April 1902 was £73 3s. 8d., in April 1945 it was £3,434 12s. 6d., and in 1996 it was of the order of £450,000. In a list of stock mixtures in 1915 there were some 77 products – typical of the demand of the time. Nowadays the number of different pharmaceutical products is over seven thousand, reflecting the development of medical treatment over the years.

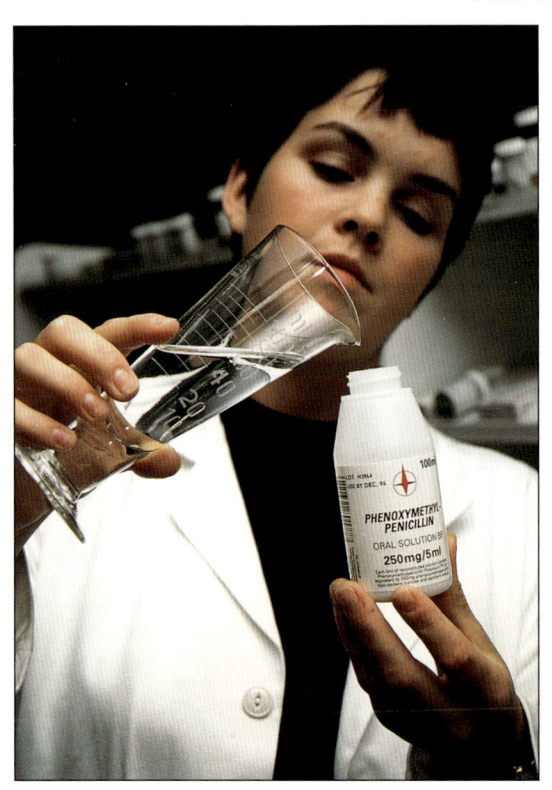

Pharmacist Róisín McCrory preparing a solution of penicillin, 1996
ROYAL VICTORIA HOSPITAL

PHYSIOTHERAPY

The origins of physiotherapy in the Royal Victoria Hospital lie in the 'Electrical Department', to which Dr John Rankin was appointed in 1903, though the department also included x-ray equipment and Finsen light treatment for skin diseases. In 1912 there were 4,682 attendances at the department and only 895 radiograms, so presumably many of the other patients were receiving some form of 'heat treatment'. During World War One large massage departments were set up all over the UK for the benefit of sick and wounded soldiers, and in 1920 the hospital annual report refers to a 'Massage Department' which had 798 new cases in the year and gave 6,459 treatments. This report comments that 'the Hospital has found the usefulness of this department in decreasing the period of disability, lessening the suffering and increasing the comfort of a large and increasing number of patients'. In this activity the hospital was following the trend throughout the UK; in 1894 a Society of Trained Masseuses had been set up, and by 1920 it had a membership of five thousand. This body became the Chartered Society of Physiotherapists in 1942.

After World War One, annual reports give specific figures for massage, electrical treatment, radiant heat and Swedish remedial exercises. In 1923 twelve cubicles with sliding curtains were provided, as well as a new radiant heat lamp and a 'new and up-to-date diathermy apparatus' for treatment of sciatica, arthritis and injuries. In 1928 Dr E.D. Rutherford (a Queen's graduate and formerly a surgeon-captain) was in charge of the department, but he retired in 1938. Annual treatment figures thereafter continue to increase and, whilst the majority of patients were from outside the hospital, about six thousand treatments were given to inpatients. The department continued to provide a service throughout World War Two, and in 1942 a gymnasium was opened in connection with the fracture clinic. Eventually, in 1948, the Northern Ireland Hospitals Authority decided to provide a new Physiotherapy Department and in the following year a School of Physiotherapy. Prior to this students had to travel to England, Scotland or the Republic of Ireland to be trained.

Two particular individuals were instrumental in the development of physiotherapy within the Royal Victoria Hospital in this era: Dr George Gregg OBE, MD, FRCPI, Dip.Phys.Med, who was the physician in charge of physiotherapy in 1953, and John Heylings MCSP, TET, TMMG, who took up the post of Principal of School and Group Superintendent in 1956. John Heylings was physiotherapy adviser to the Northern Ireland Hospitals Authority. Initially the school was based within the Physiotherapy Department, which was housed in a number of different locations across the site at different times. It originally occupied two rooms at the rear of the 'caves', and in 1950 moved to a separate building overlooking what used to be the outdoor swimming pool. The Physiotherapy School then moved into Nissen hut accommodation for a period of about four years before being relocated onto the Broadway site, which was originally Broadway Mills.

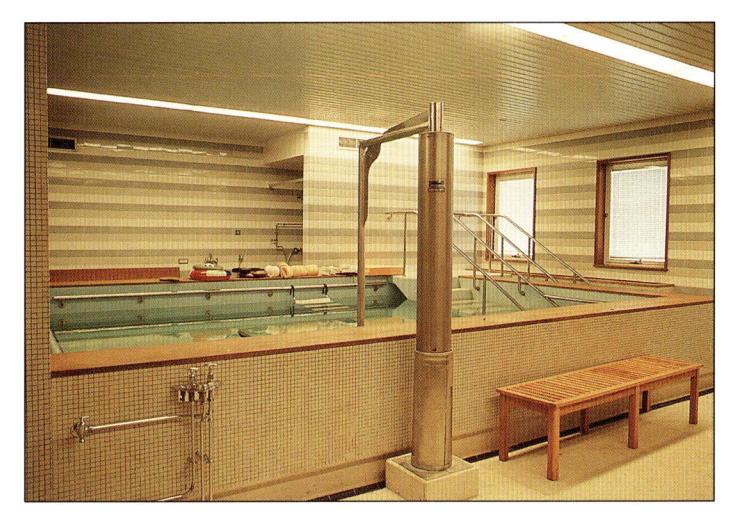

The physiotherapy pool on Level 3 of the Outpatient Building
ROYAL VICTORIA HOSPITAL

By 1953 the physiotherapy department was employing twenty physiotherapists, a number of whom were providing satellite services to other hospitals in the greater Belfast area including Belfast City Hospital, Musgrave Park Hospital, the Whiteabbey and Greenisland hospitals, Forster Green Hospital and Claremont Street Hospital.

In 1968–69 the Physiotherapy Department moved to the new Austen Boyd Outpatient Building. The new department afforded much-improved facilities including a large gymnasium, a hydrotherapy pool, and a spacious outpatient treatment department.

In 1972 the Northern Ireland School of Physiotherapy transferred from

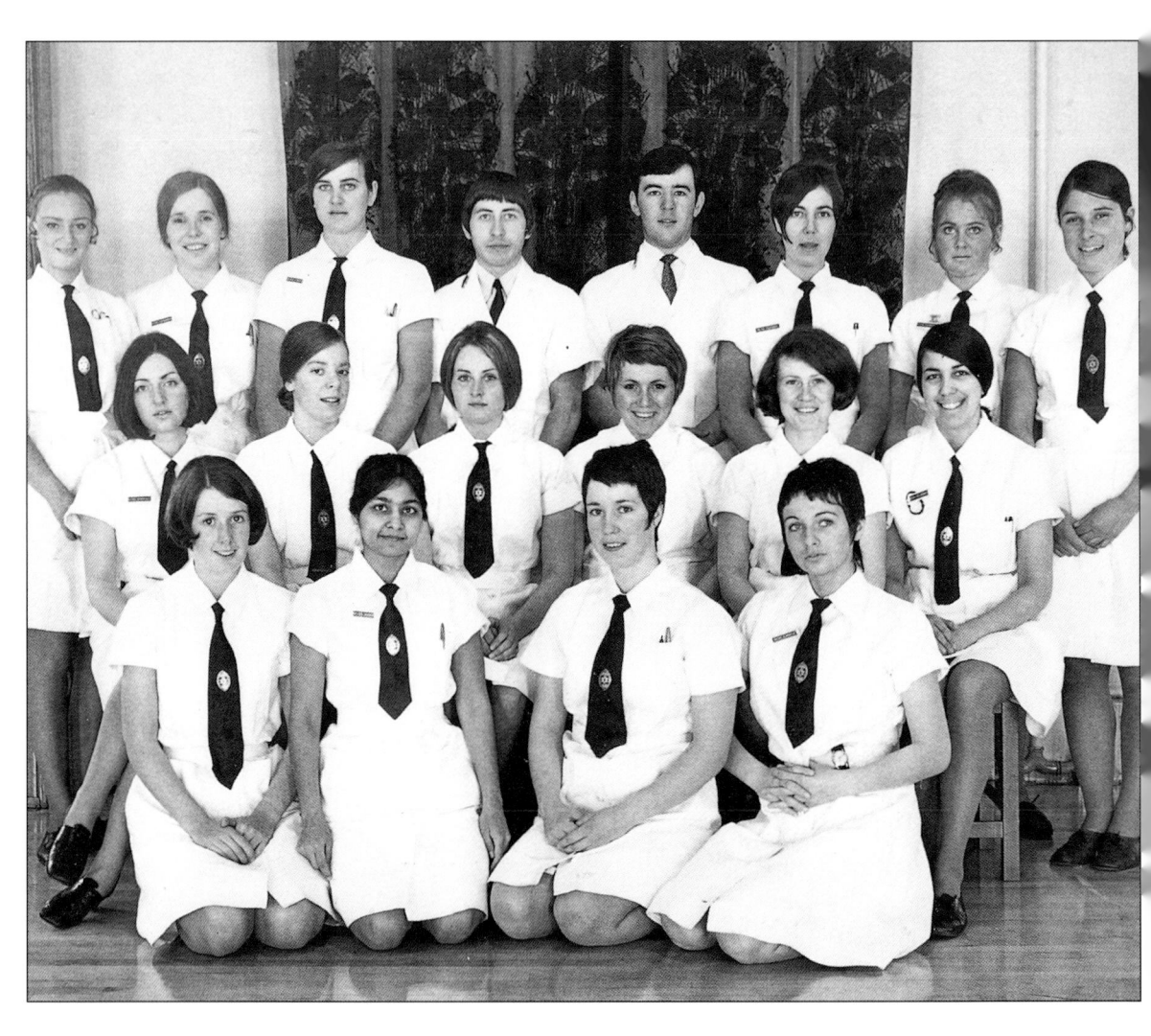

Physiotherapy students in 1969: *back row, left to right:* Barbara Cummings, Pat Drummond, Alice Lynch, Arne Baerem, Petre Goodman, Aileen Creaney, Beatrice McMordie and Hazel Wylie; *middle row:* Catherine Worrall, Meryl McDonald, Anthea Barbour, Pam Balmer, Geraldine McMillan and Doreen Henry; *front row:* Jennifer Best, Nilham Kehr, Aileen McCloud and René Larkin.
ROYAL VICTORIA HOSPITAL

the Royal site to the Ulster Polytechnic at Jordanstown (now the University of Ulster), and in 1976 it established the first degree course in the UK. The opportunity to do this arose when part of the Broadway site was demolished to make way for the new West Link road development; John Heylings was instrumental in achieving the much-desired relocation for the school.

When the new physiotherapy department opened in the Austen Boyd Outpatient Building, the Superintendent Physiotherapist in charge was Elizabeth Thompson. She had first joined the staff in 1945 and remained there until her retirement in June 1979, when she was succeeded by Muriel Patterson OBE, MCSP. Muriel Patterson in turn was succeeded by Rita Fox MBA, B.Sc., MCSP in June 1989.

Physiotherapy services in the Royal Victoria Hospital have continued to grow and develop over the years in tandem with other advances in the fields of medicine and rehabilitation. By 1996 a total of fifty-seven qualified physiotherapists were employed, providing a wide range of specialist physiotherapy services to patients throughout the renamed Royal Hospitals Trust.

OCCUPATIONAL THERAPY

Occupational therapy was preceded by diversional therapy and the latter should be mentioned here if only to emphasise the distinction. Diversional therapy started in 1946 – and some may remember Mrs Crawford Brown pushing round a trolley loaded with wool for knitting and rug making, leatherwork, et cetera – the aim essentially being to help patients to pass their time in hospital. The next personality to take on this service was Mrs Webster, mother of the well-known comedienne Leila Webster. Occupational therapy, by contrast, is carried out by trained staff and is aimed at treating the patient and remedying a specific clinical need or disability.

The occupational therapy service was established in 1968 in the newly built Austen Boyd Outpatient Building, and the department opened with a very small 'activities of daily living' unit within the Physiotherapy Department in the Department of Physical Medicine (DPM). The Consultant in Charge of the DPM was Dr George Gregg. The first Occupational Therapist to be appointed was Lindsay Farries, 1968–70; she was followed by Joan Meharry, 1969–74, and the first head Occupational Therapist was Celia Gore-Grimes, 1970–72.

In 1971 the staffing establishment increased to six and services were offered to patients in wards 1–22, the Musgrave and Clark Clinic, Outpatients and the Claremont Street Hospital. The Ulster Polytechnic opened its doors to the first Occupational Therapy students in 1972, and the RVH Occupational Therapy Department accepted its first students on clinical placement. Occupational therapy services expanded to include the geriatric medical unit, that is, Florence Elliott House and later the Catherine Dynes Unit, which included day-stay patients and a further two wards. Services were also supplied from the department to the Throne Hospital and to Haypark Hospital. In 1972, following the resignation of Mrs Gore-Grimes, a new head Occupational Therapist, Mrs Gwenda Dunlop (née Pape), was appointed. She was also designated district occupational therapist for the North and West Belfast Unit of Management and as part of that role was instrumental in establishing both the occupational therapy service in the Mater Hospital and the domiciliary/community occupational therapy service in North and West Belfast.

The Occupational Therapy Department underwent some structural changes in the 1980s, and has expanded its service in order to meet the changing demands of an ever-changing health service. Today, occupational therapy is provided across a range of specialities on the hospital site including neurosciences, general medical and surgical wards, fractures, A & E, geriatric medicine and outpatients; since 1991 the department has also provided a service to children suffering from delayed development, cerebral palsy and other congenital and acquired conditions attending the

Royal Belfast Hospital for Sick Children. The whole staffing establishment is twenty-eight, which includes eighteen qualified Occupational Therapists, occupational therapy helpers, a technician, an art therapist and therapy support workers. The present head of department is Mairead McGowan, appointed in 1993.

NUTRITION AND DIETETICS

The Dietetic Department at the Royal Victoria Hospital was opened in 1947, in response to a growing awareness of the need to respond to the nutritional requirements of the individual patient. On the recommendation of Rose Simmons who pioneered dietetics in the British Isles, Barbara Taylor was appointed to establish the Dietetic Department. A diet kitchen was set up in a bay of the main kitchen with the dietitian's office nearby. A staff of diet cooks was employed to provide the practical elements of the service. In 1948, Kathleen Acheson, a qualified nurse from the Royal Victoria Hospital, returned to the hospital having completed a Diploma in Dietetics from the Royal College of Nursing, London, and took up a post in the Dietetic Department. Later, in 1950, she became Chief Dietitian. At that time, there was a staff of three dietitians; the numbers reached a peak in the mid-eighties when the full-time equivalent dietetic staff numbered twelve. When Kathleen Acheson retired in 1983, she was succeeded by Anne Wilson, who had trained at Athol Crescent domestic science school, Edinburgh, and at the Glasgow and West of Scotland College of Domestic Science, followed by work in Oxford and Greenwich. She had returned to Belfast to become Senior Dietitian in the Sir George E. Clark Metabolic Unit. Anne Wilson retired from the post of Chief Dietitian in February 1995, and was replaced by Jennifer Holmes, formerly Deputy Chief Dietitian.

Until a course in Nutrition and Dietetics was set up at the University of Ulster at Coleraine in the eighties, it was necessary for students to complete their academic course elsewhere in the British Isles. The department has provided clinical experience for a considerable number of student dietitians and enjoys an excellent working relationship with the various colleges. For many years, the Royal Victoria Hospital was a recruiting ground for other dietetic departments in Northern Ireland.

Since its beginning, the Dietetic Department has played an integral role in the nutritional welfare of the patients. Many dietary regimes have come and gone. The education of the diabetic patients remains a fundamental part of therapy along with many other therapeutic regimes, while more recently support of the undernourished patient has become recognised as an essential element of medical care.

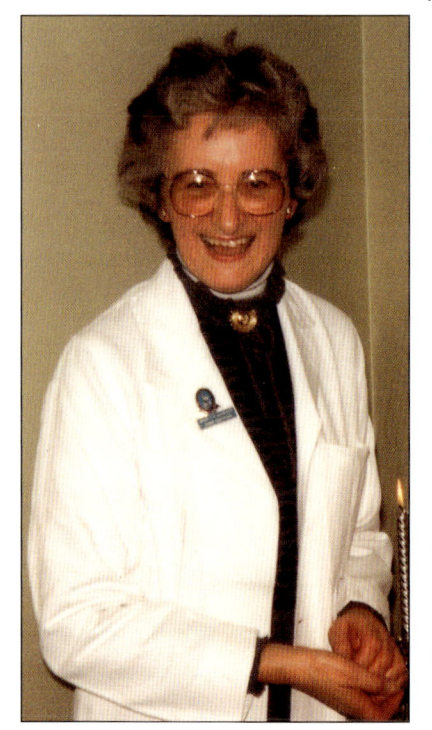

Kathleen Acheson,
Chief Dietitian, 1950–83
ROYAL VICTORIA HOSPITAL

SPEECH AND LANGUAGE THERAPY

In December 1938, Molly (Hayward) Christie, an English speech therapist, opened the speech clinic at the Belfast Hospital for Sick Children. It was the first of its kind in Ireland and she had concerns about how the medical profession would receive it. However 'they showed interest and gave every help and facility within their power'. The following year she was also appointed to the staff of the Nervous Diseases Hospital, Claremont Street. During that first year, the caseload had a predominance of stammerers, followed in numbers by 'lallers', 'retarded speakers', cleft palates, neurological disorders, the deaf, and 'lispers'. Molly Christie departed from Northern Ireland in 1945 and her post was taken by Joyce Mitchell, who had just left the Auxiliary Territorial Service at the end of World War Two. She stayed for seven years, working single-handed for some time and later with a more junior therapist.

With the opening of Quin House, neurosurgeons and neurologists referred patients to the speech clinic at the Royal Belfast Hospital for Sick Children; post-laryngectomy patients were referred by the ENT Consultants. Bettina Kay, another English therapist, came from Lincoln in 1954 to the post of Senior Speech Therapist and remained until her untimely death from leukaemia in 1977. In this period, assessment and treatment of children and adults with communication problems became well established.

In 1956 the first speech therapy joint appointment, between the Belfast Hospitals Management Committee and Belfast Corporation, was made. Later the Belfast City Hospital, Eastern Special Care, Malcolm Sinclair House (Northern Ireland Council for Orthopaedic Development) and Musgrave Park Hospital asked to have speech therapy sessions. The Northern Ireland Hospitals Authority policy in 1963 was to form a pool of therapists in the Royal Belfast Hospital for Sick Children, with the Senior Speech Therapist allocating staff to the clinics with greatest need.

The Northern Ireland Hospitals Authority had provided contracts for student speech therapists, as an aid to recruitment in Northern Ireland, but in 1968 these were abolished. Bettina Kay was reduced to working with the help of only one speech therapy aide and a secretary. In order to cope with the many patients referred, she organised group therapy for pre-school children, stammerers, laryngectomy patients and dysphasic patients, as well as being involved in the Regional Joint Cleft Palate Clinic and providing individual therapy for some children and adults.

As early as 1949, discussions were held about the viability of providing training for speech therapists in Northern Ireland; Miss Van Thal (an early pioneer of speech therapy in England) came from London to assist in these talks. Training did not begin, however, until the first students commenced their course at the Ulster Polytechnic in 1975.

The present senior course tutor in the honours-degree Speech and

Language Therapy course at the University of Ulster is Aileen Patterson, who worked with Bettina Kay in the Royal Belfast Hospital for Sick Children. Another of Miss Kay's colleagues was Eleanor (Hutchinson) Gildea, now retired from the profession but previously the area therapist for the Eastern Health and Social Services Board and very influential in the growth and development of speech and language therapy in the board area.

At present, the Royal Hospitals Trust Department of Speech and Language Therapy comprises six therapists – five full-time and one part-time – and one secretary. The therapists are hospital-based and work in the areas of paediatrics, health care of the elderly, acute and rehabilitation stroke care, neurosciences and ENT.

There is more co-operation between physicians, neurologists, laryngologists and speech therapists in the nineties than there was in the thirties and forties, and more babies and very young children are now referred. Both adults and children are seen because of feeding and swallowing difficulties as well as communication difficulty, and speech and language therapists are involved in bedside and radiological assessment of these patients. The department continues to have child patients and large numbers of adult and child outpatients with voice disorders. There has been a reversal in the ratio of inpatients to outpatients, however, with stroke and other neurological problems – many more inpatients are now seen for acute care and early-stage rehabilitation, often subsequently being referred to community therapists for follow-up.

Margaret Newman, the present head of the department, who first worked in the Royal Belfast Hospital for Sick Children with Bettina Kay, records that Molly Christie had a caseload of 68 patients in 1939, whereas in 1994–95 a total of 570 new patients were seen by the Department of Speech and Language Therapy.

CHIROPODY AND PODIATRY

The first full-time podiatrist (then known as a 'chiropodist'), was appointed in 1979 to assess, diagnose and treat foot problems in the diabetic population attending the metabolic unit at the Royal Victoria Hospital. Treatment included preventative education about general care of the feet, palliative footcare, and intensive management of those patients with limb-threatening ulceration. In 1984 an outpatient nail surgery service was introduced in the department and in April 1985 a podiatry service began at the diabetic clinic in the Royal Belfast Hospital for Sick Children with an emphasis on preventative care in the young diabetic. In the Department of Health Care for the Elderly, a podiatry service is provided for the elderly patients on an inpatient and outpatient basis at the day hospital.

Emphasis today is very much on preventative care, and on the intensive treatment of diabetic foot ulcers on an outpatient basis, thus reducing the need for hospital admission.

CLINICAL PSYCHOLOGY

There have been many changes in the fifty-year history of psychology services in the Royal hospitals, with a significant expansion during the past ten years. Clinical and educational psychology formed part of the Child Guidance Service in the hospitals, which was established in 1943, although it is uncertain when the first psychologist took up post. Other psychology staff transferred with the Department of Child Psychiatry from the Belfast City Hospital in the early 1970s to form the Regional Child Mental Health Service. Clinical psychology, however, established a wider service within the Royal Hospitals Group itself across a range of specialities.

Belfast City Hospital provided the neuropsychological service to the Royal Victoria Hospital during the early 1980s, until Alice Haller and Hazel Dusoir eventually transferred over in the late 1980s.

The role of the psychologist expanded during this period with the establishment in 1988 of a post in paediatric cardiology (Nichola Rooney), the transfer of the Regional Paediatric Child Mental Health Services from Lissue House to Forster Green Hospital (Jacqueline McMaster), and establishment of services to Paediatric Intensive Care and the general paediatric specialities.

Until 1991, clinical psychologists were organised as an area service within the Eastern Health and Social Services Board under the direction of Dr Desmond Poole, and managed by the medical administration in the Royal Victoria Hospital (Dr George Murnaghan) with the other nonmedical clinical services. The Department of Clinical Psychology was only formally established in 1991 with the appointment of a Services Manager (Patricia Donnelly), who in 1994 also became the first Clinical Director of the reorganised nonmedical specialities, now entitled the Directorate of Clinical Professions.

During the 1990s, the Department of Clinical Psychology was at the centre of trauma services to the children of Northern Ireland through treatment and research. Bereavement services were established in the Royal Belfast Hospital for Sick Children under the direction of Dr Rooney. Following a major study, psychology input to occupational health services was provided in 1996 by Wendy Losty, who also developed a role with the breast clinic and the Department of Genito-Urinary Medicine.

There has always been a strong association with Queen's University Belfast in training, teaching and research in the doctorate programme for Clinical Psychology, and in the research activity in the Royal Maternity Hospital (Donald Sykes and Elizabeth Hoy, Professor Peter Hepper) and the Belfast Monica Project for Heart Disease.

Clinical psychologists have become involved in the reorganisation of the

Royal Hospitals Group through participation in many committees and working groups. By 1996 they had a well-established service within the group, an establishment of ten posts and six external service contracts to community and acute units within Northern Ireland. For nearly two years the unit has also provided psychology services to the Dumfries and Galloway area in the west of Scotland: staff have travelled to Stranraer each week to run clinics for local general practitioners.

THE LADIES' COMMITTEE

In 1939, as the possibilities of war loomed, a group of women responded to a suggestion from the surgeon Mr A.B. Mitchell and the honorary treasurer Victor Clarendon to form a fundraising committee. It was at first called the Association of Friends of the Royal Victoria Hospital, but in 1943 the name was changed to the Ladies' Committee. The funds raised in pre-NHS days were, of course, mainly used to endow beds, but some luxuries were provided, such as a nurses' library, a patients' library and a mobile canteen for the students. The committee was also responsible for the refurbishment of the wards in 1947–59.

After 1948 all the money raised by the committee went to make the hospital more comfortable, by providing curtained cubicles, lockers, soundproofed floors, easy chairs, clocks and radios. Later items included television sets, telephone trolleys, more hygienic water jugs, patients' guides and the refurbishment of the chapel on the corridor. Since the 1980s and financial constraints, the committee has returned to helping with more expensive items for patient care, such as specialist hoverbeds fitted with airflow canopies for the treatment of serious burn victims, operating

The Ladies' Committee in the board room, King Edward Building, 1982, including Miss O'Brien, Mrs Carson, Mrs McKeown, Miss Heather Barrett (Matron), Mrs Stanfield, Dr Ingrid Allen, Lady Dunleath, Dr Terence Fulton, Mrs Calwell, Mrs Lavery, Mrs Vaugh, Mrs Moorehead and Mrs Campbell
ROYAL VICTORIA HOSPITAL

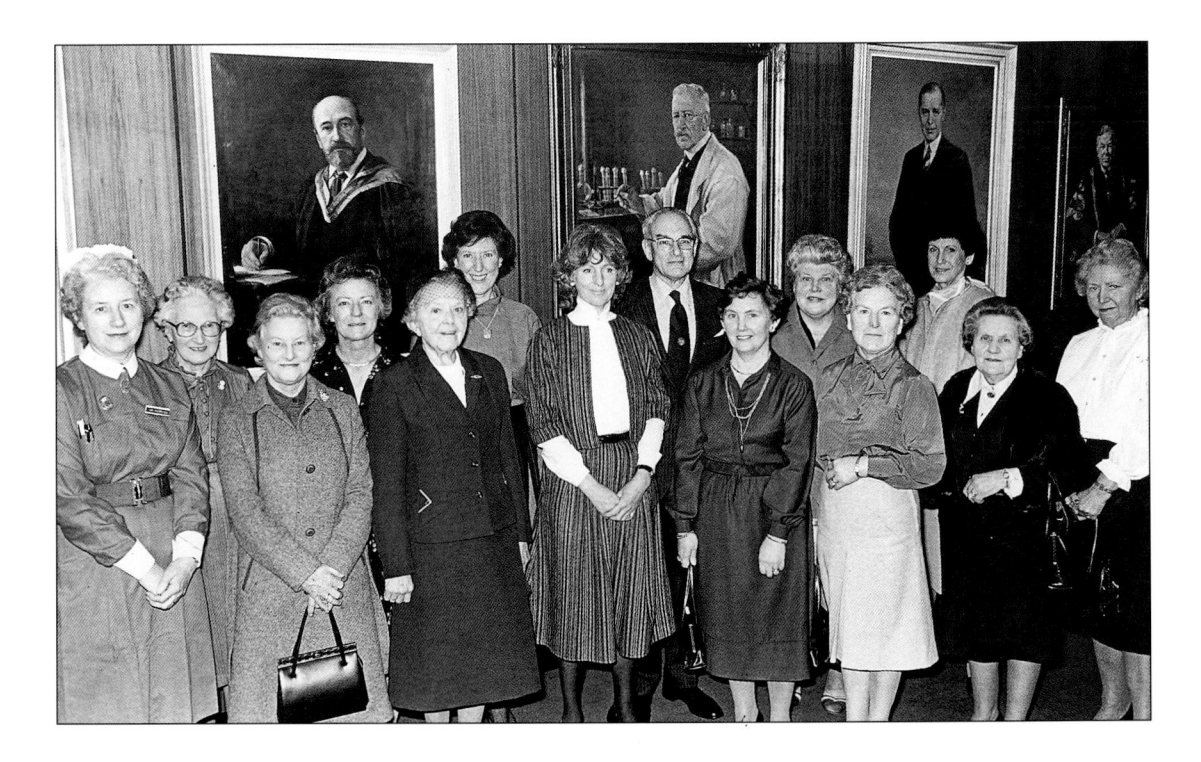

microscopes, and special lifts for paralysed patients.

Lady Dunleath is currently the president of the Ladies' Committee, Heather Calwell is chairperson, Mary Angus is vice-chairperson, Eleanor Menarry is honorary secretary, and Pamela Lewis is honorary treasurer. The committee has remained at its strength of forty to fifty members and has always managed to attract influential and energetic people to do work, so that now after more than fifty years of existence it is still playing an important part in the fundraising of the hospital.

THE EX-PATIENTS' GUILD

The Ex-Patients' Guild was inaugurated in December 1945 to attract donations from grateful patients. It was decided that every ex-patient should be entitled to become a member on paying or collecting for the guild the sum of at least £2 and on contributing ten shillings annually. A sum of over £13,000 had been raised by 1953, and the guild was still flourishing into the 1970s. The collections were used for a variety of purposes such as soundproofing the wards by reflooring (1962), and purchase of an anaesthetic ventilator and curtains for the x-ray department. The guild gradually declined during the 1970s, at least partly because of problems with the Data Protection Act, but the pharmacist George Davis was the much-valued secretary until his death in January 1996.

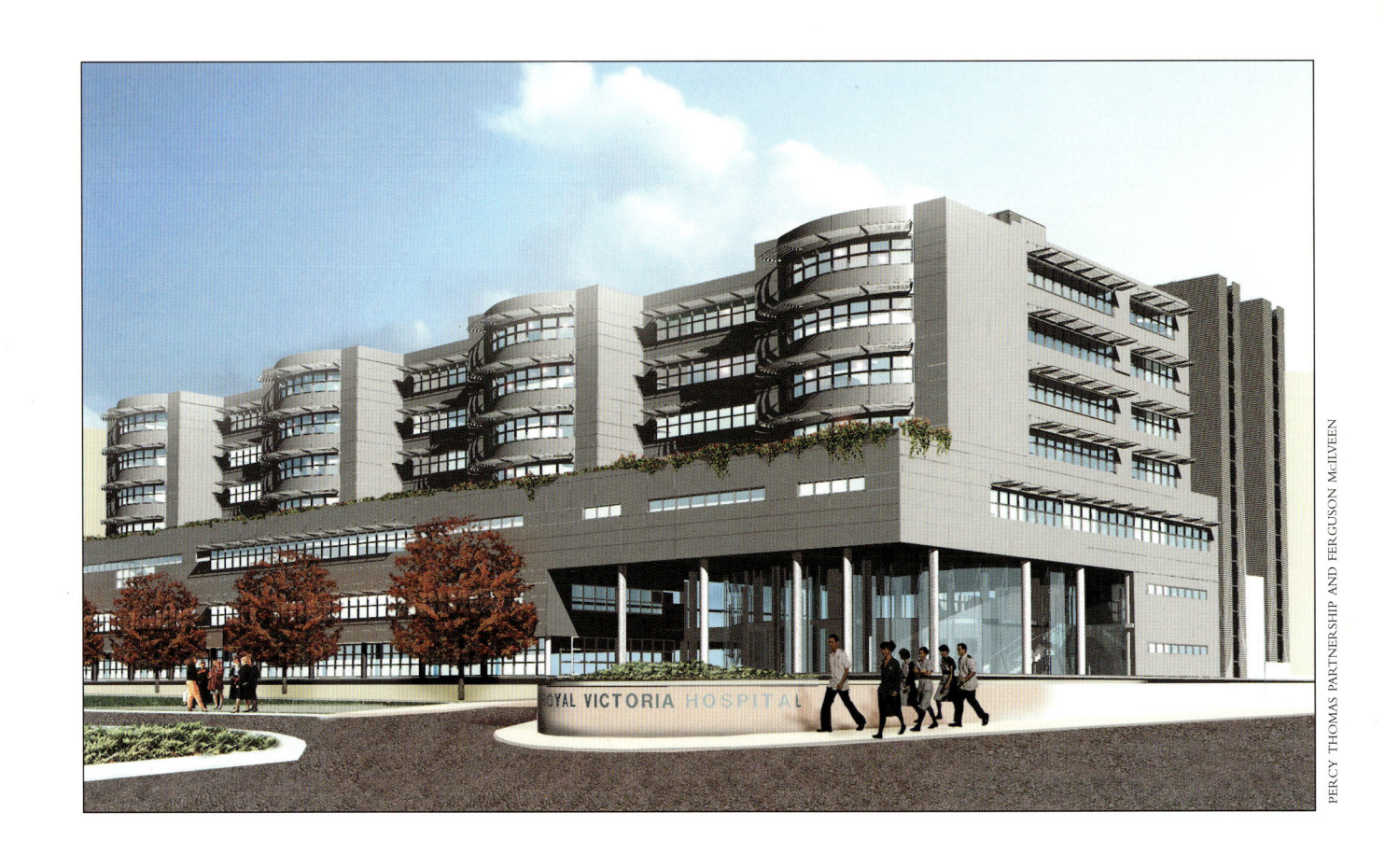

PERCY THOMAS PARTNERSHIP AND FERGUSON McILVEEN

8

TRUST STATUS AND REBUILDING

Above:
Architect's computerised drawing of the south front of the proposed new hospital

In the 1990s, the concept of 'trust' status offered hospitals new powers and freedoms to manage their own affairs. Operating independently of area health and social services boards (purchasers), hospitals – as service providers – could take advantage of wider National Health Service reforms to improve services, seek more appropriate contracts and take greater control of their futures. Direct access to government for capital development funding would end the reliance on unsatisfactory existing arrangements for such funding, which by 1990 had left much of the Royal hospitals site with badly maintained buildings and ageing equipment. Self-government would enable a trust to bring about long-overdue redevelopment plans.

As already noted, since 1972 the Royal hospitals had had a unified management structure as part of the North and West Belfast District of the Eastern Health and Social Services Board. However, from 1984 this structure changed: the Royal hospitals and Dental Hospital were separated from the Mater Infirmorum Hospital and from the social services of North and West Belfast, and three separate 'units of management' were created. Within the Royal Group of Hospitals each division (anaesthetists, surgeons, medical, laboratories, et cetera) became a directorate and its chairman elected by his or her peers was replaced by a director appointed from above. By the end of the decade the directors of the various directorates were asked to prepare shadow budgets on the basis that they controlled their own staff and expenditure. With this information they could then plan their activities. Along with this went the concept of resource management by which all was costed and managed in the most efficient way.

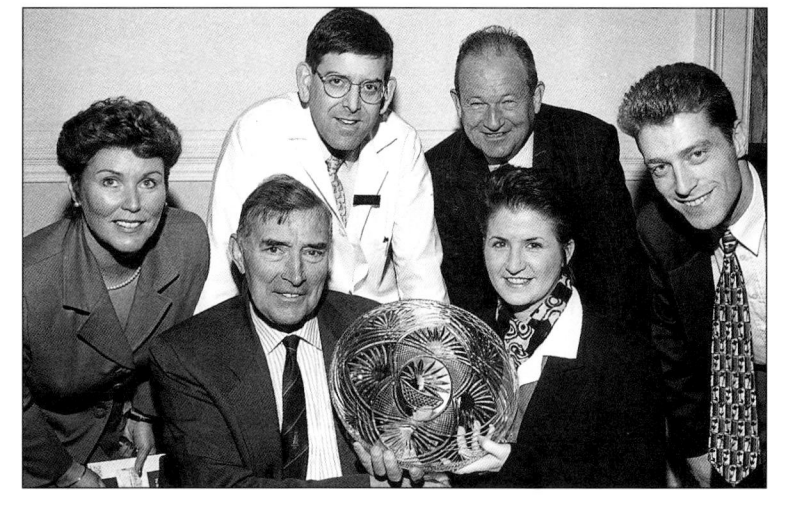

The Royal Group of Hospitals and Dental Hospital applied to the Department of Health and Social Services for trust status in April 1991. The application was accepted and the Royal Group of Hospitals and Dental Hospital Health and Social Services Trust came into operation on 1 April 1993. The chairman of the trust was the leading Northern Ireland banker and former civil service permanent secretary Sir George Quigley, who had skilfully guided the hospitals through a 'shadow trust' period. William McKee, who had chaired the Unit of Management Executive Team, was appointed chief executive. Sir George resigned as chairman in January 1996 when he was succeeded by Paul McWilliams OBE, who was already a nonexecutive trust director and has wide experience in industrial development and the computing world.

A hospital trust is not, of course, a free agent even within the financial constraints imposed by budgeting and tendering. In theory a trust can tender for any service, for example repair of an inguinal hernia or coronary artery bypass grafting, but in practice purchasers of services – area boards and general practitioners – can influence the infrastructure available in a particular hospital for a given procedure. The area board is also responsible for ensuring quality control, often guided by the royal colleges, while leaving to the hospital trust the question of how that quality is to be maintained.

The handing over of one of the commemorative pieces of Tyrone crystal to the Bicentenary Committee chairman: *left to right:* Mary Graham, Professor John Bridges, Dr Julian Johnston, Paul McWilliams (chairman of the Trust), Fidelis Ewing (Tyrone Crystal) and Peter Compton (Tyrone Crystal)
ROYAL VICTORIA HOSPITAL

Opposite:
Site plan for the redevelopment of the Royal Victoria Hospital (by the Percy Thomas Partnership and Ferguson McIlveen, architects). The dark areas in the centre are the new buildings, the part to the south (with four bays) being Phase 1 and that to the north, occupying the site of the present corridor wards, being Phase 2. The old corridor and the buildings fronting onto the Grosvenor Road (including the engine room with the fans, et cetera) are to be preserved.
ROYAL VICTORIA HOSPITAL

On the positive side, trust status should mean full financial control of expenses, costs and salaries and, provided the concept that the 'money follows the patient' means what it says, a trust should operate smoothly. However, the trust director must also take into account the hidden costs of running a tertiary referral service, a continuous emergency service, a radiological investigative service, and an intensive care service – all for the whole of Northern Ireland. In addition there are the costs of teaching undergraduates and postgraduates and of continuing research in all departments of the hospital. These costs can be difficult to quantify for any large teaching hospital, and when 'efficiency savings' are demanded they can often make life very difficult for trust board and directors.

REBUILDING THE ROYAL

Plans have been mooted for rebuilding the hospital in the space behind the wards for at least twenty-five years. Committees, architects and plans have come and gone. More particularly, the A Block and its link block with the outpatient corridor were completed, but the B Block to rehouse the general wards was never started. However, following extensive planning work during 1993–95, plans were accepted by the Department of Health and Social Services and finally some £65 million was allocated by the government for the rebuilding of the Royal Victoria Hospital.

At this stage the Royal Hospitals Trust mounted a major design competition which involved the Royal Institute of British Architects and the Royal Society of Ulster Architects, with the architect Sir Philip Powell, an international expert, as senior assessor. Applications came in from all over the world and eventually a shortlist of ten suitably experienced consortia was selected. These were supplied with a detailed brief on the project, which itself had taken a year to compile but did define very closely what was required. Finally a design submitted by a consortium led by the Percy Thomas Partnership, based in London, and the local architects Ferguson McIlveen was selected. The judges were impressed by the organisation of the winning entry, the immediately understandable layout, the large capacity for natural lighting, and the attention paid to the views out of the hospital. Externally the building will have a light, bright modern cladding system contrasting with the red brick of the old building. It will also be distinctive in having its main entrance through a cleverly

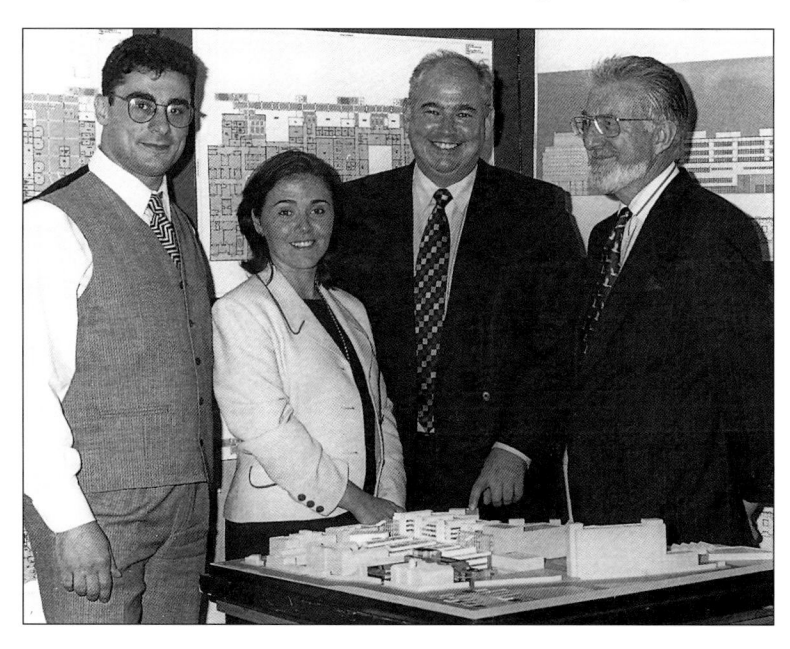

Chief Executive William McKee (*second from right*) showing the model of the new Royal Victoria Hospital to Alan McNally (*left*), Nuala McKeagney and John Comerton, members of the City Business Club
ROYAL VICTORIA HOSPITAL

GROSVENOR ROAD

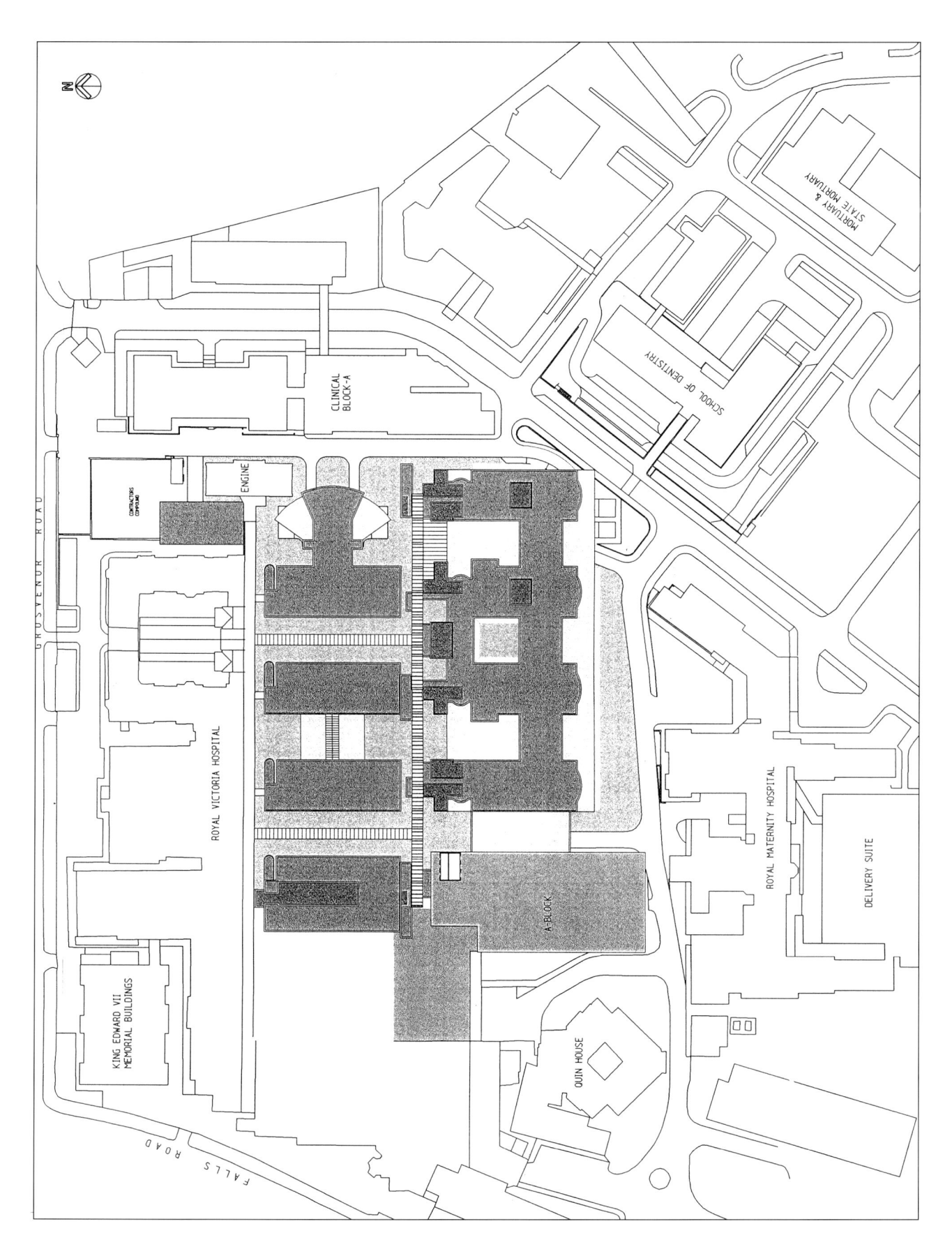

CLINICAL BLOCK-A

ENGINE

ROYAL VICTORIA HOSPITAL

SCHOOL OF DENTISTRY

MORTUARY & STATE MORTUARY

A-BLOCK

ROYAL MATERNITY HOSPITAL

DELIVERY SUITE

KING EDWARD VII MEMORIAL BUILDINGS

QUIN HOUSE

FALLS ROAD

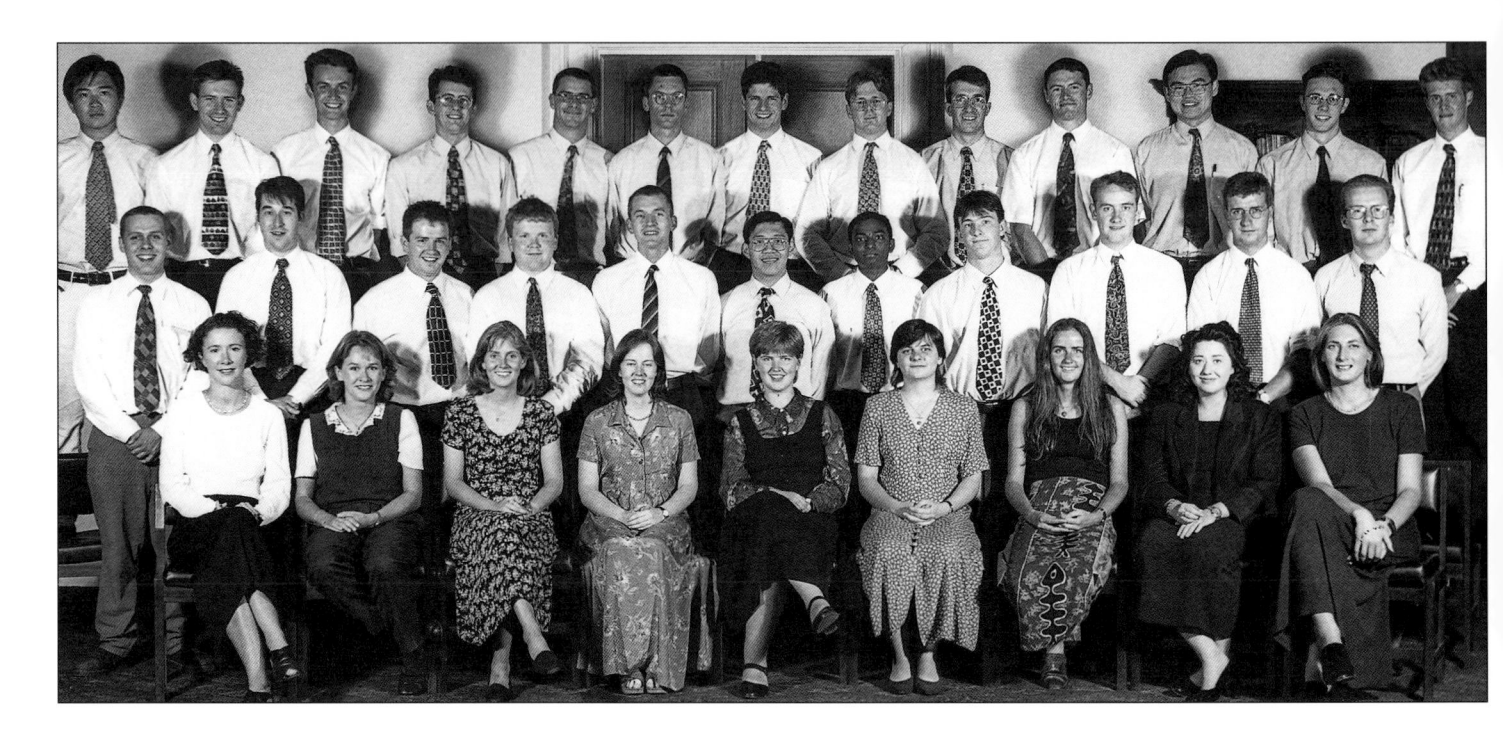

The Resident House Officers of 1997–98: these men and women, even more than the new buildings, must be our vision for the future of patient care in the next millennium.
Back row, left to right: Dr Jenn Chyuan Wang, Dr Ian McAllister, Dr John Turkington, Dr Stephen Johnston, Dr Mark Murnaghan, Dr William Humphries, Dr Julian Leggett, Dr David Craig, Dr John Gray, Dr Thomas Flannery, Dr Bing Ng, Dr Michael Crawford and Dr Jonathan Younger; *middle row:* Dr Philip Grieve, Dr Raymond McKee, Dr Turlough Farnan, Dr Brian Donnelly, Dr John O'Hare, Dr Say Pheng Quah, Dr Ramesh Pulendran, Dr Graham Turner, Dr Richard Park, Dr Peter Martin and Dr Paul Fearon; *front row:* Dr Sinead Langan, Dr Nuala Flanagan, Dr Angela Knox, Dr Tracy O'Neill, Dr Anne-Marie Cunningham, Dr Allison Freeburn, Dr Holly Robinson, Dr Clare Giles and Dr Sarah Stafford
ROYAL VICTORIA HOSPITAL

designed area, which will feature the extensive use of glass and be adjacent to the new visitor car-parking areas.

The redevelopment will take place in two phases, the first half on the grass/car-parking area to the side of the Royal Maternity Hospital, while the second-phase buildings will be on the site of the old corridor wards. Phase 1 will include new operating theatres, the intensive care unit, day procedure unit and a substantial part of the Outpatient Department. In addition, the wards that will replace the old corridor wards must be built in this phase. Phase 2 will include the remainder of the Outpatient Department, the Emergency (x-ray and scanning) Department and an education centre. One of the points in the design is that most of the outpatients will be seen on the first and second floors, and the layout has been specifically designed so that patients can easily find their way around the various facilities. In addition, airy courtyards will help visitors to identify their location in the building, give sites for the incorporation of art, and generally humanise the whole design. Money has been allocated for a large piece of sculpture outside the building which will be an additional feature of this hospital.

The loss of the old wards to accommodate the second phase of the building programme will grieve the historically minded but is essential if patients and staff are to have the environment they need in the twenty-first century. The old wards have been frequently altered from Henman's original plans, and the balcony side has lost much of the elegance it had when it was first conceived. In spite of improvements these wards no longer have a place in patient care. There have been discussions with the Listed Buildings Division of Historic Monuments and it is accepted that the wards will go, but the main corridor of the old hospital, together with the ventilation corridor and engine room at the end, will be retained. The buildings on the Grosvenor Road side of the corridor also have a unity, and once they are restored they could again provide an attractive façade.

The site works are already under way. The slow progress with former plans and the equally slow progress of other hospitals in Northern Ireland are a warning of what can happen. The project is scheduled to start in 1997 and all interested in the hospital look forward to its completion by the year 2000. It is an inspiring vision and one that Dr James McDonnell in 1797 and equally Dr John Walton Browne in 1903 would have applauded.

The future in terms of patient care is hard to predict, especially in the field of nursing, but we can be sure that there will never be enough beds and there will be increasing pressure to shorten the time spent by patients in hospital. As salaries in the medical, nursing and allied professions continue to rise slowly, there will be pressure to have more duties undertaken by less skilled helpers. This pressure is inevitable but it is to be hoped that all the professions will continue to show that they have something unique to offer and that there is no better value for money. The public want the health service to be run economically but the moment people are ill they want the best care and expertise that can be found. The Royal Group of Hospitals is certainly committed to providing this care, and its long history makes it ideally placed to do so.

APPENDICES

1

CHRONOLOGICAL LIST OF THE VISITING PHYSICIANS AND SURGEONS (CONSULTANTS AFTER 1948) OF THE DISPENSARY AND FEVER HOSPITAL, THE BELFAST GENERAL HOSPITAL, BELFAST ROYAL HOSPITAL AND ROYAL VICTORIA HOSPITAL

This list is based primarily on the names of Attending and Associate doctors in the annual reports (often grouped as Honorary Visiting Staff) between 1818 and 1947 with additions from Malcolm's history for the earlier period. The so-called auxiliary staff have been omitted. After 1948 there is no single list, but in general all consultants on the staff appointed to the Royal Victoria Hospital have been listed with their dates (whether or not they were members of the Medical Staff Committee). Some of these played no actual part in the medical care within the hospital but as far as they could be found all have been included. Inadvertent omissions are possible because of the manner of compilation and the author apologises for any of these. For those who are no longer alive, dates of birth and death have been obtained as fully as possible from obituaries and curricula vitae in the Archive Office and sometimes from the Registrar-General's records. Qualifications have been listed from the *Medical Directory* and *Medical Register*, but entries in these are not always completed by the doctor concerned. Dates of appointment are generally the first and last dates in which the doctor appears in the annual report.

DOCTOR	SPECIALITY	BORN	APPOINTED TO ASSISTANT/ ATTENDING STAFF	APPOINTMENT ENDED OR RESIGNED	DIED
Dr James McDonnell MD (Edin) 1784	Medicine	1762	1797	1837	5 Apr 1845
Dr Samuel Martin Stephenson MD (Edin) 1776	Medicine	1742	1800	1809	13 Jan 1833
Mr Robert McCluney	Surgery	1768	1801	1828	21 Jan 1837
Dr Andrew Marshall LRCP Edin 1804; MD (Glas) 1854	Surgery	24 Dec 1779	1807	1828	27 Mar 1868
Dr Samuel Smith Thomson MD (Edin) 1800	Medicine	May 1778	1810	1830	3 Apr 1849
Prof James Lawson Drummond MD (Edin) 1814	Medicine	1783	1814	1849	17 May 1853
Dr Robert Stephenson MD (Edin) 1817; LRCP Lond 1859	Medicine	1794	1818	1831	21 Sept 1869

DOCTOR	SPECIALITY	BORN	APPOINTED TO ASSISTANT/ ATTENDING STAFF	APPOINTMENT ENDED OR RESIGNED	DIED
Dr Henry Forcade MD	Surgery	1784/5	1820	1828	22 July 1835
Mr David Moore FRCSE	Surgery	1780	1821	1845	1847
Dr Benjamin Thompson	Medicine		1826		14 Nov 1826
Prof Robert Coffey LRCS Edin 1819; MD (Glas) 1833	Surgery		1827	1836	5 Jan 1847
Dr Thomas McCabe MD	Medicine	1790/1	1827		25 Nov 1828
Mr James B. McCleery LRCS Edin 1817	Surgery	1795/6	1827	1832	9 July 1847
Mr Robert McKibbin MD	Surgery		1827	1832	
Dr W.M. Wilson MD	Medicine		1827	1828	
Dr William Duncan LAH; MD	Medicine		1829	1834	
Mr William Quin	Surgery		1829	1834	1849
Prof Robert Little MD and LM (Glas) 1826; LAH 1827	Midwifery	1801	1830	1840	27 Feb 1889
Prof Henry MacCormac MD (Edin) 1824; LRCS Edin 1824	Medicine	1800	1831	1836	26 May 1886
Dr John McMechan MD (Edin) 1828; LRCS 1828	Medicine		1831	1832	
Dr Hawthorne	Medicine		1832	1836	
Dr Joseph Wallace Bryson LRCS Edin 1828; MD (Edin) 1831	Surgery	20 June 1807	1833	1836	8 Mar 1855
Dr William Mateer MD	Medicine		1834	1850	
Dr Thomas Henry Purdon FRCSI 1826; MB (TCD) 1828	Surgery	1805	1834	1851	6 Aug 1886
Dr William Johnson	Medicine		1835	1838	
Dr Thomas Thompson MD	Medicine		1835	1841	28 May 1867
Mr John Wales	Surgery		1835	1838	1 Feb 1840
Prof Thomas Andrews MD (Edin) 1835; LRCS Edin 1835	Chemistry	19 Dec 1813	1838	1846	26 Nov 1885
Dr James Maxwell Sanders MD (Edin) 1835	Surgery	24 Apr 1814	1838		26 July 1846
Prof James Seaton Reid LRCS Edin 1832; MD (Edin) 1833; LSA 1837	Materia Medica	11 July 1811	1840	1847	16 May 1896
Dr Hunter	Surgery		1841	1845	
Dr William Moffat MD (Edin)	Medicine	1813/4	1841	1852	27 Apr 1852
Dr Sheil	Medicine		1841	1842	
Prof Alexander Gordon MD; LRCS Edin 1841	Surgery	1818	1845	1873	29 July 1887
Dr Andrew George Malcolm LRCS Edin 1842	Medicine	17 Dec 1818	1846		19 Sept 1856

DOCTOR	SPECIALITY	BORN	APPOINTED TO ASSISTANT/ ATTENDING STAFF	APPOINTMENT ENDED OR RESIGNED	DIED
Dr James Moore MD (Edin) 1842; MRCSE 1842	Surgery	29 Mar 1819	1846	1877	28 Oct 1883
Mr Aeneas Lamont FRCSI 1844	Surgery		1849	1858	
Dr Patrick A. Lynch MD (Glas) 1841; LAH 1841; MRCSE 1853	Medicine		1849	1856	19 May 1864
Dr John Miller Pirrie BA and MB (TCD) 1845; LRCSI 1845; MD 1848	Medicine	30 Nov 1824	1849	1865	16 July 1873
Prof Horatio Agnew Stewart MD (Glas) 1841	Materia Medica	12 Aug 1820	1849		14 May 1857
Mr Samuel Browne RN, JP MRCSE 1851, MRCPI 1881; LKQCPI and LM 1859	Ophthalmic surgery	1809	1851	1875	26 Aug 1890
Dr Murphy	Medicine		1852	1853	
Prof John Creery Ferguson BA (TCD) 1823; MB 1827; FKQCPI 1829	Medicine	22 Aug 1802	1853		24 June 1865
Dr Henry Murney MRCSE and LM 1846; MD (Edin) 1847	Surgery	1825	1854	1882	25 Aug 1907
Prof Robert Foster Dill MRCSE 1833; MD (Glas) 1834	Midwifery	1811/2	1856	1864	20 July 1893
Dr John Swanwick Drennan BA 1831; LRCSI 1834; MB (TCD) 1838; MD 1854	Medicine	3 Oct 1809	1856	1870	1 Nov 1893
Sir William MacCormac, Bt. BA (QUI) 1855; MD 1857; FRCSI 1864; FRCSE 1871	Surgery	17 Jan 1836	1864	1870	4 Dec 1901
Dr James William Thomas Smith LRCSI 1848; MD (QUI) 1863	Medicine	1830	1864	1888	11 July 1890
Prof James Cuming BA (QUI) 1854; MD 1855; MA 1858; FKQCPI 1876	Medicine	1833	1865		27 Aug 1899
Dr Richard Ross LRCSI 1848; MD (St And.) 1850	Medicine	1827	1865		13 Nov 1895
Dr Henry Samuel Purdon LRCSI 1864; LRCP Edin 1865; MD (Glas) 1865	Dermatology	25 Dec 1843	1870	1882	21 Jan 1906
Dr John Moore MD (QUI) 1851; MRCSE 1855	Surgery		1871	1884	2 May 1887
Sir John Walton Browne BA (QUI) 1863; MRCSE 1867; MD (QUI) 1867	Surgery	1845	1875	1912	18 Dec 1923
Sir John Fagan LRCSI 1865; FRCSI 1874; LM KQCPI 1866	Surgery	16 July 1843	1877	1897	17 Mar 1930

DOCTOR	SPECIALITY	BORN	APPOINTED TO ASSISTANT/ ATTENDING STAFF	APPOINTMENT ENDED OR RESIGNED	DIED
Prof Sir William Whitla MP LRCP LRCS Edin 1873; LAH 1873; MD (QUI) 1877	Materia Medica; Medicine	13 Sept 1851	1877/1882	1918	11 Dec 1933
Dr Henry O'Neill JP MD (QUI) 1877; LAH 1877	Surgery	9 Sept 1853	1879/1882	1900	16 May 1914
Dr Charles Workman MD (QUI) 1877	Medicine		1879/1882	1883	
Mr Thomas Kennedy Wheeler MD and LM (RUI) 1879; MCh 1880	Surgery	1848	1882/1884	1902	29 Dec 1937
Prof Sir John William Byers BA (QUI) 1874; MA 1875; MD 1878; MRCSE 1879; LM KQCPI 1879	Gynaecology	1853	–/1883	1919	20 Sept 1920
Prof James Alexander Lindsay BA (QUI) 1877; MA 1878; MD (RUI) 1882; MRCP 1890	Medicine	20 June 1856	1883/1888	1923	14 Dec 1931
Dr Joseph Nelson MD (QUI) 1863; LRCSI 1863	Ophthalmic surgery	1840	–/1883	1905	31 Aug 1910
Mr James Barron BA (QUI) 1874; MD (Hons) 1879	Surgery		1884/–	1885	2 Apr 1887
Prof Thomas Sinclair CB, MP MD MCh (QUI) 1881; FRCSE 1885	Surgery	1857	1885/1897	1923	25 Nov 1940
Dr Robert Stafford Smith MD (RUI) 1882; MCh 1887	Medicine	1859/60	1888/1895	1899	5 Oct 1900
Mr Arthur Brownlow Mitchell OBE MB (RUI) 1890; FRCSI 1900	Surgery	1865	1894/1899	1930	3 Sept 1942
Dr William Calwell OBE MA 1881; MD (RUI) and LM 1883	Medicine and Dermatology	1859	1895/1900	1924	17 May 1943
Dr Thomas Sinclair Kirk BA; MB (RUI) 1893	Surgery	1869	1897/1902	1934	10 Nov 1940
Dr Henry Lawrence McKisack MB (RUI) 1887; MD 1890; FRCP Lond 1916	Medicine	1859	1899/1900	1924	26 Mar 1928
Mr Robert Campbell MB (RUI) 1892; MRCS LRCP Lond 1893	Surgery	1 Aug 1866	1900/1912		6 Sept 1920
Dr Victor George Leopold Fielden MB (RUI) 1892; MD 1912	Anaesthesia	1866	1900/1911	1932	5 June 1946
Sir Thomas Houston OBE BA 1890; MB (Hons) (RUI) 1895; MD 1899	Pathology	15 Dec 1868	1900/1916	1934	21 June 1949
Dr William Baird McQuitty MA (RUI) 1885; MD (Hons) (RUI) 1887; DPH (Camb) 1890	Medicine	1863	1900/–		30 Dec 1910
Prof James Lorrain Smith MA (Edin) 1884; MD 1889	Pathology	21 Aug 1862	–/1901	1904	18 Apr 1931

DOCTOR	SPECIALITY	BORN	APPOINTED TO ASSISTANT/ ATTENDING STAFF	APPOINTMENT ENDED OR RESIGNED	DIED
Mr James Andrew Craig MB (Hons) (RUI) 1895; MRCS LRCP Lond 1898; FRCSE 1900	Ophthalmic surgery	20 Mar 1872	1902/1905	1937	26 Nov 1958
Prof Andrew Fullerton CB, CMG MB (Hons) (RUI) 1890; MD 1893; FRCSI 1901	Surgery	20 Mar 1868	1902/1918	1933	22 May 1934
Prof Sir Robert James Johnstone MP BA 1893; MB (RUI) 1896; FRCSE 1900	Gynaecology	1872	1902/1919	1937	26 Oct 1938
Dr John Smyth Morrow OBE BA 1887; MB (RUI) 1890; MD 1895	Medicine	1865/6	1903/1918	1930	8 Apr 1942
Prof William St Clair Symmers MB (Hons) (Aber) 1887	Pathology	3 Jan 1863	–/1905	1929	4 Oct 1937
Mr Henry Hanna BA 1894; MA BSc 1896; MB (RUI) 1903	Otolaryngology	1874	1907/1925	1939	28 Sept 1946
Prof John Elder MacIlwaine BSc 1894; MB (Hons) (RUI) 1901; MD 1904	Materia Medica; Therapeutics	13 Aug 1874	1910/1921		6 Aug 1930
Dr John Campbell Rankin MB (RUI) 1900; MD 1906	Medicine	7 June 1876	1911/1916	1945	30 Nov 1954
Mr Howard Stevenson BA (RUI) 1897; MB 1900; FRCSI 1904	Surgery	15 Apr 1876	1911/1920	1941	16 Mar 1950
Prof Percival Templeton Crymble MB (RUI) 1904; FRCSE 1908	Surgery	21 Mar 1880	1918/1929	1945	28 June 1970
Dr Foster Coates BA (Hons) (RUI) 1900; MB (Hons) 1905; MD 1907; DPH 1908	Medicine	9 Oct 1880	1918/1924	1945	23 Mar 1949
Sir Samuel Thompson Irwin MP BA (RUI) 1900; MB (Hons) 1902; MCh 1906; FRCS Edin 1909	Surgery	3 July 1877	1918/1923	1945	21 June 1961
Prof William Willis Dalziel Thomson BA (Hons) (RUI) 1907; MB (Hons) 1910; BSc (Hons) 1913; MD 1916; FRCP Lond 1928	Medicine	8 Sept 1885	1918/1924		26 Nov 1950
Prof Charles Gibson Lowry MB (RUI) 1903; MD 1906; FRCSI 1918; FRCOG 1929	Gynaecology	1880	1919/1924	1945	9 Sept 1951
Mr Robert John McConnell MB (QUB) 1912; MCh 1919	Surgery	15 Feb 1884	1920/1933	1950	22 July 1956
Dr Robert Maitland Beath BA 1907; MB (Hons) (QUB) 1914; MB (Lond) 1919	Radiology	17 Oct 1886	1921/1921		21 Nov 1940
Dr Samuel Burnside Boyd Campbell MC MB (Hons) (Edin) 1912; FRCP Edin 1919; MD 1921	Medicine	1890	1921/1929	1954	28 Feb 1971
Mr Frederick Jefferson MB (QUB) 1913	Oto-laryngology	28 Aug 1887	1923/–	1933	1 Nov 1939

DOCTOR	SPECIALITY	BORN	APPOINTED TO ASSISTANT/ ATTENDING STAFF	APPOINTMENT ENDED OR RESIGNED	DIED
Mr Henry Price Malcolm MC MB (QUB) 1912; MCh 1920	Surgery	30 Aug 1885	1923/1934	1950	6 Apr 1974
Mr Henry Little Hardy Greer MB (Hons) (QUB) 1913; DPH RCSI 1920; FRCS Edin 1922; FRCOG 1929	Gynaecology	7 Nov 1890	1924/1937	1956	19 Apr 1973
Dr Robert Marshall MB (Hons) (QUB) 1912; MD 1920; FRCPI 1921	Medicine	9 Sept 1889	1924/1930	1954	20 Mar 1975
Dr John Andrew Smyth BSc; MB (Hons) (QUB) 1921; MD 1924	Medicine	1891/2	1924/1932	1958	2 June 1971
Dr Samuel Ireland Turkington MB (QUB) 1912; MD 1915	Medicine	1885	1924/1945	1950	1 Aug 1951
Sir Frank Percivale Montgomery MC MB (QUB) 1915; DMRE (Camb) 1924	Radiology	10 June 1892	1927/1929	1957	11 Aug 1972
Prof Alexander Murray Drennan MB (Hons) (Edin) 1906; FRCP Edin 1914; MD 1924	Pathology	Jan 1884	–/1929	1931	29 Feb 1984
Dr Joseph Tegart Lewis BSc 1923; MB (Hons) 1921; MD 1924; FRCP Lond 1936	Medicine	2 Sept 1897	1929/1946	1962	8 Oct 1969
Mr George Raphael Buick Purce MC MB (Hons) (QUB) 1914; MCh 1920; FRCS Edin 1921	Surgery	13 Dec 1891	1929/1941		29 June 1950
Dr Richard Sydney Allison VRD MB (QUB) 1921; MD 1924; FRCPE 1938	Neurology	15 May 1899	1930/1947	1964	27 Apr 1978
Prof John Stirling Young MC MA (Glas) 1919; BSc 1921; MB (Hons) 1923; MD (Hons) 1929	Pathology	24 Sept 1894	–/1931	1937	16 Sept 1971
Prof Charles Horner Greer Macafee MB (Hons) (QUB) 1921; FRCSI and FRCSE 1927	Gynaecology	23 July 1898	1932/1945	1963	16 Aug 1978
Dr Ivan Henry McCaw MB (Hons) (QUB) 1922; MD 1933	Dermatology	1897	1933/1939		17 Mar 1967
Mr Cecil John Alexander Woodside MB (QUB) 1917; FRSCI 1925	Surgery	30 Aug 1895	1933/1942		14 Feb 1955
Mr James Reid Wheeler MB (QUB) 1923; FRCS Edin 1929	Ophthalmic surgery	27 Dec 1898	1934/1937	1964	22 Mar 1973
Mr Cecil Armstrong Calvert MB (Hons) (QUB) 1922; FRCSI 1926	Neuro-surgery	9 May 1894	1935/1945		4 Apr 1956
Prof Sir John Henry Biggart CBE MB (QUB) 1928; MD 1931; DSc 1937	Pathology	17 Nov 1905	–/1937	1971	21 May 1979
Mr Henry Connell Lowry MB (QUB) 1924; FRCS Edin 1927; FRCOG 1940	Gynaecology	29 Jan 1898	1937/1948	1960	12 Jan 1964
Mr Francis Alexander MacLaughlin MB (Hons) (QUB) 1921; FRCSE 1926	Oto-laryngology	27 May 1899	1937/1939	1964	4 May 1984

DOCTOR	SPECIALITY	BORN	APPOINTED TO ASSISTANT/ ATTENDING STAFF	APPOINTMENT ENDED OR RESIGNED	DIED
Mr Joseph Allison Corkey MB (Hons) (QUB) 1930; MD 1933; FRCSI 1932	Ophthalmic surgery	18 Aug 1906	1939/1948	1972	7 Mar 1979
Mr Kennedy Hunter MB (Hons) (QUB) 1930; FRCS Edin 1934	Oto-laryngology	20 Nov 1907	1939/1948	1972	18 July 1975
Dr Thomas Howard Crozier MB (Hons) (QUB) 1921; MD 1924; BSc (Hons) 1934; FRCP Lond 1941	Medicine	23 Nov 1899	1945/1948	1965	18 Dec 1989
Sir Ian Fraser DSO MB (Hons) (QUB) 1923; FRCSI 1926; MCh 1927; FRCSE 1927; MD 1932	Surgery		1945/1948	1966	
Dr Reginald Hall MB (Hons) (QUB) 1936; MD 1940; FRCPI 1943	Dermatology	18 Apr 1906	1945/1948	1971	28 Sept 1996
Mr James Stevenson Loughridge MB (Hons) (QUB) 1923; BSc 1925; MD 1926; FRCSE 1928	Surgery	3 Oct 1901	1945/1948	1967	6 Apr 1980
Mr Harold Ian McClure MB (QUB) 1927; BSc 1929; FRCS Edin 1932; FRCOG 1944	Gynaecology	26 Aug 1904	1945/1948	1969	9 Jan 1982
Mr Eric Wilson McMechan MB (Hons) (QUB) 1933; FRCSE 1938	Surgery	13 Aug 1910	1945/1948	1968	13 Jan 1980
Mr Robert James Wilson Withers MB (Hons) (QUB) 1930; MD 1933; MCh 1936; FRCS Edin 1934	Orthopaedic surgery	6 June 1908	1945/1948		15 May 1965
Dr Wilfred Maurice Brown MB (QUB) 1936; DA Eng 1945; MD 1948; FFA RCSE 1953; FFA RCSI 1973	Anaesthesia	28 Sept 1912	1946/1948	1976	14 Sept 1993
Prof Maurice Gerald Nelson MB (Hons) (QUB) 1937; MD 1940; FRCPI 1955; FRCPE 1961; FRC Path. 1963	Haematology		1947/1948	1979	
Prof Harold William Rodgers OBE MRCS LRCP (St Bart's) 1931; FRCSE 1933	Surgery		1947/1948	1973	
Mr Henry Aitken MB (Aber) 1928; FRCS Edin 1938	Oto-laryngology	23 Sept 1906	1948	1972	14 Sept 1992
Dr Frederick Silvester Bonugli MB (QUB) 1937; DRCOG 1939; MD 1946	Venereology	28 June 1913	1948		28 Aug 1967
Mr Gavin Boyd MB (Glas) 1936; FRCS Edin 1947; FRCOG 1956	Gynaecology		1948	1978	
Dr John Boyd MB (QUB) 1926; MD 1933; DA RCPSI 1943; FFA RCSE 1949	Anaesthesia	19 Dec 1902	1948	1969	26 Oct 1981

DOCTOR	SPECIALITY	BORN	APPOINTED TO ASSISTANT/ ATTENDING STAFF	APPOINTMENT ENDED OR RESIGNED	DIED
Dr Brice Richard Clarke MC, CBE MB (Hons) (QUB) 1921; MD 1926	Chest medicine	12 May 1895	1948	1961	15 June 1975
Dr Stafford Geddes MB (QUB) 1915; DA Eng 1936	Anaesthesia	1892/3	1948	1956	14 May 1969
Dr Norman Clotworthy Graham MC MB (QUB) 1912	Bacteriology	19 Apr 1889	1948	1954	10 Feb 1969
Dr George Gregg OBE MB (QUB) 1938; MD 1946 FRCPI 1953	Physical medicine	16 Nov 1911	1948	1977	13 Feb 1982
Dr George Hamilton MA 1917; MB (QUB) 1927; DA RCPSI 1943	Anaesthesia	7 Mar 1887	1948	1952	7 Dec 1967
Dr Margaret Marion Vida Lemon MB (Otago) 1927; DA RCPSI 1944; FFA RCSI 1960	Anaesthesia	8 Jan 1900	1948	1964	26 Mar 1979
Dr William Lennon MB (QUB) 1922; MD 1925; MRCP 1933	Rheumatology	23 May 1901	1948	1966	2 Dec 1993
Dr John Sydney McCann MB (QUB) 1936; MD 1940; DPH 1942	Venereology	5 Jan 1912	1948	1977	16 Feb 1996
Dr Florence May McClelland MB (QUB) 1938; DRCOG 1942; DA Eng 1942	Anaesthesia	23 Oct 1903	1948	1967	1989
Mr Norman Samuel Martin MBE MB (QUB) 1935; MD 1939; FRCSE 1941	Orthopaedics	8 Aug 1912	1948	1977	27 July 1992
Prof John Edgar Morison OBE BSc (Hons) 1932; MB (Hons) (QUB) 1935; MD 1940; DSc 1952; FRC Path. 1964	Pathology		1948	1954	
Dr David Cuthbert Porter MB (Hons) (QUB) 1933; MD 1936; FFR RCSI 1961	Radiology	10 June 1910	1948	1975	30 Mar 1978
Dr Charles Reid MB (QUB) 1935; DA Eng 1941; FFA RCSE 1953; FRCPI 1954	Anaesthesia	12 Sept 1912	1948	1977	17 Feb 1981
Dr Charles Booth Robinson BA (TCD) 1938; MB 1939; MA MD 1942; FRCPI 1948	Psychiatry		1948	1969	30 Nov 1969
Prof Alan Carruth Stevenson CBE BSc (Glas) 1930; MB 1933; MD 1946; FRCP Lond 1955	Social medicine	27 Jan 1909	1948	1958	18 Sept 1995
Dr Hugh Edwin Hall VRD MB (QUB) 1916; MD 1929	Venereology	22 Aug 1894	1949	1959	22 Aug 1964
Dr James Frederick Bereen OBE BSc (Hons) (QUB) 1934; MB 1937; FFA RCSE 1953	Anaesthesia	6 July 1913	1950	1977	7 Oct 1987

DOCTOR	SPECIALITY	BORN	APPOINTED TO ASSISTANT/ ATTENDING STAFF	APPOINTMENT ENDED OR RESIGNED	DIED
Mr Walter Standish Braidwood BA (Camb) 1926; MB (QUB) 1938; FRCS Edin 1947	Surgery	21 Aug 1904	1950	1969	7 Sept 1985
Mr Rainier Campbell Connolly MRCS LRCP (St Bart's) 1941; FRCSE 1947	Neuro- surgery		1950	1952	
Mr Norman Campbell Hughes OBE MB (QUB) 1937; FRCSE 1947	Plastic surgery	15 May 1915	1950	1979	1 June 1995
Mr John Walker Sinclair Irwin MB (QUB) 1937; FRCS Edin 1947	Surgery		1950	1978	
Mr Terence Leslie Kennedy MB (Lond Hosp) 1942; FRCSE 1946; MS 1950	Surgery	12 Dec 1919	1950	1984	11 Dec 1993
Mr Ernest Morrison MB (Hons) (QUB) 1942; FRCS Edin 1948	Surgery		1950	1984	
Dr William Henry Thompson Shepherd MB (QUB) 1939; MD 1950; FFR RCSI 1962; FFR 1965; FRCR 1975	Neuro- radiology		1950	1979	
Mr John Alexander Walter Bingham MB (Hons) (QUB) 1934; FRCSE 1938; MCh 1946	Thoracic surgery	1 Feb 1911	1951	1976	1 Jan 1983
Dr John Stephens Logan MB (Hons) (QUB) 1939; MD 1946; FRCP Lond 1966	Medicine		1951	1982	
Prof Desmond Alan Dill Montgomery CBE. MB (Hons) (QUB) 1940; MD 1946; FRCP Lond 1964; FRCPI 1975; DSc (NUI) 1980	Endo- crinology		1951	1979	
Prof James Francis Pantridge CBE, MC MB (Hons) (QUB) 1939; MD 1946; FRCP Lond 1962; Hon FRCPI 1970	Cardiology		1951	1982	
Mr Thomas Boyd Smiley MC MB (QUB) 1939; FRCSE 1948	Thoracic surgery	9 May 1917	1951	1977	2 Aug 1981
Prof Sir Graham MacGregor Bull MB (Cape Town) 1939; MD 1947; FRCP Lond 1954	Medicine	30 Jan 1918	1952	1966	14 Nov 1987
Dr John Harold Dundee Millar MB (QUB) 1940; MD 1946; FRCP Lond 1963	Neurology	29 May 1917	1952	1982	6 Sept 1992
Mr Alexander Robertson Taylor MA (Aber) 1937; MB (Hons) 1941; FRCS Edin 1946	Neuro- surgery	1916/7	1952	1974	9 July 1978
Dr John Martin Beare MB (Hons) (QUB) 1942; MD 1946; FRCP Lond 1966; FRCPI 1978	Dermatology		1953	1985	
Dr Charles Finbarr Campbell MB (QUB) 1935; MD 1947	Chest medicine	13 Sept 1912	1953	1977	11 Aug 1984

DOCTOR	SPECIALITY	BORN	APPOINTED TO ASSISTANT/ ATTENDING STAFF	APPOINTMENT ENDED OR RESIGNED	DIED
Dr John Llewellyn Edgar Millen MB (QUB) 1935; MD 1939	Radiotherapy	19 Apr 1912	1953		10 May 1960
Mr Samuel Ronald Sinclair BSc (QUB) 1933; MB 1936 FRCSE 1947	Ophthalmic surgery	17 May 1912	1953		18 Jan 1960
Mr Howard Morris Stevenson MB (QUB) 1943; FRCS Edin 1948	Thoracic surgery		1953	1986	
Prof Robert Irvine Wilson MBE MB (QUB) 1938; FRCS Edin 1947	Orthopaedic surgery		1953	1982	
Dr James Elliott MB (QUB) 1938; MD 1941; FFA RCSE 1954	Anaesthesia	25 Mar 1915	1954	1980	18 Oct 1983
Dr Thomas Terence Fulton OBE MD (Cincinnati) 1943; MB (Hons) (QUB) 1945; MD (QUB) 1951; FRCP Lond 1967; FRCPI 1977	Medicine		1954	1986	
Dr William Robert Gilmore MB (QUB) 1945; DA Eng 1949; FRCA 1953	Anaesthesia		1954	1987	
Dr Samuel Harold Swan Love MB (QUB) 1945; DA RCPSI 1949; MD 1952; FRCA 1953	Anaesthesia		1954	1984	
Dr James Edmund Reid MB (QUB) 1946; DA RCPSI 1949; DA Eng 1952	Anaesthesia		1954	1986	
Dr Richard Arthur Womersley MB (Camb and Middlesex) 1944; MA (Camb) 1946; MD 1954; FRCP Lond 1968	Medicine		1954	1984	
Prof George Williamson Auchinvole Dick MB (Edin) 1938; BSc (Hons) 1939; MD 1949; FRCP Edin 1955; DSc 1955; FRC Path. 1964; FRCP Lond 1966	Virology		1955	1966	
Mr Reginald Hamilton Livingston MB (Hons) (QUB) 1946; FRCSE 1952; MD 1955	Surgery	15 Jan 1923	1956		7 Dec 1980
Dr Howard Hilton Stewart MB (QUB) 1923; MD 1926; FRCP Edin 1951	Neurology	3 Dec 1900	1956		25 Nov 1961
Dr David Maurice Surrey Dane MRCSE LRCP Lond 1951; MB (Camb and St Thom) 1955; FRC Path. 1972; FRCP Lond 1980	Virology		1957	1966	
Prof John George Gibson MB (QUB) 1942; MD 1947; FRCP Lond 1964; FRC Psych 1971	Mental health	14 Apr 1920	1957		15 June 1974

DOCTOR	SPECIALITY	BORN	APPOINTED TO ASSISTANT/ ATTENDING STAFF	APPOINTMENT ENDED OR RESIGNED	DIED
Mr Colin Allan Gleadhill MB (Edin) 1939; MD 1941; FRCS Edin 1948	Neuro-surgery	1 Mar 1914	1957	1979	20 July 1991
Prof Owen Lyndon Wade MA (Camb) 1945; MB (Camb and UCH) 1945; MD 1951; FRCP Lond 1964; FRCPI 1970	Therapeutics		1957	1971	
Prof Richard Burkewood Welbourn BA (Camb) 1940; MB 1942; FRCSE 1945; MA MD 1953; DSc (QUB) 1985	Surgery		1957	1963	
Mr Willoughby Wilson OBE MB (QUB) 1946; FRCS Edin 1962; FRCSI 1969	Surgery		1957	1987	
Dr James Camac Clarke MB (QUB) 1949; DA RCPSI 1951; FRCA 1953	Anaesthesia		1958	1982	
Mr William Robert Dickie MB (QUB) 1940; FRCS Edin 1948	Plastic surgery		1958	1980	
Prof John Wharry Dundee OBE MB (QUB) 1946; MD 1951; FFA RCSE 1953; PhD (Liverp) 1957; FFA RCSI 1959; FRCP Lond 1984	Anaesthesia	8 Nov 1921	1958	1988	1 Dec 1991
Prof Archibald David Mant Greenfield BSc 1937; MB (St Mary's) 1940; DSc 1953; FRCP Lond 1973	Physiology		1958	1964	
Prof Elizabeth Florence McKeown MB (Hons) (QUB) 1942; MD 1945; FRC Path. 1964; FRCP Lond 1974	Pathlogy		1958	1984	
Prof John Pemberton MB (UCH Lond) 1936; MRCS LRCP Lond 1936; MD 1940; FRCP Lond 1964; FFCM 1974	Social medicine		1958	1976	
Prof John Joseph Pritchard BSc (Adelaide) 1934; MA (Oxf) 1941; BM (Oxf) 1941; DM 1951; FRCSE 1964	Anatomy	9 Feb 1916	1958	1977	10 Apr 1979
Dr Richard Stanley Crone MB (TCD) 1949; MD 1954; MA 1957; FFR RCSI 1963	Radiology	6 Aug 1925	1959	1989	19 Aug 1991
Dr Peter Cardwell Elmes BM (Oxf) 1945; MD (Cleveland) 1947 FRCP Lond 1967	Therapeutics, Medicine		1959	1976	
Dr Frederick Searle Grebbell MB (QUB) 1947; MD 1957; FFR RCSI 1964	Radiology		1959	1988	
Mr Robert Samuel McCrea MB (QUB) 1943; FRCS Edin 1950	Oto-laryngology	19 June 1920	1959	1982	14 June 1983

DOCTOR	SPECIALITY	BORN	APPOINTED TO ASSISTANT/ ATTENDING STAFF	APPOINTMENT ENDED OR RESIGNED	DIED
Dr William Reynolds Macartney Morton MB (QUB) 1930; MD 1934; MA (Camb) 1937	Embryology	4 Nov 1906	1959		5 Feb 1968
Dr William Eric Bruneton Scott MB (QUB) 1949; FFA RCSE 1954	Anaesthesia		1959	1963	
Dr John Andrew Weaver MB (QUB) 1950; MD 1954; FRCP Lond 1970	Medicine		1959	1989	
Dr James Owen Young Cole MB (QUB) 1938; MD 1948; FFR RCSI 1962	Radiology	18 June 1914	1960	1979	15 June 1991
Mr Eric Cecil Cowan MB (QUB) 1952; FRCS Edin 1959; MCh 1972; FACS 1977; FRCSI 1981	Ophthalmology		1960	1992	
Mr Derek Stanley Gordon CBE MB (Hons) (QUB) 1948; FRCS Edin 1954; MCh 1957	Neuro- surgery		1960	1989	
Dr Arnold Richard Lyons OBE MB (QUB) 1940; MD 1947; FFR RCSI 1962; FRCP Lond 1969	Radio- therapy		1960	1983	
Dr David Desmond Burrows MB (QUB) 1953; MD 1957; FRCP Edin 1969; FRCPI 1981	Dermatology		1961	1995	
Dr Eileen Oliver Bartley MB (Hons) (QUB) 1921; MD 1930; FRC Path. 1963	Bacteri- ology	5 Mar 1898	1962	1963	4 Apr 1984
Dr Gerald Wilson Black MB (QUB) 1949; FRCA 1955; MD 1959; FFA RCSI 1961; PhD 1969; FRCPI 1971	Anaesthesia		1962	1990	
Dr Robert Bell Brown MB (QUB) 1929	Oto- laryngology	6 Jan 1900	1962	1966	Jan 1981
Dr George Lees Gibson MB (Glas) 1949; MD 1961 FRC Path. 1974	Bacteri- ology		1962	1970	
Dr James Blackburn Gibson OBE MB (Edin) 1943; MD 1958; FRCP Edin 1961; FRC Path. 1966	Pathology		1962	1963	
Dr Robert Cecil Gray MB (TCD) 1949; MD 1961; FFA RCSI 1962	Anaesthesia		1962	1987	
Prof James MacDougall Graham Harley CBE. MB (QUB) 1953; MD 1961; FRCOG 1967; FRCPI 1986	Gynaecology		1962	1992	
Dr Lewis John Hurwitz MB (QUB) 1949; BSc 1952; MD 1953; FRCP Edin 1963	Neurology	9 Feb 1926	1962		19 Oct 1971

DOCTOR	SPECIALITY	BORN	APPOINTED TO ASSISTANT/ ATTENDING STAFF	APPOINTMENT ENDED OR RESIGNED	DIED
Dr Gerard Lynch MB (QUB) 1948; FFR 1962; FFR RCSI 1963	Radiotherapy	26 Feb 1925	1962		21 May 1988
Dr William Thomas Elliott McCaughey MB (QUB) 1950; MD 1954; MRC Path. 1964	Pathology		1962	1964	
Prof Mary Graham McGeown CBE MB (Hons) (QUB) 1946; MD 1950; PhD 1953; FRCP Edin 1969; FRCP Lond 1978; FRCPI 1982	Nephrology		1962	1988	
Dr William Anderson Norris OBE MB (QUB)1948; MD 1952; FRCPI 1981; FRC Psych 1982	Psychiatry		1962	1990	
Prof Andrew Harry Garmany Love CBE BSc (Hons) 1955; MB (Hons) (QUB) 1958; MD 1963; FRCPI 1972; FRCP Lond 1973	Medicine		1963		
Prof Thomas Kenneth Marshall CBE MB (Leeds) 1948; MD 1959; FRC Path. 1970	Forensic medicine		1963	1989	
Dr John William George Nixon MB (QUB) 1935; MRCPI 1961	Psychiatry		1963	1971	
Prof John Henry McKnight Pinkerton CBE. MB (QUB) 1943; MD 1948; FRCOG 1960; FRCPI 1977	Gynaecology		1963	1985	
Mr Robert Hamilton Baird MB (QUB) 1939; FRCSE 1955	Ophthalmology		1964	1981	
Dr Sheila Margaret Bell MB (QUB) 1950; FRCA 1955; FFA RCSI 1971	Anaesthesia		1964	1992	
Dr Douglas Priestley Bell Boyd MB (QUB) 1931; FFR RCSI 1962	Radiology		1964	1971	
Dr Alastair McCrae Connell BSc (Hons) (Glas) 1941; MB 1954; MRCP Edin 1954	Gastro-enterology		1964	1971	
Mr David Hanna Craig MB (QUB) 1931; FRCS Edin 1937; FRCSI 1968	Oto-laryngology	9 May 1909	1964	1974	29 Aug 1992
Dr John Kennedy Addison Dorman MB (QUB) 1940; DA Eng 1941; MD 1951; FRCA 1953	Anaesthesia		1964	1977	
Dr James Mellis Dunbar BSc (St And.) 1943; MB 1946; MD (Hons) 1951; FRC Path. 1971	Microbiology		1964	1977	
Mr Victor Alexander Faris Martin MB (QUB) 1936; FRCS Edin 1947; DO (Oxf) 1948	Ophthal-mology	10 Dec 1912	1964	1978	11 Mar 1983

DOCTOR	SPECIALITY	BORN	APPOINTED TO ASSISTANT/ ATTENDING STAFF	APPOINTMENT ENDED OR RESIGNED	DIED
Dr Robert Joseph Skelly MB (UCD) 1949; MD 1955; FRCPI 1971; FRCP Lond 1974	Medicine	12 Mar 1925	1964		7 Nov 1981
Mr Gordon Dill Long Smyth MB (QUB) 1953; FRCSE 1959; MD 1961; DSc 1971; MCh (Hons) 1976	Oto-laryngology	2 May 1929	1964		20 May 1992
Dr Michael William Swallow MB (Westminster) 1952; FRCP Lond 1972	Neurology		1964	1989	
Dr David Wilson Barron MB (QUB) 1948; FRCA 1954; MD 1961; FFA RCSI 1971	Anaesthesia		1965	1988	
Dr Dennis McCord Boyle MB (QUB) 1957; MD 1960; FRCP Lond 1976	Cardiology		1965		
Prof Richard Samuel Jessop Clarke BSc (Hons) 1951; MB (QUB) 1954; MD 1958; FRCA 1961; PhD 1969; FFA RCSI 1971	Anaesthesia		1965	1994	
Col Thomas Eglinton Field MBE MB (QUB) 1939; DTM&H 1951; MD 1963; FRC Path. 1975	Medical Super-intendent	24 Sept 1915	1965	1969	24 July 1992
Dr William Ormsby McCormick MB (Camb and St Mary's) 1953; MRCP Lond 1961; MRC Psych 1971	Psychiatry		1965	1976	
Dr Edwin Maynard McIlrath MB (QUB) 1956; FFR 1962	Radiology		1965		
Mr Paul Harald Osterberg BA; MB (TCD) 1953; FRCSI 1959; FRCSE 1961	Orthopaedics		1965	1989	
Prof Ian Campbell Roddie BSc (Hons) 1950; MB (QUB) 1953; MD 1957; DSc 1962; FRCPI 1965	Physiology		1965	1987	
Prof John Moore Bridges CBE MB (QUB) 1954; MD 1958; FRCP Edin 1970; FRC Path. 1979; FRCP Glas 1988	Haematology		1966	1994	
Mr Stewart Desmond Clarke MB (QUB) 1955; MCh (Hons) 1960; FRCS Edin 1960; FRCSE 1961	Surgery		1966	1974	
Dr George Joseph Alexander Edelstyn MB (QUB) 1954; MD 1961; FFR 1963; FRCR 1975	Radiotherapy	13 Sept 1930	1966		20 May 1979
Prof Kenneth Boyd Fraser MC MB (Aber) 1940; MD 1950; DSc 1961	Microbiology		1966	1982	

DOCTOR	SPECIALITY	BORN	APPOINTED TO ASSISTANT/ ATTENDING STAFF	APPOINTMENT ENDED OR RESIGNED	DIED
Sir Peter Froggatt MB (TCD) 1952; MD 1958; PhD (QUB) 1967; FFCM 1972; FRCPI 1973; FRCP Lond 1980	Epidemiology		1966	1976	
Dr Alan Denis Gough MB (QUB) 1956; FFR RCSI 1975; FRCR 1975	Radiology		1966	1993	
Prof Thomas James Harrison MB (Hons) (QUB) 1942; MD 1949; PhD 1957	Anatomy		1966	1984	
Prof George Weir Johnston MB (Hons) (QUB) 1956; FRCSE 1962; MCh 1965; FRCSI 1977	Surgery		1966	1995	
Dr John Harold Jones MB (QUB) 1953; MD 1959; LDS RCSE 1962; FRC Path. 1974; FFD RCSI 1977	Dental pathology		1966	1967	
Mr Joseph Aloysius Kennedy MB (QUB) 1955; FRCS Edin 1959; MCh 1962	Urology		1966	1996	
Mr John Henry Lowry MB (QUB) 1954; FRCS Edin 1959	Orthopaedics		1966	1988	
Mr Reginald Arthur Edward Magee CBE, MP. MB (QUB) 1937; FRCSI 1947; FRCOG 1963	Gynaecology	18 Aug 1914	1966	1979	16 Dec 1989
Prof James Moore MB (QUB) 1952; FRCA 1957; MD (Hons) 1961; PhD 1974	Anaesthesia		1966	1992	
Dr Robert Martin Nicholl MB (QUB) 1952; FRCA 1958; MD 1965; FFA RCSI 1971	Anaesthesia		1966	1992	
Dr Stanley Desmond Roberts OBE MB (QUB) 1956; MD 1960; FRCPI 1975; FRCP Lond 1975	Rheumatology		1966		
Mr Harold Walter Henry Shepperd MB (QUB) 1947; FRCSE 1954	Oto-laryngology		1966	1986	
Prof John Vallance-Owen MB (Camb) 1946; MD 1951; FRCP 1970	Medicine		1966	1982	
Dr Charles Richard Whitfield MB (QUB) 1950; MD 1965; FRCOG 1969; FRCP Glas 1981	Gynaecology		1966	1974	
Dr Jacob Willis MB (QUB) 1956; MD 1960; FRC Path. 1978	Cytology		1966	1995	
Prof Ingrid Victoria Allen CBE MB (Hons) (QUB) 1957; MD (Hons) 1963; FRC Path. 1977; DSc 1985; FRCP Glas 1987	Neuro-pathology		1967	1997	

DOCTOR	SPECIALITY	BORN	APPOINTED TO ASSISTANT/ ATTENDING STAFF	APPOINTMENT ENDED OR RESIGNED	DIED
Dr William Bingham MB (QUB) 1941; DA RCPSI 1947; MD 1951; FRCA 1953	Anaesthesia		1967	1981	
Dr Peter Fletcher Binnion BSc 1952; BM (Oxf) 1956; PhD 1963	Physiology		1967	1970	
Dr Peter Alexander Henry McConnell Foster MB (QUB) 1942; MD 1947	Medicine		1967	1970	
Dr Walter Ernest Glover MB (QUB) 1955; MD 1960	Physiology		1967	1969	
Prof David Robert Hadden MB (Hons) (QUB) 1959; MD 1963; FRCP Edin 1970; FRCPE 1987	Endocrinology		1967		
Dr James Kenneth Houston MB (QUB) 1956; MD 1968; FRCOG 1974	Gynaecology		1967	1968	
Dr Michael Alan Lewis MB (TCD) 1959; FFA RCSI 1969	Anaesthesia		1967	1997	
Dr Joseph McEvoy MB (Hons) (QUB) 1959; MRCP Lond 1962; MD 1965	Nephrology		1967	1975	
Mr Charles James Frederick Maguire MB (QUB) 1954; FRCSE 1966	Ophthalmology		1967	1994	
Prof Norman Cummings Nevin BSc (Hons) 1957; MB (QUB) 1960; MD 1965; FRCP Edin 1976; FRC Path. 1981; FRCP Lond 1990	Medical genetics		1967	1975	
Mr William Harford Rutherford OBE MB (TCD) 1944; FRCS Edin 1951 FRCSE 1985	A and E surgery		1967	1986	
Prof Robert Gray Shanks CBE BSc 1955; MB (Hons) (QUB) 1958; MD (Hons) 1963; DSc 1969; FRCP Edin 1979	Therapeutics		1967		
Dr Derek John Lockhart Carson MB (QUB) 1957; MD (Hons) 1963; FFPath. RCPI 1982	Forensic medicine		1968		
Mr John Colville MB (QUB) 1955; DRCOG 1958; FRCS Edin 1962; FRCSI 1981	Plastic surgery		1968	1990	
Prof John Henry Connolly MB (QUB) 1954; MD 1958; FRCPI 1975; MRC Path. 1966	Virology		1968	1993	
Dr Alfred Kenneth Irvine MB (QUB) 1952; MRCPI 1964	Physical medicine		1968	1988	
Mr Alan Grainger Kerr MB (QUB) 1958; DRCOG 1961; FRCSE 1964	Oto-larnygology		1968		

DOCTOR	SPECIALITY	BORN	APPOINTED TO ASSISTANT/ ATTENDING STAFF	APPOINTMENT ENDED OR RESIGNED	DIED
Dr Robert Lannigan MB (Glas) 1945; MD 1957; PhD (Birm) 1967; MRC Path. 1967	Pathology		1968	1970	
Dr Samuel Morrell Lyons OBE BSc (Hons) (QUB) 1957; MB 1960; FRCA 1965; FFA RCSI 1971; MD 1975	Anaesthesia		1968		
Dr John Desmond Howard Mahony MB (QUB) 1945; MD 1961	Venereology		1968	1972	
Mr Patrick John Molloy MB (Otago) 1952; FRCSE 1960	Cardiac surgery		1968	1973	
Mr John Daniel Alexander Robb MB (QUB) 1957; FRCSE 1961	Surgery		1968	1970	
Dr Paul Sandby Thomas MB (QUB) 1958; FRCR 1975; FFR RCSI 1977	Radiology		1968		
Prof Keith Deans Buchanan MB (Glas) 1958; MD 1969; PhD (QUB) 1973; FRCP Edin 1973; FRCP Lond 1977	Medicine		1969		
Dr Thomas Alexander McNeill BSc (Hons) (QUB) 1956; MB (Hons) 1959; MD 1965; DSc 1982; FRC Path. 1982	Micro-biology		1969	1994	
Dr William Frank Keith Morrow MB (QUB) 1948; DA RCPSI 1952; FFA RCSI 1961; FRCP Edin 1971	Anaesthesia	23 Aug 1923	1969		28 May 1982
Dr George Charles Patterson MB (QUB) 1950; MD 1955; PhD 1968	Cardiology		1969	1991	
Dr Thomas John Ryan MRCSE LRCP Lond (St Mary's) 1943; MSc 1962; FRCPI 1980	Geriatrics		1969	1982	1 Nov 1988
Dr John Denis Biggart MB (QUB) 1961; FRC Path. 1962; MD 1965	Pathology		1970		
Dr Dennis Leslie Coppel MB (QUB) 1960; FFA RCSI 1967	Anaesthesia		1970		
Dr John Alexander Lyttle MB (QUB) 1957; MD 1963; FRCP Lond 1979	Neurology		1970	1996	
Dr William Andrew Gordon MacCallum MB (QUB) 1954; FRCPI 1972; FRC Psych 1974	Psychiatry		1970	1989	
Dr Edmund Eric Richey MB (QUB) 1962; LAH (Dub) 1964; FFA RCSI 1969	Anaesthesia		1970	1977	
Prof William Thompson BSc (Hons) (QUB) 1958; MB (Hons) 1961; MD 1975; FRCOG 1980	Gynaecology		1970		

DOCTOR	SPECIALITY	BORN	APPOINTED TO ASSISTANT/ ATTENDING STAFF	APPOINTMENT ENDED OR RESIGNED	DIED
Prof Agnes Anne Jennifer Adgey MB (Hons) (QUB) 1964; MD (Hons) 1975; FRCP Lond 1978	Cardiology		1971		
Dr Grace Elvira Allen MB (QUB) 1958; MD 1971; FRCPI 1973	Dermatology		1971		
Mr John Cleland MB (Hons) (QUB) 1958; FRCS Edin 1962; FRCSE 1963	Cardiac surgery		1971	1995	
Prof Dugald Lindsay Gardner MB (Edin and Camb) 1948; MA 1950; MD 1958; FRCP Edin 1963; FRCP Lond 1975; FRC Path. 1975	Pathology		1971	1976	
Dr John Stafford Geddes BSc (QUB) 1960; MB 1963; MD 1966; MRCP Lond 1967	Cardiology		1971	1987	
Dr John Craig Hunter MB (QUB) 1963; FFR 1969	Radiology		1971	1976	
Prof William George Irwin MB (QUB) 1948; DRCOG 1951; MD 1969; FRCGP 1972	General practice		1971	1989	
Prof Denis Gordon McDevitt MB (Hons) (QUB) 1962; MD 1968; FRCPI 1977; FRCP Lond 1978; DSc 1978; FRCP Edin 1985	Therapeutics		1971	1978	
Dr James Dunn Morrison BSc (QUB) 1959; MB 1962; FRCA 1966; MD 1969	Anaesthesia		1971	1974	
Prof Thomas George Parks MB (QUB) 1959; FRCS Edin 1963; MCh 1966; FRCS Glas 1981; FRCSI 1983	Surgery		1971		
Dr James Thomas Quinn BSc; MB (QUB) 1961; DPM RCPSI 1964; MD 1967	Psychiatry		1971	1974	
Mr Ronald MacCallum Slater MB (QUB) 1955; DRCOG 1957; FRCS Edin 1964	Plastic surgery		1971	1991	
Prof Desmond Brian Archer MB (Hons) (QUB) 1959; FRCS Edin 1963; FRCSE 1968	Ophthalmology		1972		
Dr Francis Robert Bell Browne MB (QUB) 1954; DPM RCSI 1961; MRC Psych 1972; FRCPI 1986	Psychiatry		1972	1980	
Dr David Beatty Crawford MB (QUB) 1965; FFR 1972	Radiology		1972	1974	

DOCTOR	SPECIALITY	BORN	APPOINTED TO ASSISTANT/ ATTENDING STAFF	APPOINTMENT ENDED OR RESIGNED	DIED
Prof John Harold Elwood MB (QUB) 1962; DPH 1966; DIH (Eng) 1967; MD (Hons) 1969; MFCM 1972	Social medicine		1972	1985	
Mr Robert Gibson MB (Hons) (QUB) 1957; FRCS Edin 1962; FRCSE 1964	Oto-laryngology		1972		
Dr Harith Mohamed Nasser Lamki LRCPI and LM LRCSI and LM 1961; FRCOG 1980	Gynaecology		1972		
Mr William Gordon Gault Loughridge MA MB (Camb) 1963; MD 1966; FRCS Edin 1969	Urology		1972		
Dr Elizabeth Emily Mayne MB (QUB) 1962; MD 1968; FRC Path. 1982; FRCP Glas 1986	Haematology		1972		
Dr John Barcroft MB (Camb) 1963; DCH (Eng) 1965; MPhil (Lond) 1970; MRC Psych 1972	Child psychiatry		1973	1977	
Dr Margaret Haire MB (QUB) 1943; MD 1966; FRC Path. 1980	Immunology		1973	1986	
Dr Thomas Horner MB (QUB) 1950; MD 1961	Venereology		1973	1993	
Mr Stewart Samuel Johnston MB (QUB) 1957; DO 1962; FRCSI 1965	Ophthalmology		1973	1993	
Dr John Owen Manton Mills MB (QUB) 1964; DRCOG 1966; FFR 1973	Radiology		1973		
Mr Hugh Oliver O'Kane BSc (Hons) (QUB) 1957; MB 1960; FRCS Edin 1963; MCh 1970	Cardiac surgery		1973		
Prof Arthur Douglas Roy MB (Glas) 1947; FRCSE 1952; FRCS Edin 1952; FRCPS Glas 1963; FRCSI 1976	Surgery		1973	1985	
Mr Ian Campbell Bailey BA 1951; MB (TCD) 1953; FRCSI 1959; FRCSE 1963	Neuro-surgery		1974	1995	
Dr Hoshang Bharucha MB (Vellore) 1965; MD (Madras) 1970; FRC Path. 1986	Pathology		1974		
Dr Eileen Sylvia Browne MB (QUB) 1952; DA Eng 1956; FFA RCSI 1972	Anaesthesia		1974	1990	
Mr Hugh Alan Crockard MB (QUB) 1966; FRCS Edin 1970; FRCSE 1971	Neuro-surgery		1974	1978	

DOCTOR	SPECIALITY	BORN	APPOINTED TO ASSISTANT/ ATTENDING STAFF	APPOINTMENT ENDED OR RESIGNED	DIED
Mr Alan Robert Gurd MB (QUB) 1964; FRCS Edin 1967; MCh 1969	Orthopaedic surgery		1974	1976	
Dr Jack Henneman MRCSE LRCP Lond 1943; MB (St Thom) 1945; MRCP Lond 1948; FRCGP 1970	General practice	23 Mar 1919	1974		29 Apr 1976
Prof William Sidney Blair Lowry MSc (QUB) 1957; MB 1963; FRCPI 1968; FRCR 1975	Oncology		1974	1993	
Mr Samuel Thomas Donnan McKelvey MB (QUB) 1962; DRCOG 1965; FRCS Edin 1967; FRCSE 1968; MCh 1971	Surgery		1974	1985	
Dr George Anthony Murnaghan MB (NUI) 1962; MAO 1969; FRCOG 1981	Gynaecology		1974		
Mr George William Odling-Smee MB (Durham) 1959; FRCSE 1968	Surgery		1974		
Dr James Martin Sloan MB (QUB) 1964; DRCOG 1966; MD 1969; FRC Path. 1984	Pathology		1974		
Dr Ian Wellington Carson MB (QUB) 1968; FFA RCSI 1972; MD (Hons) 1974	Anaesthesia		1975		
Mr William Caskey Logan MB (QUB) 1953; DRCOG 1956; FRCS Edin 1962; FRCSE 1963	Ophthalmology		1975	1994	
Dr Helen Mawhinney MB (QUB) 1967; MRCP UK 1970; MD 1973	Immunology		1975	1981	
Dr Peter Gerald Nelson MB (Hons) (QUB) 1966; FRCP Lond 1984	A&E medicine	28 Feb 1943	1975		20 Apr 1991
Dr Michael Denis O'Hara BSc (Hons) (QUB) 1963; MB 1966; MRC Path. 1973	Pathology		1975		
Mr John Edward Thomas Byrne MB (TCD) 1961; FRCSI 1971	Oto-laryngology		1976		
Prof Michael James Cinnamond MB (QUB) 1967; FRCS Edin 1974	Oto-laryngology		1976	1996	
Dr James Frederick Douglas MB (QUB) 1969; BM (Oxf) 1969; FRCP Lond 1986;	Nephrology		1976		
Prof Robert Reid Gillies MB (Edin) 1947; DPH 1952; MD 1959; MRC Path. 1963; FRCP Edin 1971	Pathology	31 May 1924	1976		2 July 1983

DOCTOR	SPECIALITY	BORN	APPOINTED TO ASSISTANT/ ATTENDING STAFF	APPOINTMENT ENDED OR RESIGNED	DIED
Dr Hugh Connor Mulholland BSc (Hons) (QUB) 1959; MB 1962; FRCP Edin 1979	Cardiology		1976		
Dr Herbert Kenneth Wilson MB (QUB) 1965; FRCR 1975; FFR RCSI 1983	Radiology		1976	1985	
Mr Ian Victor Adair MB (QUB) 1965; FRCS Edin 1968	Orthopaedic surgery		1977		
Mr John Robert Pelham Gibbons MBE, TD. MB (Leeds) 1954; MRCGP 1958; FRCSE 1960; FRCS Edin 1960; FRCSI 1988	Thoracic surgery		1977	1993	
Dr Mark McClean Reid MB (QUB) 1962; DCH RCPS Glas 1965; FRCP Glas 1978	Neonatology		1977		
Dr Varavoor Kaplinghat Narayanan Unni MB (Kerala) 1961; FFA RCSI 1969; PhD 1972	Anaesthesia		1977		
Dr Hugh Shaun Alister Young MB (QUB) 1968; FFA RCSI 1972	Anaesthesia	18 May 1944	1977		12 Aug 1990
Mr John Howard Bryars MB (Hons) (QUB) 1969; FRCS Edin 1974; MD (Hons) 1977	Ophthalmology		1978		
Dr Jocelyn Roger Corbett MB (QUB) 1970; FRCP 1988	Dermatology		1978		
Mr Aires Agnelo Barnabe Barros D'Sa MB (QUB) 1965; FRCS Edin 1969; FRCSE 1970; MD (Hons) 1975	Surgery		1978		
Prof George Dennis Johnston MB (QUB) 1971; DCH RCPSI 1975; MD 1978; PhD 1985; FRCP Edin 1985	Medicine		1978		
Mr Patrick Beaumont Johnston BSc (Hons) (QUB) 1968; MB 1971; FRCS Edin 1976; FCO 1989	Ophthalmology		1978		
Dr Richard John McBride MB (QUB) 1971; FFA RCSI 1975; MPhil 1994	Anaesthesia		1978		
Mr Robert Millar BSc (Hons) (QUB) 1964; MB 1967; FRCS Edin 1971	Plastic surgery		1978		
Dr James Whiteford Knox Ritchie MB (QUB) 1968; MD (Hons) 1975; MRCOG 1972	Gynaecology		1978	1984	
Dr Bharat Bhushan Sawhney MB (Amritsar) 1961; MD 1965; DM (Delhi) 1972	Neuro- physiology		1978		

DOCTOR	SPECIALITY	BORN	APPOINTED TO ASSISTANT/ ATTENDING STAFF	APPOINTMENT ENDED OR RESIGNED	DIED
Dr Charles Frederick Stanford MB (QUB) 1966; MD 1974; FRCP Lond 1983	Medicine		1978	1990	
Dr Grace Varghese MB (Madras) 1962; DCH 1964; FRCP Lond 1989	Medicine		1978		
Dr Samuel Wilson Webb BSc (Hons) (QUB) 1963; MB 1966; MRCP UK 1970; MD 1974	Cardiology		1978		
Mr Michael David Brennen MB (QUB) 1968; FRCS Edin 1972	Plastic surgery		1979		
Mr Dermot Patrick Byrnes MB (NUI) 1963; FRCS Edin 1967; FRCSI 1969	Neuro-surgery		1979		
Dr Norman Paul Stanton Campbell MB (QUB) 1969; MRCP 1972; MD 1976	Cardiology		1979		
Mr Francis Gerard D'Arcy MB (NUI) 1965; FRCS Edin 1969 and 1977; FRCSI 1970; MSc (Manch) 1981	Oto-laryngology		1979		
Prof Alun Estyn Evans MB (QUB) 1968; MD 1984; FFCM 1987; FRCPI 1989	Social medicine		1979		
Mr Thomas Francis Fannin MB (QUB) 1962; MD 1967; FRCS Edin 1969	Neurosurgery		1979		
Dr Hilary Margaret Leeburn Johnston MB (QUB) 1969; FFA RCSI 1975	Anaesthesia		1979		
Dr James Dunn Laird MB (QUB) 1963; DRCOG 1965; FFR 1969	Radiology		1979		
Mr Alan Gerald Leonard MB (QUB) 1967; FRCS Edin 1972	Plastic surgery		1979		
Dr Raymond Douglas Maw MB (QUB) 1973; FRCP Lond 1992	Genito-urinary medicine		1979		
Prof Raymond Alexander Boyce Mollan MB (Hons) (QUB) 1969; DRCOG 1971; FRCS Edin 1974; MD 1981; FRCSI 1985	Orthopaedic surgery		1979	1995	
Dr Cyril Charles Mitchel Morrison MB (TCD) 1967; FRCR 1976; FFR 1994	Radiology		1979	1983	
Dr James Gray Riddell BSc 1964; MB (QUB) 1972; MRCP 1975; MD 1979	Therapeutics		1979		
Mr William Frederick Ian Shepherd MB (QUB) 1979; DO RCPSI 1974; FRCS Edin 1976	Ophthalmology		1979	1989	

DOCTOR	SPECIALITY	BORN	APPOINTED TO ASSISTANT/ ATTENDING STAFF	APPOINTMENT ENDED OR RESIGNED	DIED
Mr John Templeton MB (QUB) 1961; FRCSC 1970; FRCSE 1991; FRCS Glas 1993	Orthopaedic surgery		1979	1988	
Prof Albert Brew Atkinson BSc (Hons) (QUB) 1970; MB (Hons) 1973; MD 1980; FRCP Glas 1987; FRCP Lond 1990; FRCP Edin 1990	Endocrinology		1980		
Dr Egerton Brian Bond MB (QUB) 1968; MD 1976; FRCOG 1992	Gynaecology		1980		
Dr David Dorrington Boyle MB (Edin) 1968; FRCOG 1986	Gynaecology		1980		
Dr Henry Jeremy Lee Craig MB (QUB) 1955; FRCA 1961; MD 1968; FFA RCSI 1971	Anaesthesia		1980	1995	
Dr Paul Mervyn Darragh TD MB (QUB) 1971; FRCPI 1975; MSc (Edin) 1976; MD 1978; FFCM 1980	Social medicine		1980		
Dr Stanley Ian Dempsey MB (QUB) 1970; MRCP UK 1973; FRC Path. 1991	Haematology		1980		
Dr Claire Margaret Hill MB (QUB) 1968; MD 1977; FRCPI 1985; FRC Path. 1992	Pathology		1980		
Dr Allan Laurence Kennedy MB (QUB) 1972; FRCP Edin 1989; FRCP Lond 1990	Endocrinology		1980	1992	
Prof Rajinder Kumar Mirakhur MB (Jammu and Kashmir) 1967; MD (Delhi) 1971; FRCA 1976; PhD (QUB) 1977; FFA RCSI 1984	Anaesthesia		1980		
Mr Trevor Arthur Stanley Buchanan MB 1972; FRCS Edin 1978	Ophthalmology		1981		
Miss Yvonne Mary Canavan MB 1970; FRCS Edin 1975; MD 1979	Ophthalmology		1981		
Dr Stanley Arthur Hawkins BSc (Hons) (QUB) 1969; MB (Hons) 1972; MRCP UK 1975	Neurology		1981		
Dr Roslyn Jane Hutchison MB (QUB) 1973; FRCR 1979	Radiology		1981	1986	
Dr David Bennett Wilson MB (QUB) 1971; DRCOG 1973; FFA RCSI 1977	Anaesthesia		1981		
Dr Michael Edwin Callender MB (KCH Lond) 1973; MA (Camb) 1974; FRCP Lond 1990	Medicine		1982		

DOCTOR	SPECIALITY	BORN	APPOINTED TO ASSISTANT/ ATTENDING STAFF	APPOINTMENT ENDED OR RESIGNED	DIED
Prof John Patrick Howard Fee MB (QUB) 1972; FFA RCSI 1976; MD 1980; PhD 1990	Anaesthesia		1982		
Dr David Hugh Gilmore MB (QUB) 1972; MRCP UK 1977	Geriatrics		1982		
Mr John Metcalf Hood MB 1970; FRCS Edin 1974	Surgery		1982		
Dr Mazhar Muhammad Khan MB (Punjab) 1962; MRCP UK 1976	Cardiology		1982		
Dr Hilary Anne Lavery MB (QUB) 1975; MRCP UK 1978; MD (QUB) 1980	Genito-urinary medicine		1982	1985	
Miss Elizabeth Morrison MB (QUB) 1974; FRCS Edin 1979	Ophthalmology		1982		
Mr Colin Frederick James Russell BDS 1966; MB (QUB) 1971; FRCS Edin 1976	Surgery		1982		
Prof David Ian Hewitt Simpson MB (QUB) 1959; MD 1971; FRC Path. 1983	Microbiology		1982		
Dr Ian Christie Taylor BSc (Hons) 1972; MB (QUB) 1975; MD 1980; FRCP Glas 1993; FRCP Edin 1994	Geriatrics		1982	1985	
Mr Alfred Edward Wood MB (NUI) 1971; FRCSI 1975	Cardiac surgery		1982	1983	
Dr William Paul Abram BSc (Hons) (QUB) 1972; MB 1975; FFR RCSI 1980; FRCR 1980	Radiotherapy		1983		
Dr Brian Denis Burrows MB (QUB) 1960; FFR 1968; FRCR 1975	Radiotherapy		1983		
Dr Julian Rowland Johnston MB (QUB) 1975; FFA RCSI 1979; MD 1982	Anaesthesia		1983		
Dr Richard William Kendrick MB (QUB) 1977; FDS RCPS Glas 1980; FFD RCSI 1980	Maxillo-facial surgery		1983		
Dr Arthur Kerr MB (QUB) 1954; FRCPI 1972; FRC Psych 1980	Psychiatry		1983	1991	
Dr Emer Mary McAteer MB (QUB) 1975; FFA RCSI 1979	Anaesthesia		1983	1986	
Mr Charles Joseph McClelland MB (QUB) 1972; FRCS Edin 1976	Orthopaedic surgery		1983		
Dr Ian Alexander Orr MB (QUB) 1975; FFA RCSI 1978; MD (Hons) 1981	Anaesthesia		1983	1986	

DOCTOR	SPECIALITY	BORN	APPOINTED TO ASSISTANT/ ATTENDING STAFF	APPOINTMENT ENDED OR RESIGNED	DIED
Mr Anthony Peter Walby MB (QUB) 1974; FRCS Edin 1979	Oto-laryngology		1983		
Mr David Alexander Adams BSc 1971; MB (QUB) 1974; FRCS Edin 1979; MSc (Manch) 1982	Oto-laryngology		1984		
Mr James William Calderwood MB (QUB) 1966; FRCS Edin 1970	Orthopaedics		1984		
Prof Alfred Michael Emmerson BSc (Hons) 1962; MB (UCH) 1965; FRC Path. 1984; FRCP Glas 1988	Bacteriology		1984	1989	
Dr David Thomas Graham MB (QUB) 1959; FRCR 1980	Radiology		1984	1986	
Mr Samuel Robinson Johnston MB (QUB) 1971; FRCS Edin 1976	Urology		1984		
Dr David Rolande McCluskey MB (QUB) 1976; MD (Hons) 1983; FRCP Edin 1989	Medicine		1984		
Dr David Paul Nicholls MB (Manch) 1969; MD 1984; FRCP Lond 1991	Medicine		1984		
Dr Victor Howard Patterson MB (Camb) 1973; FRCP Lond 1990	Neurology		1984		
Dr Edward Thomas Martin Smyth MB (QUB) 1976; MD 1993; FRC Path. 1995	Microbiology		1984		
Dr Allister James Taggart MB (QUB) 1975; MD 1982; FRCP Edin 1989; FRCP Lond 1994	Rheumatology		1984		
Prof Peter Gilmour Toner MB (Hons) (Glas) 1965; DSc 1972; FRC Path. 1984; FRCP Glas 1984	Pathology		1984		
Dr Anthony Ivor Traub MB (QUB) 1972; MD (Hons) 1980; FRCOG 1989	Gynaecology		1984		
Dr Timothy Richard Orr Beringer MB (QUB) 1977; MD 1985; FRCPI 1990; FRCP Glas 1991; FRCP Lond 1993	Geriatrics		1985		
Dr Elizabeth Ann Bingham MB (QUB) 1973; FRCP Lond 1993	Dermatology		1985		
Dr Roger Blaney MB (QUB) 1957; DPH 1961; MD 1965; FFCMI 1977; FFCM 1979	Community medicine		1985	1987	
Prof Jack Crane MB (QUB) 1977; MRC Path. 1984; FFPath. RCPI 1985	Forensic medicine		1985		

DOCTOR	SPECIALITY	BORN	APPOINTED TO ASSISTANT/ ATTENDING STAFF	APPOINTMENT ENDED OR RESIGNED	DIED
Dr Joseph Graham Crothers MB (QUB) 1973; DRCOG 1976; FRCR 1982; FFR RCSI 1988	Radiology		1985		
Dr Peter Elliott MB (QUB) 1977; FRCA 1981; MD 1984	Anaesthesia		1985		
Dr Avril McNeill MB (QUB) 1977	Radiology		1985	1994	
Dr John Randolph Press MB (TCD) 1960; FFPath. RCPI 1982	Forensic medicine		1985		
Dr Louise Evelyn Sweeney MB (QUB) 1976; DCH RCPS Glas 1978; FRCR 1983	Radiology		1985		
Mr Alan James Wilkinson MB (QUB) 1973; FRCS Edin 1978; MD 1984	Surgery		1985		
Dr Patrick Michael Bell MB (QUB) 1977; MD 1984; FRCP Glas 1988; FRCPI 1991; FRCP Edin 1992	Medicine		1986		
Dr Linda Margaret Caughley MB (QUB) 1976; MRC Path. 1983	Cytology		1986		
Dr Brian George Craig MB (QUB) 1977; MD 1986; FRCP Lond 1994	Cardiology		1986		
Dr Christine Hazel Dearden MB (QUB) 1973; FRCS Edin 1980	A&E medicine		1986		
Dr James Connor Dornan MB (QUB) 1973; MD (Hons) 1981; MRCOG 1978	Gynaecology		1986		
Dr Anne Catherine Mary Fay MB (QUB) 1977; MRC Path. 1984; MD 1987	Immunology		1986	1989	
Mr William John Primrose MB (QUB) 1977; FRCSI 1981	Oto-laryngology		1986		
Prof Brian James Rowlands MB (Guy's) 1968; FRCSE 1973; MD (Sheff) 1978; FACS 1983; FRCSI 1988	Surgery		1986	1997	
Dr Maureen Yvonne Walsh MB (QUB) 1978	Pathology		1986		
Dr Aubrey Leathem Bell MB (QUB) 1976; MRCP UK 1981; MD 1984	Rheumatology		1987		
Dr Brendan Joseph Collins BSc (Hons) 1976; MB (Hons) (QUB) 1978; MRCP UK 1980; MD 1984	Medicine		1987	1990	

DOCTOR	SPECIALITY	BORN	APPOINTED TO ASSISTANT/ ATTENDING STAFF	APPOINTMENT ENDED OR RESIGNED	DIED
Dr Peter Valentine Coyle MB (QUB) 1979; MRC Path. 1986; MD 1993	Virology		1987		
Dr Wilbert Wallace Dinsmore MB (QUB) 1978; MD 1984; FRCP Lond 1993	Genito-urinary medicine		1987		
Dr Fiona Mary Gibson MB (QUB) 1978; MD 1987; FFA RCSI 1982	Anaesthesia		1987		
Mr Dennis John Gladstone BSc (Hons) 1968; MB (Westm); FRCSE 1976	Cardiac surgery		1987		
Dr Brian Gorman MB (TCD) 1977; MRCPI 1979; FRCR 1984	Radiology		1987		
Dr Kenneth William Harper BSc (Hons) 1971; MB (QUB) 1976; FRCA 1981; MD 1986	Anaesthesia		1987		
Dr Gerard Gavin Lavery MB (Hons) (QUB) 1979; FFA RCSI 1983; MD 1987	Anaesthesia		1987		
Dr Kenneth Gilmour Lowry MB (Manch) 1978; FFA RCSI 1982; M Med Sci 1990	Anaesthesia		1987		
Dr Charles Steven McKinstry MB (QUB) 1979; FRCR 1984	Radiology		1987		
Dr Terence Joseph McMurray MB (QUB) 1977; FRCA 1980; MD 1984	Anaesthesia		1987		
Dr John Edward McNulty MB (QUB) 1978; FFR RCSI 1985	Radiology		1987		
Mr Robert John Maxwell MB (QUB) 1974; DRCOG 1978; FRCS Edin 1979; FRCSE 1980; MD 1984	Surgery		1987		
Prof Elisabeth Ruth Trimble MB (QUB) 1967; MD 1975; MRCP UK 1971	Clinical chemistry		1987		
Dr Kathleen Elizabeth Bell MB (QUB) 1980; FRCR 1986; FFR RCSI 1993	Radiology		1988		
Dr John Mark Gibson MB (TCD) 1976; MD 1985; FRCP Lond 1994	Neurology		1988		
Mr James Adrian McGuigan MB (QUB) 1976; FRCS Edin 1980	Thoracic surgery		1988		
Mr Hugh John Dennis Mawhinney MB (QUB) 1974; FRCS Edin 1979 and 1986; MD 1991	Orthopaedic surgery		1988		

DOCTOR	SPECIALITY	BORN	APPOINTED TO ASSISTANT/ ATTENDING STAFF	APPOINTMENT ENDED OR RESIGNED	DIED
Dr Meenakshi Mirakhur MB (Lucknow) 1968; MD (Chandigarh) 1974; MRC Path. 1978	Neuro- pathology		1988		
Dr Thomas Daniel Emmett Sharpe MB (QUB) 1978; FFA RCSI 1983	Anaesthesia		1988		
Dr Patrick Clifford Hoey Watt MB (QUB) 1977; FRCS Edin 1981	Pathology	18 Feb 1953	1988		28 Dec 1990
Dr Cecil Hugh Webb BDS (QUB) 1971; MB (QUB) 1985; FFPath. RCPI 1990; FRC Path. 1991	Microbiology		1988		
Dr Malcolm David Crone MB (QUB) 1979; FRCR 1986	Radiology		1989		
Dr Michael Brendan Finch MB (QUB) 1975; MRCP UK 1979; MD 1986	Rheumatology		1989		
Mr William John Gray MB (QUB) 1976; FRCSI 1981	Neurosurgery		1989		
Dr John Patrick McCann MB (QUB) 1977; MRCP UK 1981; MD 1986	Rehabilitation		1989		
Dr James Irvine Morrow MB (Hons) (QUB) 1980; MD 1993; FRCP Lond 1993	Neurology		1989		
Dr Ann Jacinta O'Doherty MB (NUI) 1981; MRCPI 1983; FRCR 1987; FFR RCSI 1995	Radiology		1989		
Mr Albert Brian Page MB (QUB) 1974; DRCOG 1978; MRCGP 1981; FRCS Edin 1984; MD 1988	Ophthalmology		1989		
Dr Kathleen Branigan Bamford MB (QUB) 1982; MRC Path. 1988; MD 1997	Microbiology		1990		
Dr John Samuel Andrew Collins MB (QUB) 1976; MD 1988; FRCP Lond 1994; FRCP Edin 1991	Medicine		1990		
Dr Joseph Hill Gaston MB (QUB) 1967; FRCA 1973	Anaesthesia		1990		
Mr Gerald Francis Mary McCoy MB (QUB) 1976; FRCSI 1980; MD 1985	Orthopaedics		1990		
Dr Graeme Harding McDonald MB (QUB) 1981; MRC Psych 1985	Psychiatry		1990		
Dr Kevin Robert Milligan MB (QUB) 1980; FFA RCSI 1984; MD 1988; PhD 1996	Anaesthesia		1990		

DOCTOR	SPECIALITY	BORN	APPOINTED TO ASSISTANT/ ATTENDING STAFF	APPOINTMENT ENDED OR RESIGNED	DIED
Mr James Oliver Small MB (NUI) 1976; FRCSI 1980	Plastic surgery		1990	1991	
Dr James Clive Stanley MB (QUB) 1978; FFA RCSI 1983	Anaesthesia		1990		
Dr Robert Henry Taylor MB (QUB) 1982; FFA RCSI 1986	Anaesthesia		1990		
Dr Carol Mildred Wilson MB (QUB) 1979; MD 1986; FRCP Edin 1995	Cardiology		1990		
Dr Kathryn Moyna Bill MB (Edin) 1980; FFA RCSI 1984	Anaesthesia		1991		
Dr Peter Allen Farling MB (QUB) 1980; FFA RCSI 1985	Anaesthesia		1991		
Mr David George Frazer BSc (Hons) 1979; MB (QUB) 1982; FRCS Glas 1988; FRCOphths 1990	Ophthalmology		1991		
Dr Philip Joseph McGarry MB (QUB) 1982; MRC Psych 1986	Psychiatry		1991		
Dr Robert George Peter Watson BSc (Hons) 1974; MB (QUB) 1977; MRCP UK 1981; MD 1985	Medicine		1991		
Dr Susan Atkinson MB (QUB) 1981; FFA RCSI 1987; MD 1994	Anaesthesia		1992		
Mr John Gordon Brown MD (QUB) 1979; FRCS Edin 1983	Orthopaedics		1992		
Dr Gavin William Noel Dalzell MB (QUB) 1981; MRCP UK 1984; MD 1987	Cardiology		1992		
Dr Francis George Charles Jones MB (QUB) 1972; MRCP UK 1976; FRCPS Glas 1992; FRC Path. 1993	Haematology		1992		
Mr Laurence Gilmore Rocke MB (QUB) 1971; FRCS Edin 1975	A&E medicine		1992		
Dr Claire Maureen Thornton MB (QUB) 1983; MRC Path. 1990	Pathology		1992		
Dr Reginald John Barr MB (QUB) 1982; FRCS Edin 1986; MD 1993	Orthopaedic surgery		1993		
Mr David Shammuah Brooker MB (QUB) 1976; FRCS Edin 1982	Oto-laryngology		1993		
Mr Gianfranco Campalani DMS (Bari) 1975	Cardiac surgery		1993		
Dr Una Attracta Carabine MB (QUB) 1983; FFA RCSI 1988; MD 1991	Anaesthesia		1993		

DOCTOR	SPECIALITY	BORN	APPOINTED TO ASSISTANT/ ATTENDING STAFF	APPOINTMENT ENDED OR RESIGNED	DIED
Dr David Robert McCance BSc (Hons) 1979; MB (QUB) 1982; DCH RCSI 1984; MRCP UK 1985; MD 1990	Medicine		1993		
Mr Francis Gerard McGinnity MB (QUB) 1980; FRCS 1986; MD 1990; FRCOphths 1990	Ophthalmology		1993		
Dr Kevin Joseph McGrath MB (NUI) 1981; FFA RCSI 1988	Anaesthesia		1993		
Mr Kieran Gerard McManus MB (Tasmania) 1980; FRCSI 1985	Thoracic surgery		1993		
Mr John Bryson Martin MB (QUB) 1984; FRCS Edin 1989 and 1990	A&E medicine		1993	1996	
Mr Mazen Abdullah Sarsam MB (Mosul, Iraq) 1974; FRCSE 1981; FRCS Edin 1981	Cardiac surgery		1993		
Dr Anthony Baxter Stevens MB (QUB) 1982; MRCP UK 1985	Occupational health		1993		
Dr Alan Johnston Black MB (QUB) 1981; MRCP UK 1984	Occupational health		1994		
Prof Henry Lewis Halliday MB (QUB) 1970; DRCOG 1972; MD (QUB) 1980; FRCP Edin 1982; FRCP Lond 1988	Neonatology		1994		
Prof Philip John Lamey BSc (Hons) (Edin) 1975; MB (Glas) 1982; DDS Edin 1982; FDS RCPS Glas 1985	Oral medicine		1994		
Dr Michael Oliver McBride MB (QUB) 1986; MRCP UK 1989	Genito-urinary medicine		1994		
Dr Gerard James McCarthy MB (QUB) 1983; FFA RCSI 1987; MD 1992	Anaesthesia		1994	1995	
Dr John Martin McGovern BSc (UU) 1977; MSc (Aber) 1978; MB (QUB) 1985; FRCR 1992	Radiology		1994		
Dr Anne Sarah Phillips MB (QUB) 1984; FFA RCSI 1988; MD 1993	Anaesthesia		1994		
Dr Ciaran Vincent Rafferty MB (QUB) 1985; FFA RCSI 1989	Anaesthesia		1994		
Mr James Anthony Mary Sharkey MB (QUB) 1985; FRCS Glas 1989	Ophthalmology		1994		
Miss Giuliana Silvestri MB (QUB) 1983; MRCP UK 1987; FRCS Edin 1989; FRCOphths 1990; MD 1994	Ophthalmology		1994		

DOCTOR	SPECIALITY	BORN	APPOINTED TO ASSISTANT/ ATTENDING STAFF	APPOINTMENT ENDED OR RESIGNED	DIED
Dr Stephen Stranex MB (QUB) 1977; FFR RCSI 1984	Radiotherapy		1994		
Mr Paul Henry Beaumont Blair MB (QUB) 1982; FRCS Edin 1986; MCh 1995	Surgery		1995		
Dr Declan James Fogarty MB (QUB) 1983; FFA RCSI 1988; MD 1994	Anaesthesia		1995		
Mr Keith Reginald Gardiner MB (QUB) 1983; FRCSI 1987; FRCS Edin 1987; MD 1990	Surgery		1995		
Dr Barry Eoin Kelly MB (QUB) 1984; FRCS Edin 1988; FRCR 1993; FFR RCSI 1993	Radiology		1995		
Dr Ian Michael Giles Kelly BA 1981; MB (TCD) 1983; MRCPI 1986; FRCR 1993	Radiology		1995		
Mr Richard Stephen Cooke MB (QUB) 1986; FRCSI 1990	Neurosurgery		1996		
Dr Thomas Francis Grattan Esmonde MB (TCD) 1984; MRCPI 1987; MRCP UK 1987	Neurology		1996		
Dr Paul Brereton Loan MB (QUB) 1986; MRCP UK 1989; FRCA 1991	Anaesthesia		1996		
Dr William Thomas McBride BSc (Hons) (QUB) 1984; MB 1987; FRCA 1992; FFA RCSI 1992; MD 1996	Anaesthesia		1996		
Dr Eamon Paul McCoy MB (NUI) 1986; FFA RCSI 1990; MD (QUB) 1995	Anaesthesia		1996		
Mr Simon William MacGowan MB (NUI) 1983; BSc 1985 FRCSI 1987; MCh 1993	Cardiac surgery		1996		
Mr Brian Peter Gerald McNicholl MB (NUI) 1985; MRCPI 1987; FRCS Edin 1989; MCh 1996; FFAEM 1996	A&E medicine		1996		
Dr Michael Watt BSc 1982; MB (QUB) 1985; MRCP UK 1988	Neurology		1996		

2

CHAIRMEN OF THE MEDICAL STAFF COMMITTEE

1880–1899	Professor J Cuming		1958–1960	Mr F.A. MacLaughlin
1899–1912	Dr J.W. Browne		1960–1961	Mr I. Fraser
1912–1915	Sir William Whitla		1961–1963	Mr J.R. Wheeler
1915–1918	Sir John Byers		1963–1965	Mr J.A. Corkey
1918–1921	Professor J.A. Lindsay		1965–1967	Mr J.S. Loughridge
1921–1923	Professor T. Sinclair		1967–1968	Mr H.I. McClure
1923–1928	Mr A.B. Mitchell		1969–1970	Dr W.M. Brown
1928–1931	Surgeon T.S. Kirk		1971–1972	Dr M.G. Nelson
1931–1933	Professor A. Fullerton		1972–1973	Professor H.W. Rodgers
1933–1936	Professor R.J. Johnstone		1973–1975	Mr J.W.S. Irwin
1936–1937	Mr J.A. Craig		1975–1977	Professor D.A.D. Montgomery
1937–1939	Mr H. Hanna		1977–1979	Dr J.H.D. Millar
1939–1940	Dr J.C. Rankin		1979–1981	Mr E. Morrison
1940–1941	Mr H. Stevenson		1981–1983	Dr T.T. Fulton
1941–1942	Mr S.T. Irwin		1983–1985	Mr W. Wilson OBE
1942–1945	Professor P.T. Crymble		1985–1987	Dr J.A. Weaver
1945–1948	Professor W.W.D. Thomson		1987–1989	Professor J.M.G. Harley
1948–1950	Mr H.P. Malcolm		1989–1991	Dr E.M. McIlrath
1950–1952	Mr H.L.H. Greer		1991–1993	Professor J.M. Bridges
1952–1954	Dr J.A. Smyth		1993–1995	Professor G.W. Johnston
1954	Dr Robert Marshall		1995–1997	Mr R. Gibson
1954–1956	Dr J.T. Lewis		1997–	Dr E.E. Mayne
1956–1958	Dr R.S. Allison			

3

HONORARY SECRETARIES OF THE MEDICAL STAFF COMMITTEE

1875–1880	Dr H. Murney		1959–1960	Mr S.R. Sinclair
1880–1883	Sir John Fagan		1960–1961	Dr J. Elliott
1883–1899	Dr W. Whitla		1961–1963	Dr J.F. Bereen
1899–1900	Dr A. Lindsay		1963–1965	Dr D.A.D. Montgomery
1900	Dr R.S. Smith		1965–1967	Mr H.M. Stevenson
1900–1905	Dr W. Calwell		1967–1968	Dr R.A. Womersley
1905–1909	Dr H.L. McKisack		1968–1970	Dr G.L. Gibson
1909–1919	Mr R.J. Johnstone		1970–1972	Dr A.H.G. Love
1919–1921	Mr A. Fullerton		1972–1974	Dr E.M. McIlrath
1921	Dr J.E. MacIlwaine		1974–1976	Dr S.M. Lyons
1921–1927	Mr H. Stevenson		1976–1978	Dr D.R. Hadden
1927–1932	Dr F. Coates		1978–1980	Dr D.D. Burrows
1932–1937	Dr R.M. Beath		1980–1982	Dr D.L. Coppel
1937–1942	Dr S.I. Turkington		1982–1984	Mr R. Gibson
1942–1944	Dr F.P. Montgomery		1984–1986	Dr J.M. Sloan
1944–1946	Mr C.J.A. Woodside		1986–1988	Mr S.S. Johnston
1946–1948	Dr R.S. Allison		1988–1990	Dr J.O.M. Mills
1948–1950	Mr J.S. Loughridge		1990–1992	Mr I.V. Adair
1950–1953	Mr J.A. Corkey		1992–1994	Dr N.P.S. Campbell
1953–1956	Dr M.G. Nelson		1994–1996	Dr J.R.J. Johnston
1956–1957	Dr D.C. Porter		1996–	Dr P.M. Bell
1957–1959	Dr J.M. Beare			

4
ORATORS OF THE ANNUAL WINTER ORATION
UNTIL THE MID-1880s IT IS LIKELY THAT THE SPEAKER WAS SIMPLY GIVING THE FIRST LECTURE OF THE SEASON, RATHER THAN A FORMAL ORATION.

YEAR	ORATOR	TITLE OF ORATION
1827	Dr J. McDonnell	Systematic Medicine
1852	Dr A.G. Malcolm	
1856	Dr J. Ferguson	
1864	Dr W. MacCormac	
1865	Dr R. Ross	
1866	Prof. A. Gordon	
1867	Dr J.S. Drennan	
1875	Dr J. Moore	
1883	Dr J. Moore	
1884	Dr J. Cuming	
1885	Dr J.W. Browne	
1886	Dr J. Byers	
1887	Dr H. Burden	
1888	Dr J. Fagan	
1889	Dr J.A. Lindsay	
1890		
1891		
1892	Dr J. Nelson	
1893		
1894	Dr T.K. Wheeler	
1895	Mr A.B. Mitchell	
1896	No oration given	
1897	Dr L. Smith	
1898	Dr W. Calwell	
1899	Surgeon T.S. Kirk	
1900	Dr H.L. McKisack	
1901	Mr R. Campbell	
1902	Dr W.B. McQuitty	
1903	Dr J.W. Browne	
1904	Mr A. Fullerton	
1905	Dr J.S. Morrow	
1906	Mr J.A. Craig	
1907	Mr R.J. Johnston	
1908	Prof W. St C. Symmers	
1909	Dr H. Hanna	
1910	No oration given (Sir William Whitla declined)	
1911	Dr J.E. MacIlwaine	
1912	Dr T. Houston	
1913	Dr J.C. Rankin	
1914	Dr V.G.L. Fielden	
1915	Sir John Byers	
1916	Prof J.A. Lindsay	

YEAR	ORATOR	TITLE OF ORATION
1917	Dr W. Calwell	
1918	Mr T. Sinclair	
1919	Mr A.B. Mitchell	
1920	Surgeon T.S. Kirk	
1921	Dr H.L. McKisack	
1922	Marquess of Londonderry	
1923	Prof A. Fullerton	
1924	Prof W.W.D. Thomson	
1925	Prof C.G. Lowry	
1926	Name of orator not known	
1927	Prof P.T. Crymble	Defence of the Voluntary System
1928	Judge H.M. Thompson	Doctors in the Courts
1929	Mr R.J. McConnell	
1930	Dr S.B. Boyd Campbell	
1931	Dr R.M. Beath	
1932	Mr H.P. Malcolm	
1933	Mr H.L.H. Greer	
1934	Dr J.A. Smyth	Biochemistry
1935	Dr R. Marshall	Traditions of the Royal Victoria Hospital
1936	Dr S.I. Turkington	Students of Medicine
1937	Dr F.P. Montgomery	Some Aspects of Medicine and Literature
1938	Dr J.T. Lewis	Peaks of Clinical Medicine
1939	The Vice-Chancellor, QUB	
1940	Mr G.R.B. Purce	Medicine in the Army
1941	Dr R.S. Allison	Medicine and the Navy
1942	Prof C.H.G. Macafee	Medical Students and the Teaching of Midwifery
1943	Mr C.J.A. Woodside	Possible Worlds
1944	Dr I.H. McCaw	A Synopsis of the History of Dermatology
1945	Mr J.R. Wheeler	A Synopsis of the History of Ophthalmology
1946	Mr C.A. Calvert	The Development of Neurosurgery
1947	Mr H.C. Lowry	Some Landmarks in Surgical Technique
1948	Mr F.A. MacLaughlin	The Patient and his Doctor
1949	Prof J.H. Biggart	Parergon
1950	Mr J.A. Corkey	Vision and Medicine
1951	Mr J. Hunter	A Short History of Otolaryngology
1952	Mr I. Fraser	The Heritage of the Royal Victoria Hospital
1953	Mr J.S. Loughridge	Aspects of Human Heredity in Health and Disease
1954	Mr H.I. McClure	The Church and Medicine
1955	Mr E.W. McMechan	A Tribute to our Surgical Pioneers
1956	Dr T.H. Crozier	Folklore and Medicine
1957	Dr R. Hall	The Doctor's Visit
1958	Mr R.J.W. Withers	Rest and Exercise
1959	Dr W.M. Brown	The Conquest of Pain
1960	Prof H.W. Rodgers	Whither Medicine?
1961	Dr M.G. Nelson	Science and the Progress of Medicine
1962	Dr D.C. Porter	The New Photography
1963	Dr G. Gregg	The State of Medicine at the Time of the Crusades
1964	Dr J.F. Bereen	Quo Vadis
1965	Mr J.W.S. Irwin	Razors to Autoclaves
1966	Mr W.H.T. Shepherd	Hospital Relationships

YEAR	ORATOR	TITLE OF ORATION
1967	No oration given	
1968	Mr N.C. Hughes	A Short History of Plastic Surgery
1969	Mr E. Morrison	Crude Craftsmen
1970	Mr T.L. Kennedy	Communication in Medicine
1971	No oration given	(Professor J.F. Pantridge declined)
1972	Dr D.A.D. Montgomery	Clinical Research in Hospital
1973	Dr J.S. Logan	The Working Man of the Profession
1974	Mr T.B. Smiley	Medical Students and their Education
1975	Dr J.H.D. Millar	The Medical Library
1976	Mr R.I. Wilson	Sticks and Stones
1977	Dr J.M. Beare	Industrial Dermatitis and the Law in Northern Ireland
1978	Dr J. Elliott	The Rod and the Staff
1979	Dr T.T. Fulton	The Making of a Doctor
1980	Mr R.H. Livingston	They Comfort Me
1981	Mr W. Wilson	Old Ethics – New Dilemmas
1982	Mr H.M. Stevenson	Patients – A Virtue
1983	Dr J.A. Weaver	A Hospital for all Seasons
1984	Mr D.S. Gordon	The Changing Face of Medicine
1985	Prof J.W. Dundee	The Last of the Fifty – A Time for Change
1986	Dr F.S. Grebbell	Shadows
1987	Dr D.D. Burrows	Not Strangers but Pilgrims
1988	Prof A.H.G. Love	Serving Two Masters
1989	Mr P.H. Osterberg	The Lure and Love of Surgery
1990	Mr G.W. Johnston	The Enjoyment of Life Depends on the Liver
1991	Prof J.M.G. Harley	Cinderella had a Champion
1992	Dr E.M. McIlrath	An Image for Tomorrow
1993	Prof R.S.J. Clarke	A Corridor to the Past
1994	Dr S.D. Roberts	Membership by Examination
1995	Prof I. Allen	The Clinician Scientist – An Endangered Species
1996	Prof D.R. Hadden	Health and Education: The Metabolism of a Teaching Hospital

5

MEDICAL SUPERINTENDENTS AND RELATED POSTS

YEARS	NAME	TITLE
1875–1878	Commander F. Cox RN	Medical Superintendent
1878–1880	Lieutenant-Colonel Clavell Blount RN	Medical Superintendent
1880–1901	Colonel John Glancy MD	Medical Superintendent
1901–1920	Colonel Andrew Deane MD	Medical Superintendent
1921–1931	Colonel John Vincent Forrest MD	Medical Superintendent
1931–1944	Colonel James William Langstaff DSO, LRCP, MRCS	Medical Superintendent
1946–1965	Brigadier Thomas Walker Davidson MD	Medical Superintendent
1965–1968	Colonel Thomas Eglinton Field MBE, MD	Medical Superintendent
1968–1973	Mr James Stevenson Loughridge MD, FRCS	Medical Superintendent
1973–1977	Mr Bertram Leslie Ardill BSc, MD, FRCS	Group Medical Administrator
1979–1984	Mr Reginald Arthur Edward Magee MP, FRCS	Group Medical Administrator
1984–1987	Dr Samuel Harold Swan Love MD, FRCA	Group Medical Administrator
1987–	Dr George Anthony Murnaghan MB, FRCOG	Director of Medical Adminstration

6

MATRONS (AND RELATED POSTS)

YEARS	NAME	TITLE
1832–1851	Miss Ann Marshall	Matron/Head Nurse
1851–1854	Mrs Gihon	Matron and housekeeper
1855–1865	Miss Kate Mewha	Matron and housekeeper
1865–1868	Miss Olpherts	Matron and housekeeper
1868–1875	Miss Jane Nelson	Matron and housekeeper
1875–1886	Mrs Irwin	Matron and housekeeper
1886–1887	Miss Aisbitt	Matron and housekeeper
1887–1901	Mrs Waters	Matron and housekeeper
1901–1922	Miss Mary Frances Bostock	Matron
1922–1946	Miss Anne Elizabeth Musson MBE	Matron
1946–1966	Miss Florence Eileen Elliott OBE	Matron
1966–1973	Miss Mary Kathleen Robb OBE	Matron (District Administrative Nursing Officer N&W Belfast 1973–1984)
1973–1975	Miss Mary Ann McFarland	Principal Nursing Officer
1975–1984	Miss Heather Marion Barrett	Divisional Nursing Officer
1984–1997	Miss Elizabeth Duffin	Director of Nursing Services, Royal Group

7

PRESIDENTS OF THE HOSPITAL
(PRE-1948)

1792–1799	The 1st Marquess of Donegall
1799–1844	The 2nd Marquess of Donegall
1844–1883	The 3rd Marquess of Donegall
1883	W.B.T. Lyons Esq, JP, DL
1884–1886	Lord Ashley, later 8th Earl of Shaftesbury
1890–1914	The 6th Marquess of Londonderry
1915–1935	Lady Pirrie, later Viscountess Pirrie
1939–1948	The Rt Hon Sir J. Milne Barbour, Bt

8

HONORARY TREASURERS OF THE HOSPITAL
(PRE-1948)

1817–1818	William Clarke
1818–1829	John Barnett
1829–1843	John Clarke
1843–1846	Robert Wright
1846–1847	John Coleman
1847–1848	William Bottomley
1849–1854	Gustavus Heyn
1854–1873	James Girdwood
1873–1877	Elias H. Thompson
1878–1881	William Bell
1881–1898	William F. MacElheran
1898–1907	James Davidson
1908–1919	John Tate
1919–1933	Henry Berrington
1933–1948	Victor F. Clarendon

9

HONORARY SECRETARIES OF THE HOSPITAL (PRE-1948) AND SENIOR ADMINISTRATIVE OFFICERS AFTER 1948

YEARS	NAME	TITLE
1846–1847	Dr William Moffat and James McIntyre	
1847–1853	——	
1853–1859	Rev William Anderson and James M. Thompson	
1859–1860	James M. Thompson and Plato Oulton	
1860–1878	A.J. Macrory	
1878–1879	James A.M. Heyn	
1879–1881	H.H. Bottomley	
1881–1887	R.W. Murray	
1887–1890	John Marsh	
1890–1896	William Agnew	
1896–1898	E. O'Rorke Dickey	
1898–1903	Joseph C. Marsh	
1903–1908	Joshua Pim	
1908–1925	Robert M. Young	
1925–1938	F.A. Heron	
1938–1945	J.S. Rodgers	
1945–1948	William McKinney	
1949–1958	Lieutenant-Colonel W.M. Knatchbull	Administrative Officer
1953–1957	Lieutenant-Colonel V.D. Gordon	Secretary and Superintendent
1957–1962	Brigadier Thomas Davidson	Medical Superintendent and Secretary
1962–1974	Robert T. Spence	Group Secretary
		District Administrative Officer
1974–1984	J.C. Girvan Jackson	District Administrative Officer
1984–1988	Samuel C. Haslett	Group Adminstrator
1988–	William McKee	Acting Group Administrator
		Unit Manager
		Chief Executive

SOURCES & BIBLIOGRAPHY

PRIMARY SOURCES

The main unpublished sources for the history of the Royal Victoria Hospital and its predecessors consist in the minutes of the board of management of the hospitals in the Office of Archives of the Royal Victoria Hospital. These are in manuscript and date from 1818, shortly after the opening of the Belfast Fever Hospital, covering the period up to 1948 when the National Health Service took over management. From 1865 there are also the minutes of the Medical Staff Committee and for the period 1896–1904 there are the minutes for the 'New Hospital Scheme', a number of committees specifically concerned with the opening of the new Royal Victoria Hospital. Most of this material is in manuscript and it must be said that the most convenient source for the whole pre-1948 period is the collection of printed annual reports, dating from 1818 and also preserved in the Office of Archives.

For the period from 1948 onwards we have the minutes of the Belfast Hospitals Management Committee (1949–73), of its Royal Victoria Hospital subcommittee (1949–64), and of the Group Medical Advisory Committee (1953–71). We also have the minutes of the Eastern Health and Social Services Medical Executive (1971–90), of the District Executive Team (1973–84), and of the Royal Group of Hospitals Unit of Management (1984–91), and from 1972 we have minutes of most of the divisional and directorate committees.

Finally, among the primary sources is the collection of personal material about senior medical staff of all periods, which has been gathered by the honorary archivists down the years. This includes applications, CVs, photographs, collections of published papers, and obituaries. With this material may be grouped lengthy memoirs of the pathology department by Professor M.G. Nelson and Dr Margaret Haire.

PRINTED SOURCES

The years up to 1948 have been described in three invaluable sources: Dr A.G. Malcolm's *The History of the General Hospital, Belfast* covering the early years to 1850, Dr R.S. Allison's *The Seeds of Time* covering 1850–1903, and Dr R. Marshall's *Fifty Years on the Grosvenor Road* covering 1903–53. The period from 1948 is inevitably more difficult because of the absence of any previous overview, but also because of the diversity of subspecialities that have developed and because of the radical reorganisations that occurred around 1972, 1984 and 1993. However, many useful articles have been published in the *Ulster Medical Journal*, many being the texts of the hospital's annual winter oration, which take us well into the second half of the twentieth century. For the sake of completeness all the texts of the winter orations are listed below in the published articles.

BOOKS

Addison, W.I. *A Roll of the Graduates of the University of Glasgow from 31 December 1727 to 31 December 1897.* Glasgow, 1898.
Allison, R.S. *The Very Faculties.* Belfast, 1969.
   The Seeds of Time. Belfast, 1972.
   The Surgeon Probationers. Belfast, 1979.
Bardon J. *A History of Ulster.* Belfast, 1992.
Barton, B. *The Blitz: Belfast in the War Years.* Belfast, 1989.
Boyd, A. *Holy War in Belfast.* Tralee, Ireland, 1969.
Boyd, F.I. *Social Work in the Royal Victoria Hospital, 1938–1988.* Belfast, 1988.
Brown, W.M. *While There is Life.* Belfast, 1988.
Burtchaell, G.D. and Sadleir, T.U. *Alumni Dublinenses.* London, 1924.
Chart, D.A. *The Drennan Letters: Being a Selection of the Correspondence Which Passed between William Drennan MD and his Brother-in-law and Sister, Samuel and Martha McTier, During the Years 1776–1819.* Belfast, 1951.
Clarke, R.S.J. *Gravestone Inscriptions, Belfast,* Vol. 3. Belfast, 1986.
Clarkson, L.A. and Litvic, M. *The Working Men's Committee of the Royal Victoria Hospital, Belfast, 1888–1992.* Belfast, 1996.
Craig, D.H. *Belfast and Its Infirmary: The Growth of a Hospital.* Belfast, 1985.
Deane, A. *The Belfast Natural History and Philosophical Society: Centenary Volume, 1821–1921.* Belfast, 1924.
Dictionary of National Biography. Articles on the Revd S.M. Stephenson (1742–1833), Sir James Murray (1788–1871) and Dr James Lawson Drummond (1783–1853).
Donaldson, M. *Yes, Matron.* Belfast, 1989.
Fisher, J.R. and Robb, J.H. *Royal Belfast Academical Institution: Centenary Volume, 1810–1910.* Belfast, 1913.
Fraser, I. *Blood, Sweat and Cheers.* Cambridge, 1989.

Jefferson, H. *Viscount Pirrie of Belfast*. Belfast [*c.* 1948].

MacCormac, W. *Notes and Recollections of an Ambulance Surgeon, Being an Account of Work Done under the Red Cross During the Campaign of 1870*. London, 1871.

McCreary, A. *Survivors*. Belfast, 1976.

Malcolm, A.G. *The History of the General Hospital, Belfast*. Belfast, 1851. Reprinted with a biography by H.G. Calwell as *Andrew Malcolm of Belfast, 1818–1856, Physician and Historian*. Belfast, 1977.

Marshall, R. *Fifty Years on the Grosvenor Road: An Account of the Rise and Progress of the Royal Victoria Hospital, Belfast, During the Years 1903–1953*. Belfast [1953].

Medical Directory, The. Published annually from 1844. London.

Merrick, A.C.W. and Clarke, R.S.J. *Old Belfast Families and the New Burying Ground*. Belfast, 1991.

Moody, T.W. and Beckett, J.C. *Queen's Belfast, 1845–1949: The History of a University*. London, 1959.

Moss, M. and Hume, J.R. *Shipbuilders to the World: 125 years of Harland and Wolff, Belfast, 1861–1986*. Belfast, 1986.

Odling-Smee, W. and Crockard, A. *Trauma Care*. London, 1981.

Owen, D.J. *History of Belfast*. Belfast, 1921.

Pantridge, J.F. *An Unquiet Life*. Antrim, 1989.

Rutherford, W.H., Nelson, P.G., Weston, P.A.M. and Wilson, D.H. *Accident and Emergency Medicine*. Tunbridge Wells, 1980.

Strain, R.W.M. *Belfast and Its Charitable Society*. London, 1961.
Les Neiges d'Antan. Belfast, 1982.

Swallow, M. *Selected Papers of Lewis J. Hurwitz*. Belfast, 1975.

Symington, J. and Rankin, J.C. *An Atlas of Skiagrams, Illustrating the Development of the Teeth*. London, 1908.

Toner, P.G. (ed.). *Pathology at the Royal: The First Hundred Years, 1890–1990*. Belfast, 1990.

Ulster Museum, Belfast. *James Moore, 1819–1883*. Belfast, 1973.

PUBLISHED ARTICLES

Allen, I.V. 'The clinician scientist – an endangered species?' *Ulster Medical Journal*, 1996; 65: 61–7.

Anon. 'Sir Robert James Johnstone'. *Ulster Medical Journal*, 1939; 8: 48–50.

Beare, J.M. 'Industrial dermatitis and the law in Northern Ireland'. *Ulster Medical Journal*, 1978; 47: 29–38.

Beath, R.M. 'Radiology: its background and its future'. *Ulster Medical Journal* 1937; 6: 99–109.

Bereen, J.F. 'Quo vadis'. *Ulster Medical Journal*, 1964; 33: 83–9.

Biggart, J.H. 'Parergon'. *Ulster Medical Journal*, 1949; 18: 116–28.
'Cnidos v. Cos'. *Ulster Medical Journal*, 1972; 41: 1–9.

Brown, W.M. 'The conquest of pain'. *Ulster Medical Journal*, 1959; 28: 101–17.

Burrows, D. 'Not strangers, but pilgrims'. *Ulster Medical Journal*, 1988; 57: 11–21.

Calvert, C.A. 'The development of neurosurgery'. *Ulster Medical Journal*, 1946; 15: 123–40.

Calwell, H.G. 'The development of neurology in Belfast'. *Ulster Medical Journal,* 1979; 48: 123–36.

Campbell, W.S. 'The life and work of Robert Campbell'. *Ulster Medical Journal,* 1963; 32: 168–85.

Clarke, R.S.J. 'A corridor to the past'. *Ulster Medical Journal,* 1994; 63: 76–98.

Corkey, J.A. 'Vision and medicine'. *Ulster Medical Journal,* 1950; 19: 142–51.

Crockard, H.A. 'The severe head injury: methods of assessment'. *Ulster Medical Journal,* 1973; 42: 45–56.

Crozier, T.H. 'Folklore and medicine'. *Ulster Medical Journal,* 1956; 25: 41–61.

Dundee, J.W. 'The last of the fifty – a time of change'. *Ulster Medical Journal,* 1986; 55: 15–22.

Elliott, J. 'The rod and the staff'. *Ulster Medical Journal,* 1979; 48: 32–42.

Esler, R. 'Early history of medicine in Belfast'. *Transactions of the Ulster Medical Society,* 1884; 158–69.

  'Sketch of the Ulster Medical Society and its presidents'. *Transactions of the Ulster Medical Society,* 1886; 75–84.

Fraser, I. 'The heritage of the Royal Victoria Hospital'. *Ulster Medical Journal,* 1952; 21: 114–29.

  'Great teachers of surgery in the past: Andrew Fullerton (1868–1934)'. *British Journal of Surgery,* 1964; 51: 401–5.

  'Father and son, a tale of two cities, 1800–1901'. *Ulster Medical Journal,* 1968; 37: 1–39.

  'The Campbell heritage lives on'. *Ulster Medical Journal,* 1973; 42: 111–35.

  'The first three professors of surgery'. *Ulster Medical Journal,* 1976; 45: 12–46.

  'The Belfast Medical School and its surgeons'. *Ulster Medical Journal,* 1981; 50, supplement.

  'The personalities and problems of sixty years ago'. *Ulster Medical Journal,* 1987; 56, supplement: S15–S30.

Froggatt, P. 'The foundation of the "Inst" medical department and its association with the Belfast Fever Hospital'. *Ulster Medical Journal,* 1976; 45: 107–45.

  'The first medical school, 1835–1849'. *Medical History,* 1978; 22: 237–66.

  'Dr James MacDonnell, MD (1763–1845)'. *The Glynns,* 1981; 9: 17–31.

  'The early medical school: foundation and first crisis – the "college hospital" affair'. *Ulster Medical Journal,* 1987; 56, supplement: S5–S14.

Froggatt, P. and Wheeler, W.G. 'Robert Little MA MD LAH LM, Professor of Midwifery and diseases of women and children, Royal Belfast Academical Institution, 1835–40: A biographical note'. *Ulster Medical Journal,* 1983; 52: 58–66.

Fulton, T. 'The making of a doctor'. *Ulster Medical Journal,* 1980; 49: 23–36.

  'Through the artist's eyes'. *Ulster Medical Journal,* 1982; 51: 1–22.

Gallagher, H.W. 'Sir William Thomson, physician'. *Ulster Medical Journal,* 1973; 42: 15–27.

  'W.B. McQuitty'. *Ulster Medical Journal,* 1975; 44: 15–27.

Gordon, D.S. 'The changing face of medicine'. *Ulster Medical Journal,* 1985; 54: 20–29.

  'Advances in the treatment of trauma'. *Ulster Medical Journal,* 1987; 56, supplement: S91–S94.

Gordon, D.S. and Blair, G.A.S. 'Titanium cranioplasty'. *British Medical Journal,* 1974; 2: 478–81.

Gray, R.C., Dundee, J.W. and Clarke, R.S.J. 'Intensive respiratory care: a survey of 350 consecutive cases'. *Ulster Medical Journal,* 1967; 36: 145–50.

Grebbell, F.S. 'Shadows'. *Ulster Medical Journal,* 1987; 56: 30–38.

Gregg, G. 'The state of medicine at the time of the Crusades'. *Ulster Medical Journal,* 1963; 32: 141–50.

Hall, R. 'Medical ethics'. *Ulster Medical Journal,* 1957; 26: 108–21.

'History of dermatology in Northern Ireland'. *British Journal of Dermatology,* 1970; 83: 690–7.

Harley, J.M.G. 'Cinderella had a champion'. *Ulster Medical Journal,* 1992; 61: 75–85.

Heney, J.W. 'Premedication as an aid to anaesthesia'. *Ulster Medical Journal,* 1934; 3: 23–30.

Hewitt, J.C. and Dundee, J.W. 'Development of anaesthesia in Northern Ireland'. *Ulster Medical Journal,* 1970; 39: 97–107.

Hughes, N.C. 'A short history of plastic surgery'. *Ulster Medical Journal,* 1969; 38: 55–61.

Hunter, K. 'A short history of otolaryngology'. *Ulster Medical Journal,* 1951; 20: 106–17.

Hunter, R.H. 'A history of the Ulster Medical Society'. *Ulster Medical Journal,* 1936; 5: 107–23 and 178–95.

Irwin, J.W.S. 'Razors to autoclaves'. *Ulster Medical Journal,* 1965; 34: 66–73.

Irwin, S.T. 'Thomas Sinclair'. *Ulster Medical Journal,* 1941; 10: 61–4.

Johnston, G.W. 'Enjoyment of life depends on the liver'. *Ulster Medical Journal,* 1991; 60: 10–20.

Johnstone, R.J. 'Frederick Street'. *Ulster Medical Journal,* 1940; 9: 3–5.

Kennedy, T.L. 'Communication in medicine'. *Ulster Medical Journal,* 1971; 40: 43–53.

Larmour P. *et al.* 'A revolution in hospital design: the revolution continues'. *Perspective,* 1996, Jan./Feb.: 1–9.

Leman, R.M. 'Fifty years – a radiographic retrospect'. *Ulster Medical Journal,* 1966; 35: 1–11.

Lewis, J.T. 'Peaks of clinical medicine'. *Ulster Medical Journal,* 1939; 8: 14–28.

Livingston, R.H. 'They comfort me: the history of nursing in Belfast'. *Ulster Medical Journal,* 1981; 50: 33–45.

Logan, J.S. 'The working man of the profession'. *Ulster Medical Journal,* 1974; 43: 22–32.

'Trench fever in Belfast and the nature of the "relapsing fevers" in the United Kingdom in the nineteenth century'. *Ulster Medical Journal,* 1989; 58: 83–8.

'Dr Sanders' silver lancet case'. *Ulster Medical Journal,* 1991; 60: 93–5.

Logan, Mary S.T. 'The centenary of the admission of women students to the Belfast Medical School'. *Ulster Medical Journal,* 1990; 59: 200–203.

Loughridge, J.S. 'Aspects of human heredity in health and disease'. *Ulster Medical Journal,* 1953; 22: 100–112.

Love, A.H.G. 'Serving two masters'. *Ulster Medical Journal,* 1989; 58: 13–28.

Lowry, C.G. 'Robert Maitland Beath'. *Ulster Medical Journal,* 1941; 10: 63–7.

Lowry, H.C. 'Some landmarks of surgical technique'. *Ulster Medical Journal,* 1947; 16: 102–13.

Macafee, C.H.G. 'The history of the Belfast School of Obstetrics'. *Ulster Medical Journal,* 1942; 11: 20–50.

'Medical students and the teaching of midwifery'. *Ulster Medical Journal,* 1943;

12: 24–40.

'The history of the Chair of Midwifery and Gynaecology in the Queen's University of Belfast'. *Ulster Medical Journal,* 1975; 44: 93–115.

MacArthur, W. 'Famine fevers in England and Ireland'. *Ulster Medical Journal,* 1948; 17: 28–33.

McCaw, I.H. 'A synopsis of the history of dermatology'. *Ulster Medical Journal,* 1944; 13: 109–22.

McClure, H.I. 'The church and medicine'. *Ulster Medical Journal,* 1954; 23: 89–101.

McCoy, G.F., Orr, J.F. and Templeton, J. 'External fixation in contemporary fracture management'. *Ulster Medical Journal,* 1987; 56: 81–9.

McIlrath, E.M. 'An image for tomorrow'. *Ulster Medical Journal,* 1993; 62: 79–86.

MacLaughlin, F.A. 'The patient and his doctor'. *Ulster Medical Journal,* 1948; 17: 127–39.

McMechan, E.W. 'A tribute to our surgical pioneers'. *Ulster Medical Journal,* 1955; 24: 81–91.

Marshall, R. 'Royal Victoria Hospital, Belfast'. *Ulster Medical Journal,* 1936; 5: 14–24.

'The open window'. *Ulster Medical Journal,* 1948, 17: 188–99.

Millar, J.H. 'The medical library'. *Ulster Medical Journal,* 1976; 45: 47–55.

Mitchell, A.B. 'Sir William Whitla'. *Ulster Medical Journal,* 1934; 3: 84–6.

Montgomery, D.A.D. 'Royal Victoria Hospital research fellowships'. *Ulster Medical Journal,* 1973; 42: 28–44.

Montgomery, F.P. 'Some aspects of medicine and literature'. *Ulster Medical Journal,* 1938; 7: 18–34.

Morrison, E. 'Crude craftsmen'. *Ulster Medical Journal,* 1970; 39: 30–42.

Murney, M. 'Statistical report of the injuries sustained during the riots in Belfast from 8th to 22nd August 1864'. Reprinted in R.S. Allison, *The Seeds of Time.* Belfast, 1972.

Nelson, M.G. 'Science and the progress of medicine'. *Ulster Medical Journal,* 1961; 30: 73–85.

'Thomas Houston and the founding of clinical pathology at the Royal Victoria Hospital, Belfast'. *Ulster Medical Journal,* 1994; 63: 223–34.

Osterberg, P. 'The lure and lore of surgery'. *Ulster Medical Journal,* 1990; 59: 11–16.

Pantridge, J.F. and Wilson, C. 'A history of prehospital coronary care'. *Ulster Medical Journal,* 1996; 65: 68–73.

Pinkerton, J.H.M. 'John Creery Ferguson, 1807–1865, physician and fetologist'. *Ulster Medical Journal,* 1981; 50: 10–20.

Porter, D.C. 'The new photography'. *Ulster Medical Journal,* 1962; 31: 117–27.

Purce, G.R.B. 'Some aspects, historical and otherwise, of surgery of the thorax'. *Ulster Medical Journal,* 1947; 16: 87–101.

Roberts, S.D. 'Membership by examination'. *Ulster Medical Journal,* 1995; 64: 72–84.

Rodgers, H.W. 'Whither medicine'. *Ulster Medical Journal,* 1960; 29: 102–16.

Shanks, R.G. 'The legacies of Sir William Whitla'. *Ulster Medical Journal,* 1994; 63: 52–75.

Shepherd, W.H.T. 'Hospital relationships'. *Ulster Medical Journal,* 1967; 36: 13–22.

Simms, S. 'The founder of the Belfast Medical School'. *Ulster Medical Journal,*

1932; 1: 34–8.

Smiley, T.B. 'Medical students and their education'. *Ulster Medical Journal,* 1975; 44: 28–38.

Smiley, T.B. and Cheeseman, E.A. 'Cancer of the lung in Northern Ireland'. *Ulster Medical Journal,* 1956; 25: 62–74.

Smyth, J.A. 'Biochemistry'. *Ulster Medical Journal,* 1935; 4: 39–61.

Smyth, J.C. 'The poor relation'. *Ulster Medical Journal,* 1959; 28: 85–100.

Stevenson, H.M. 'Patients – a virtue?' *Ulster Medical Journal,* 1983; 52: 19–30.

Stewart, R. 'A memoir of the late Samuel Smith Thomson'. *Ulster Medical Journal,* 1963; 32: 3–9.

Stoy, P.J. 'A history of the Queen's University of Belfast Dental School'. *Ulster Medical Journal,* 1951; 20: 118–30.

'Early dentistry in Belfast'. *British Dental Journal,* 1966, 120: 253–8 and 297–300.

Strain, R.W.M. 'University Square – a sentimental retrospect'. *Ulster Medical Journal,* 1969; 38: 1–33.

'The foundations of Belfast medicine'. *Ulster Medical Journal,* 1971; 40: 17–42.

Turkington, S.I. 'Students of medicine'. *Ulster Medical Journal,* 1937; 6: 1–19.

'The historical development of the resident pupil system'. *Ulster Medical Journal,* 1938; 7: 241–50.

Weaver, J.A. 'A hospital for all seasons'. *Ulster Medical Journal,* 1984; 53: 18–32.

'John Henry Biggart, 1905–1979 – a portrait in respect and affection'. *Ulster Medical Journal,* 1985; 54: 1–19.

Wheeler, J.R. 'A synopsis of the history of ophthalmology'. *Ulster Medical Journal,* 1945; 14: 73–84.

Wilson, R.I. 'Sticks and stones'. *Ulster Medical Journal,* 1977; 46: 14–21.

Wilson, W. 'Old ethics: new dilemmas'. *Ulster Medical Journal,* 1982; 51: 23–34.

Withers, R.J.W. 'Rest and exercise'. *Ulster Medical Journal,* 1958; 27: 117–29.

Woodside, C.J.A. 'Andrew Fullerton'. *Ulster Medical Journal,* 1934; 3: 147–8.

'Possible worlds'. *Ulster Medical Journal,* 1943; 12: 81–8.

INDEX

NOTE: page numbers in italics refer to illustrations.

A Block, *143*, *148*, 148–9, 246
Abercorn Restaurant, *178*, 221–2, 226–7
Abernethy, Dr C., 166
Abram, Dr William P., 166, 273
Accident and Emergency Department, *146*, 217, 219–20, *220*, *221*; *see also* Casualty Department
Acheson, Kathleen, 238, *238*
Adair, Mr Ian V., 184, 185, 270, 281
Adams, Mr C. Philip, 202–3, 204
Adams, Mr David A., 191, 274
Adgey, Professor A.A. Jennifer, 157, 267
Agnew, William, 287
Aisbitt, Miss, 285
Aitken, Mr Henry, 189, 256
Albert Foundry, 97
Albert Victor, Prince, 82
Alexandra, Queen, 74, 82
Alldritt, Professor W.A.S., 203, 205
Allen, Dr Grace E., 267
Allen, Professor Ingrid V., 168, *187*, *242*, 264, 284
Allison, Dr Richard S., 101, *102*, 139, 203, 214, 255, 281
 career, 102
 neurology, 160, 191
 retirement, 161
 Seeds of Time, 51
Allworthy, Dr Samuel, 103
almoners, 227–9
ambulances, 11
Amelioration Society, 20
Anacreontic Society, 7
anaesthesia, 34–7, 206–9
 surgery prior to use of, 14–16
 20th c., 123–6
Anaesthesia, Theatre and Intensive Care Directorate, 217
anaesthetists, 123–5, 199–200, 209–14
Anderson, Dr Alfred, 77
Anderson, Dr Olive Margery, 124
Anderson, Dr William, 146
Anderson, Reverend William, 287
Andrew, W.B.S., 122
Andrews, Professor Thomas, 19, *19*, 21, 251
Anglesey, Marquess of, 7
Angus, Deaconess Mary, 226, 243
antibiotics, 117, 150–1
antisepsis, 38–9
apothecaries, 5, 7–8, 11, 46, 231–2
Apothecaries' Hall, Dublin, 40, 231
Arbuthnot, Reverend James, *225*, 226
Archer, Professor Desmond B., 188, 267
Ardill, Mr B. Leslie, 141, 285
Ards Hospital, 170, 184, 186
Arnold, Irene, 222
Arrott, Surgeon, 10
asepsis, 39–40, 107
Ashley, Lord, 286
Asiatic cholera, 11
Association of Anaesthetists of Great Britain and Ireland, 199
Association of Hospital Almoners, 227
Association of Surgeons of Great Britain and Ireland, 180

Atkinson, Professor A. Brew, 159, 272
Atkinson, Dr Susan, 206, 213, 278
Austen Boyd Outpatient Building, 142, *143*, *143*, 144, *146*, 177
 construction, *146*, 147–8
 occupational therapy, 237
 physiotherapy, 235–6

B Block, 148, 246
bacteriology, 170–1
Baerem, Arne, *236*
Bailey, Mr Ian C., 193, 268
Baird, Mr Robert H., 262
Balmer, Pam, *236*
Bamford, Dr Kathleen B., 170, 277
Bamford, Margaret, 230
Banbridge, Dromore and South Armagh Group, 153, 213
Barbour, Anthea, *236*
Barbour, John, 14
Barbour, Rt Hon Sir J. Milne, 83, 146, 286
Barcroft, Dr John, 268
Barnett, John, 286
Barr, Mr Reginald J., 185, 278
Barrett, Miss Heather M., 141, 175, *242*, 285
Barron, Dr David W., 212, 263
Barron, Mr James, 253
Barros D'Sa, Mr Aires, 182, *183*, 270
Bartley, Dr Eileen O., 130, 131, 170, 261
Bateman, Dr S., *101*
Beare, Dr John M., 151, 155, 258, 281, 284
Beath, Dr R. Maitland., 127, 128, 254, 281, 283
Beck, Dr Neill, *101*
Beeches, The, Hampton Park, 175
Belfast, map of (1822), 7
Belfast Academical Institution, *1*, 6–7, 16–17, *17*, 18; *see also* Royal Belfast Academical Institution
 Medical School, 20–1
Belfast Castle, 80
Belfast Charitable Institute, 52
Belfast Charitable Society, 2, 4, 54, 55
Belfast City Hospital, 12, 119; *see also* Union Fever Hospital
 anaesthesia, 212
 Belfast and its Infirmary, 190
 child psychiatry, 241
 dermatology, 104, 155
 neurology, 161
 oral surgery, 204
 pathology, 131, 167
 physiotherapy, 235
 radiology, 127, 164
 speech therapy, 239
 surgery, 182, 183
Belfast Clinical and Pathological Society, 41
Belfast Co-operative Society, 83–4
Belfast Corporation, 51, 68, 239
Belfast Dispensary and Fever Hospital, 3–4, *9*, 53, 55
 becomes General Hospital, 12–13
 Dispensary Districts, 10–11
 fever epidemics, 8–10, 11–14
 finances of, 8–9
 medical staff, 4–7, 16–20
 nursing, 22–4
 students, 20–1

surgery, 14–16
Belfast Fever Hospital, *1*, 3
Belfast Fixator, 184, *184*
Belfast General Hospital, 3, *12*, 12–13, 24–6, *25*, 75, 77
 building programme, 51–3
 dispensary, 232
 finances
  donors, 27–9, 79–82
  expenditure, 31
  sources of finance, 27–31
 General Committee, 29–30
 medical practice, 32–40, 53–8
 medical staff, 26
 medical students, 44–6
 students, 40
Belfast Health Journal, 51
Belfast Hospital for Sick Children, 190
 dentistry, 206
 diabetes, 240
 speech clinic, 239, 240
Belfast Hospitals Management Committee (BHMC), 138, 139, 140, 239
Belfast Literary Society, 17
Belfast Lunatic Asylum, 7, 18, *68*
Belfast Lying-In Hospital, 47, 53–5
Belfast Maternity Hospital, 55
Belfast Medical Society, 6, 7, 17, 24, 41, 47
Belfast Medical Students' Association, 51
Belfast Monica Project for Heart Disease, 241
Belfast Natural History Society, 17
Belfast News-Letter, 13, 61, 225
Belfast Ophthalmic Hospital, 56
Belfast People's Magazine, 20
Belfast Philharmonic Society, 7
Belfast Public Health Laboratories, 130
Belfast Reading Society, 5
Belfast Royal Hospital, 3, *27*, *34*, 44, *52*, 56, 75, 77, 118
 becomes RVH, 70–1
 charter, 52–3, *53*
 finances
  donors, 80
  sources of income, 86
 and Maternity Hospital, 55
 need for expansion, 65–7
 rebuilding, 67–70
Belfast Working Classes' Association, 19–20
Bell, Dr Aubrey L., 275
Bell, Sir Charles, 49
Bell, Elizabeth, 46
Bell, J., 167
Bell, Dr Kathleen E., 163, 276
Bell, Louis, 168
Bell, Margaret, 46
Bell, Mr Millar, 206, 212
Bell, Dr Patrick M., 155, 275, 281
Bell, Dr Sheila M., 212, 262
Bell, William, 286
Benn, Mr Edward, 59, 147
Benn EENT Hospital, 56, 120, 121, 146, 147, 188, 189, 190
Benn Hospital for Diseases of the Skin, 47, 103, 114, 144
Bennett, Cecil, 168
Bennington, Professor Ian C., 203, 205
Benson, Mr J.K.H., 203
Benson, Sister, 177

295

Benton, Dr Frank, 166
Bereen, Dr James F., 151, 209, 222, 257, 281, 283
Bereen, Janet, 222
Beringer, Dr Timothy R.O., 155, 274
Berrington, Henry, 286
Best, Jennifer, 236
Betty, Miss Florence, *176*, 177
Beveridge, Lord, 138
Bharucha, Dr Chitra, 167
Bharucha, Dr Hoshang, 167, 268
Bicentenary Committee, 245
Biggart, Dr John D., 167, 266
Biggart, Professor Sir John H., 119, *130*, 130–1, 167, 170, 171, 255, 283
Biggart House, 147
Bill, Dr K. Moyna, 199, 278
Bingham, Dr Ann, 155, 195, 274
Bingham, Mr John A.W., 151, 195, 213, 258
Bingham, Mr W., 20
Bingham, Dr William, 195, 213, 265
Binnion, Dr Peter F., 265
Birch, C.B., 30
Black, Dr Alan J., 279
Black, Dr Gerald W., 197, 211, 261
Black, Sir James, 151
Black, Mr, 53
Black, Wilfie, 232
Blackmore, Sir Charles, 188
Blackwood, Mr S., 205
Blair, Sister Eleanor, 217
Blair, Mr George A.S., 192, 205
Blair, Mr Paul H.B., *183*, 183, 280
Blaney, Dr Roger, 274
blood transfusion, 117, 129, 194
Blood Transfusion Service, 167
Blount, Lt-Colonel Clavell, 53, 285
Board of Management, 71, 77, 115
  and nursing staff, 61
  rebuilding, 89, 93
  replaced (1949), 138
  women students, 46
  and Working Men's Committee, 85–6
Boden, Reverend Derek J., 227
Boer War, 191
Bond, Dr Egerton B., 272
Bonugli, Dr Frederick S., 104, 159, 256
Bostock, Miss Mary F., 78, *132*, 133, 135, 172, 285
Bostock House, *92*, 142–4, *143*, 147, 175, 226
Bottomley, H.H., 287
Bottomley, William, 286
Boyd, Mr Austen, 138, 147
Boyd, Dr Douglas P.B., 262
Boyd, Mr Gavin, 185–6, 256
Boyd, Dr John, 125, 126, 209, 256
Boyd, René, 229
Boyle, Dr David D., 187, 272
Boyle, Dr Dennis M., 157, *187*, 263
Braidwood, Mr Walter S., 151, 184, 258
Brennen, Mr Michael D., 201–2, 271
Bridges, Professor John M., *154*, 169–70, *245*, 263, 281
Bristow, Reverend William, 4
British Association of Plastic Surgeons, 201
British Dental Association, 203
British Legion, 124
British Medical Association, 59, 116, 117, 119
British Medical Journal, 131
British Pharmaceutical Codex, 150

British Society for Surgery of the Hand, 201
Broadway Housing Association, 147
Broadway Presbyterian Church, 225
Broadway Tower, 147, *147*, 176, 235, 236
Brooker, Mr David S., 278
Brown, Mrs Crawford, 237
Brown, Mr John G., 278
Brown, Dr Robert B., 261
Brown, Dr Wilfred Maurice, 196, 197, 206, 209, *209*, 210, 256, 281, 283
Brown, Mr William A.B., 204
Browne, Dr Eileen S., 268
Browne, Dr Francis R.B., 267
Browne, Sir John Walton, 45, *45*, 50, 79, 105, 147, 249, 252, 281, 282
  career, 56
  knighted, 87
  retirement, 107
  royal visit, 74
Browne, Dr Samuel, 55–6, *56*, 147, 252
Browne, Dr Sylvia, 206, 211
Bryars, Mr John H., 188, 270
Bryson, Surgeon-Major Allen, 28
Bryson, Dr Joseph W., 251
Buchanan, Professor Keith D., 154, 266
Buchanan, Mr Trevor A.S., 188, 272
Bull, Professor Graham M., 150, 153, *153*, 154, 258
Burden, Mr Donald, 204
Burden, Dr Henry, 54, 58, 282
Burgess, Enid, *183*
Burnett, Mr C.A., 205
burns treatment, 200–2
Burrows, Dr Brian D., 166, 273
Burrows, Dr David Desmond, 155, *181*, *187*, 261, 281, 284
Byers, F.M.R., 138
Byers, Sir John W., 45, 54, 79, 253, 281, 282
  career, 55
  construction committee, 69, 70
  retirement, 117
Byers, Margaret, 54
Byrne, Mr John E.T., 269
Byrne, Father Paul, 227
Byrnes, Mr Dermot P., 193, 271

Cairns, Sir Hugh, 115, 191
Calderwood, Mr James W., 274
Callaghan, Sydney, 227
Callender, Dr Michael E., 155, 206, 272
Calvert, Mr Cecil A., 111, 112, 115, *115*, 139–40, 191, 255, 283
Calvert Room, 115
Calwell, Mrs Heather, *242*, 243
Calwell, Dr William, 59, 79, 97, 253, 281, 282, 283
  career, 48
  dermatology, 58, 103
  retirement, 99, 103
Campalani, Mr Gianfranco, 198, 278
Campbell, Agnes, 173
Campbell, Dr Charles F., 152, 258
Campbell, Mr George, 57
Campbell, Dr Margaret, 174
Campbell, Mrs, *242*
Campbell, Dr Norman P.S., *154*, 157, 271, 281
Campbell, Mr Robert, 105–6, 107, 253, 282
Campbell, Dr S.B. Boyd, *100*, 100–1, 254, 283
  retirement, 156

Campbell, Dr Wilfred, 100–1
Canavan, Miss Yvonne M., 188, 272
cancer, 110–11, 162–5, 166
  cytology, 168
  lung cancer, 194
Carabine, Dr Una A., 213, 278
cardiac surgery, 196–200
  open-heart surgery, 196–200
Cardiac Surgical Intensive Care Ward, 199
cardiology, 96–7, 156–8
Carr, Professor Katherine, 167
Carrickmannon Appeal, 163
Carson, Dr Derek J.L., 160, 265
Carson, Dr Ian W., 199, 269
Carson, J.C., 126
Carson, Mrs, *242*
Carville, W.J., 177
case records, 90
Casson, Sir Hugh, 145
Casualty Department, 219–20; *see also* Accident and Emergency Department
Cathcart, Dr J., *98*
Catherine Dynes Unit, 149, 237
Caughley, Dr Linda M., 168, *187*, 275
Caves, Helen, 224
'caves, the', 143
Central Registry, 142, 229
Central Sterile Supplies Department, 179
chapel, 227, *227*
chaplains, 225–7
Chapman, Alexander, 232
Chartered Society of Physiotherapists, 235
Charters, John, 49, 50, 52, 59, 81
Charters, Katherine Maria, 50
Charters family, 28
Charters Wing, 52, *52*
child abuse, 37
Child Guidance Service, 241
Children's Hospital, 103
chiropody, 240–1
chloroform, 35–7, 125
cholera, 11–12, 18
Christian Medical Fellowship, 116
Christie, Molly, 239, 240
Church of Ireland, 185
Cinnamond, Professor Michael J., 190, 269
City Business Club, 246
Claremont Street Hospital, 102, 138, 160
  neurology, 161
  occupational therapy, 237
  physiotherapy, 235
  speech therapy, 239
Clarendon, Victor F., 138, 242, 286
Clark, Sir George, 93, 144
Clark, Captain H.D., 144
Clarke, Dr Brice R., 152, 257
Clarke, Dr James C., 211, 260
Clarke, John (1785), 3
Clarke, John (1829), 286
Clarke, John, Ltd, 126
Clarke, Mr John A., 205
Clarke, Mr John Clough, 57
Clarke, Professor Richard S.J., *187*, 197, 210–11, 214, *215*, 263, 284
Clarke, Mr Stewart D., 182, 263
Clarke, William, 286
Clarkson, Professor Leslie, 87
Cleland, Mr John, 198, *198*, 267
Clifford, Mr Thomas, 205
Clifton House, *1*
clinical biochemistry, 132, 171–2

clinical psychology, 241–2
Clothing Society, 9
Coates, Dr Foster, 99–100, 254, 281
Coates, Dr Stanley, 99
Coffey, Professor Robert, 15, 16, 21, 251
Cohen, Ronald, 18
Cole, James 'Matt', *34*, 232
Cole, Dr James O.Y., 163–4, 206, 261
Coleman, John, 286
College Hospital, 13, 21, 22
College of Technology, 167
Collins, Dr Brendan J., 155, 275
Collins, Dr John S.A., 155, 277
Colville, Mr John, 201, 265
Comerton, John, *246*
Committee of Management, 20, 24, 26, 31, 225, 227
Community Management Unit, 141
Compton, Peter, *245*
Computed Tomography (CT) scanning, 162
Connell, Dr Alastair McCrae, 262
Connolly, Professor John H., 170, 265
Connolly, Mr Rainier C., 192, 258
Conor, William, 108
Consumptive Hospital, 135
Cooke, Mr Richard Stephen, 193, 280
Cooper, Thomas, 70
Coppel, Dr Dennis L., 213, 215, *215*, 266, 281
Corbett, Dr J. Roger, 155, *187*, 270
Corkey, Mr Joseph A., 121, 188, 256, 281, 283
Coronation Extension Fund, 93
Corran, Ann, 3
Cotton, G. Lennox, 146
Coulter, Mr John, 172
Coulter, Dr John G., 46
Cowan, Mr Eric C., 188, 261
Cowan, Mr G.C., 204
Cox, Commander F., 53, 285
Coyle, Dr Peter V., 276
Coyle, Dr Seamus, 206
Craig, Dr B.G., 275
Craig, Dr David, *248*
Craig, Mr David H., 189, 190, 262
Craig, Dr Henry J.L., 213, 272
Craig, Mr James A., 120, 187, 254, 281, 282
Craigavon Area Hospital, 174, 199
Crane, Professor Jack, 160, 206, 274
Crawford, Dr David B., 267
Crawford, Elizabeth, 3
Crawford, Dr Michael, *248*
Crawford, Sir William, 69, 77, 89
Creaney, Aileen, *236*
Crimean War, 39
Cripples' Institute, 181
Crockard, Mr Alan, 183, 192, 193, 268
Croker, Dr Walter B., 77
Crone, Dr Malcolm P., 277
Crone, Dr Richard S., 164, 260
Crothers, Dr J. Graham, 165, 275
Crozier, Dr T. Howard, 102–3, 174, 256, 283
Crymble, Professor P.T., 111, 116, 124, 254, 281, 283
Cullen, Dr William, 5
Cuming, Professor James, 33, 41–2, *42*, 69, 70, 81, 252, 281, 282
Cummings, Barbara, *236*
Cunningham, Dr Anne-Marie, *248*
Cunningham, James, 69
Cunningham, Reverend Robert, 226

Curry, Mr Rodney, 206
cytology, 168

D'Abreu, Professor Alphonsus, 197
Dalzell, Dr Gavin W.N., 278
Dane, Dr David M.S., 170, 259
D'Arcy, Mr Francis G., 190–1, *271*
Darragh, Dr Paul M., 272
Data Protection Act, 243
Davidson, James, 286
Davidson, Brigadier Thomas W., 78, 140, *140*, 225, 285, 287
Davis, George, 243
Davison, Dr S., *98*
Deane, Colonel Andrew, 53, 77–8, 285
Dean's Birthday Party, 131
Dearden, Dr Christine H., 220, 275
Dempsey, Dr Stanley I., 272
Dental Hospital, 147, *147*, 245
dentistry, 57, 89, 145, 202–6
 dental pathology, 168–9
 dental surgery, 121–3
Department of Conservative Dentistry, 205
Department of Genito-Urinary Medicine, 241
Department of Health Care for the Elderly, 240
Department of Neurology, 102, 128, 160–1
Department of Neurosurgery, 128, 160
Department of Physical Medicine, 237
Department of Vaccine Therapy and Haematology, 89
Department of Venereology, 159–60
dermatology, 58, 103–4, 155–6
Devlin, Richard, 231
Dick, Professor George W.A., 170, 259
Dickens, Charles, 23
Dickey, E. O'Rorke, 287
Dickie, Mr William R., 201, 260
Dickson, Belle, 165, *165*
Dickson, Ruth, 113
dietetics, 238
Dill, Professor Robert F., 54, *54*, 252
Dimmer, Mrs Anne, 205
Dinsmore, Dr Wilbert W., 160, 276
Dispensary Districts, 10–11, 19, 26
District Lunatic Asylum, *5*
Dixon, Sir Daniel, 69
Dobbin, Mrs, 22
Dr Steevens' Hospital, Dublin, 2
Dodds, Sister Hadessa, 176
Doherty, Rae, *149*
Doll, Richard, 194
Dolly's Brae, 38
Domestic Mission to the Poor of Belfast, 20
Donaldson, Peggy, 22n, 113–14, 172, 174
Donegall, 1st Marquess of, 286
Donegall, 2nd Marquess of, 9, 286
Donegall, 3rd Marquess of, 24, 80, 286
Donegall, 5th Earl of, 2
Donnelly, Dr Brian, *248*
Donnelly, Patricia, 241
Dorman, Dr John K.A., 212, 262
Dornan, Dr James C., 187, 275
Douglas, Dr James F., 269
Dowling, Beatrice, 113
Drennan, Professor Alexander M., 130, 255
Drennan, Dr John S., 47, 252, 282
Drennan, Dr William C., 5, 47
Drew, Thomas, 38
Drew Memorial Church of Ireland, 225
Drummond, James, 7

Drummond, Professor James Lawson, 7, *16*, 16–17, 20, 21, 250
Drummond, Pat, *236*
Drummond, William, 16
Dufferin and Ava, Marquess of, 80
Duffin, Miss Elizabeth, 141, 175, *187*, 285
Duffin, Emma, 114
Dugdale Report, 158
Dunbar, Dr James M., 170, 262
Duncan, Dr William, 251
Dundee, Professor John W., 124, 150, *187*, *210*, 214, *215*, 260, 284
 career, 210
 retirement, 215
Dunleath, Lady, *242*, 243
Dunlop, Mrs Gwenda, 237
Dunn, Sister Lorna, 177
Dunville, Robert, 65
Dunville, William, 59
Dunville Park, *65*
Dusoir, Hazel, 241
Dynes, Sister Catherine, 133–4, *134*, 149, 173

ear, nose and throat, 189–91
Earls, Miss Nora, 172, *225*
East Wing, *65*, 72–3, 77, 230
Eastern Health and Social Services Board, 140–1, 241, 245
Eastern Special Care, 239
Eccles, Mr John D., 205
Edelstyn, Dr George J.A., 166, 263
Edward VII, King, 74, 82, 89, 124
Electrical Department, 89, 234
electrocardiograph, 96–7, *100*
Elkin, Sister Edna, *176*
Elliott, David, 232
Elliott, Miss Florence E., 149, 172, *172*, 175, 229, 285
 career, 133, 173, 174
 retirement, 140
Elliott, Dr James, 199, 206, 209–10, 259, 281, 284
Elliott, Dr Peter, 199, 275
Elliott, Mr Robert H., 206
Elmes, Professor Peter C., 214, 260
Elwood, Mr Herbert, 122, 203
Elwood, Professor John H., 268
Emmerson, Professor A. Michael, 170, *187*, 201, 284
Enniskillen bombing, 176
entertainments, 86
Esmonde, Dr Thomas F.G., 280
Evans, Professor Alun E., 271
Ewing, Fidelis, *245*
Ex-Patients' Guild, 200, 243
Eye, Ear, Nose and Throat Hospital, *146*, 146–7, 188
eye, ear, nose and throat surgery, 120–1

Faculty of Medicine, QUB, 154, 211
 chairs, 90, 111, 168, 185, 188, 190
 clinical psychology, 241
 Dental School, 123, 202–5
 first DPH, 100
 honorary degrees, 173, 182
 Institute of Pathology, 90, 92, 130
 neurology, 160
 part-time professors, 99
Fagan, Sir John, 50, 252, 281, 282
Fannin, Mr Thomas F., 193, 271
Farling, Dr Peter A., 213, 278

Farnan, Dr Turlough, *248*
Farrar, Thomas, 21
Farries, Lindsay, 237
Fay, Dr Anne C.M., 275
Fearon, Dr Paul, *248*
Fee, Professor J.P. Howard, *187*, 211, 215, 273
Fenton, Sister Margaret, 217
Ferguson, J.A., 177
Ferguson, Professor John C., 41, *41*, 252, 282
Ferguson McIlveen, 246
fever epidemics, 32
Field, Colonel Thomas E., 140, 263, 285
Fielden, Dr Victor G.L., 123–4, *124*, 125, 253, 282
Finance and General Purposes Committee, 138
Finch, Dr Michael B., 277
Finlay, Mr Ian A., 203
First Presbyterian Congregation, 7
Flanagan, Dr Nuala, *248*
Flannery, Dr Thomas, *248*
Florence Elliott House, 149, 173, 237
Fogarty, Dr Declan J., 214, 279
Forcade, Dr Henry, 10, 17, 251
Ford, Father Peter, 226
forensic pathology, 160
Forrest, Colonel John V., 78, 285
Forrest, Sir Patrick, 163
Forster Green Hospital, 100, 127, 235, 241
   anaesthesia, 210, 211
   enlarged, 136
   established, 59
   TB, 194
Foster, Dr Peter A.H.M., 265
Foster, Vere, 66–7
Fox, Rita, 236
Franco-Prussian War, 38, 50
Fraser, Sir Ian, 50, 84, 112, *116*, 172, 256, 281, 283
   Campbell Oration, 106, 108–9
   career, 115–16
Fraser, Professor Kenneth B., 170, 263
Frazer, Mr David G., 188, 278
Freeburn, Dr Allison, *248*
Freeman, Dr Ruth, 206
Friendly Societies, 229
Friers, Rowel, 212
Froggatt, Sir Peter, 264
Fuller, Mr Bartholomew, 6
Fullerton, Professor Andrew, 106, *108*, 127, 133, 179, 254, 281, 282, 283
   career, 108
   neurosurgery, 191
   retirement, 111
Fulton, Dr Thomas T., 153, *242*, 259, 281, 284

Galbraith, Kate, 177
Galbraith, Sister Mary, 177
Gallagher, Reverend Eric, *225*, 226
Gallaher, Ruby, 83
Gallaher, Thomas, 83
Gardiner, Mr Keith R., 183, 280
Gardner, Professor Dugald L., 167, 267
Garibaldi, Giuseppe, 57
Gaston, Dr Joseph H., 213, 277
Gaw, Hazel, 173, 176
Geddes, Dr John S., 125, 157, 267
Geddes, Dr Stafford, 125, 157, 257
Geddis, Dr S., *98*

General Committee, 24, 71
General Dental Council, 203
General Medical Council, 131
genito-urinary medicine, 159–60
George, Barbara, *183*
George VI, King, 93
Geriatric Medical Unit, 143, 149
Gibbons, Mr John R.P., *187*, 195, 270
Gibson, Colin, 92
Gibson, Dr Fiona M., 199, 276
Gibson, Dr George L., 170, 261, 281
Gibson, Dr James B., 261
Gibson, Professor John G., 166, 259
Gibson, Dr John M., 161, 276
Gibson, Sister Noelle, 176, 216, 217, *217*
Gibson, Mr Robert, 190, 268, 281
Gibson, Dr T.J., *85*
Gihon, Mrs, 22, 285
Giles, Dr Clare, *248*
Gillespie, Reverend Wilbur, 226
Gillies, Professor Robert R., 170, 269
Gilmore, Dr David H., 273
Gilmore, Dr Robert W., 211, 259
Ginty, John, 85
Girdwood, James, 30, *30*, 53, 77, 286
Gladstone, Mr Dennis J., 198, 276
Glancy, Colonel John, 53, 285
Gleadhill, Mr Colin A., 192, 260
Gleadhill, Dr Valerie, 192
Glover, Dr Walter E., 265
Good Samaritan window, 44, 75–6, *76*, 142
Goodman, Petre, *236*
Goodsir, Professor, 49
Goodwin Report, 158
Gordon, Professor Alexander, *42*, 42–3, 251, 282
Gordon, Mr Derek S., *187*, 192–3, *193*, 261, 284
Gordon, Lt-Colonel V.D., 287
Gore-Grimes, Celia, 237
Gorman, Dr Brian, 276
Gorman, Mr John, 204
Gough, Dr A. Denis, 165, 206, 264
Gough, Elinor, 227–8, 229, 230
Government Rehabilitation Scheme, 151
Graham, Dr David T., 274
Graham, Dr Hugh, *101*
Graham, Mary, 245
Graham, Dr Norman C., 129–30, 166, 170, 257
Grant, Albert, 138
Grant, Katherine, *164*
Gray, Dr John, *248*
Gray, Mr John, 193
Gray, Dr Robert C., *187*, 211, *212*, 213–15, 215, 261
Gray, Sara, 199
Gray, Mr William J., 277
Graymount Hospital, 112
Great Famine, 13–14, 31, 32
Grebbell, Dr Frederick S., 163, 260, 284
Green, Forster, 59
Greener, Hannah, 35
Greenfield, Professor A. David M., 260
Greenisland Hospital, 112, 235
Greer, Mr H.L. Hardy, 118–19, 255, 281, 283
Gregg, Dr George, 151, 152, 235, 237, 257, 283
Grieve, Dr Philip, *248*
Grosvenor Hall Methodist Mission, 225–6
Grosvenor Tower, 147

Group Medical Advisory Committee (GMAC), 139
Group Medical Staff Committee, 139
Gunn, Sir James, 118
Gurd, Mr Alan R., 185, 269
gynaecology *see* obstetrics and gynaecology

Hadden, Professor David R., 159, 265, 281, 284
Hadden, Dr Diana, 159
haematology, 160
Haire, Dr Margaret, 128, 170–1, 268
Hall, Betty, *228*, 229, 230
Hall, Dr H.P., *98*
Hall, Dr Hugh (Hugo) E., 104, 159, 257
Hall, Noel, 233
Hall, Dr Reginald, 103–4, 256, 283
Hall, Dr Robert, 104
Hall, Surgeon Commander Robin, 104
Haller, Alice, 241
Halliday, Dr Alexander Henry, 5
Halliday, Professor Henry L., 279
Hamilton, Dr George, 125, 257
Hamilton, Dr Peggy, 209–10
Hamilton, Dr Trevor, 125
Hanna, Mr Henry, 120, 121, 254, 281, 282
Harden, Marianne, *62*
Harland, Sir Edward James, 84
Harland and Wolff, 47, 67, 71, 82, 84, 98
Harley, Professor J.M. Graham, 186, *187*, 261, 281, 284
Harper, Hazel, 199
Harper, Dr Kenneth W., 213, 276
Harrison, Professor Thomas J., 264
Haslett, Samuel C., 141, 287
Hawkins, Dr Stanley A., 161, *187*, 272
Hawthorne, Dr, 251
Haypark Hospital, 138, 229, 237
Health, Department of, 174, 176–7
Health and Social Services, Department of, 245, 246
Health Service Act (NI) (1948), 138
Hearts of Steel, 5
Heney, Dr James W., 125, 126
Henman, William, 69–70, 73, 248
Henneman, Dr Jack, 269
Henry, Doreen, *236*
Hepper, Professor Peter, 241
Herald, Thomas Gordon, 84
Heron, Francis A., 149, 287
Heron Clinic, 149, 158
Heylings, John, 235, 236
Heyn, Gustavus, 24, 30, 286
Heyn, James A.M., 287
High Dependency Unit, 199
Hill, Dr Claire M., 167, 272
Hilson, Miss, 135
Historic Monuments, 248
Holmes, Jennifer, 238
Home, Maria Glenny, 20
Home for the Blind, 188
Hood, Mr John M., 182, *183*, 273
Hooke, Richard, 20, 54
Horner, Dr Thomas, 159, 268
Hospital for Diseases of the Nervous System, Paralysis and Epilepsy *see* Claremont Street Hospital
Hounsfield, G.W., 162
House of Industry, 9
Houston, Dr James K., 265
Houston, Dr John, 211

Houston, Sir Thomas, 89, 96, 97, 104, *129*, 253, 282
  career, 129
  retirement, 130
  verse, 218
Hoy, Elizabeth, 241
Hughes, Mr Norman C., 151, 200, 201, 204, 258, 284
Hull, Mr, 231
Humphries, Dr William, *248*
Hunter, Dr J. Craig, 165, 251, 267, 283
Hunter, Jane, 3
Hunter, Mr Kennedy, 121, 189, 256
Hunter, Mr W. Muirhead, 122, 203
Hurwitz, Dr Lewis J., 160–1, 261
Hussey, Mr David, 205
Hutchison, Dr Roslyn J., 163, 272

Ibsen, Dr, 214
Imrie, William, 82
industrial accidents, 14–15, 37, 120
Infectious Disease Acts, 39
influenza, 11, 32
Institute of Clinical Science, 116, 145, 210
Institute of Medical Laboratory Sciences, 167
Institute of Pathology, 90, *91*, 92, 129, 143, 171
insulin, 97
intensive care, 214–17
Irish Preserve and Confectionery Company, 84
Irish Republican Army (IRA), 176
Irvine, Dr Kenneth, 155, 265
Irwin, Dr Christopher, 206
Irwin, Mr J.W. Sinclair, 113, 180, *180*, *181*, 199, 258, 281, 283
  retirement, 182
Irwin, Lesley, 165
Irwin, Lorna, 199
Irwin, Mrs, 285
Irwin, Sir Samuel T., 110, *111*, 124, 152, 180, 254, 281
  career, 111, 112–13
Irwin, Professor William G., 267
Ismay, Thomas Henry, 81–2
isolation block, 70

J.A. Smyth Endocrine Laboratory, 144
Jackson, J.C. Girvan, 141, 287
Jaffe, Otto, 69
Jefferson, Mr Frederick, *98*, 254
Jefferson, Dr Jonathan, 103
Jervis Street Hospital, Dublin, 2
Johnson, Dr William, 251
Johnston, Professor G. Dennis, 270
Johnston, Professor George W., 182, *187*, 264, 281, 284
Johnston, Dr Hilary M.L., 202, 213, 271
Johnston, Dr Julian R., 213, 215, *245*, 273, 281
Johnston, Lady, 55, 59
Johnston, Mr Patrick B., 188, 270
Johnston, Mr Samuel R., 274
Johnston, Dr Stephen, *248*
Johnston, Mr Stewart S., 188, 268, 281
Johnston, Sir William, 55
Johnstone, Sir Robert J., 117–18, 123, 254, 281, 282
Johnstone House, 118
Joint Nursing and Midwives' Council, 173
Jones, Dr Francis G.C., 170, 278

Jones, Dr John Harold, 168, 264
Jones, Mark, *183*
Joy, Bruce, 89
Joy, Robert, 2
Junker's inhaler, *36*

Kamerkar, Mr D., *183*
Kay, Bettina, 239, 240
Kehr, Nilham, *236*
Kelly, Dr Barry E., 165, *183*, 280
Kelly, Dr Ian M.G., 165, *183*, 280
Kelvin School, 143, 172
Kendrick, Dr Richard W., *201*, 204, 273
Kennedy, Dr Allan L., 272
Kennedy, Dr John, 205
Kennedy, Mr Joseph A., 182, 264
Kennedy, Mr Terence L., 180–1, *181*, 182, 258, 284
Kernohan, Mr D.C., 206
Kerr, Mr Alan G., 190, 265
Kerr, Dr Arthur, 167, 273
Kerr, Reverend David J., 227
Khan, Dr Mazhar M., 157, 273
Kielty, Dr Samuel, 187
Killowen Hospital, 138
Kinder, Mr Patrick, *181*
King Edward Building, *89*, 120, *122*, 129, 136, 165, 166
  board room, *242*
  construction, 89–90
  dentistry, 89, 121, 123, 145, 147, 202
  Dining Club, 143
  outpatients, 120, 159
  Pathology Department, 132
King's Fund, 230
Kingsley, Charles, 15
Kinirons, Mr Martin, 206
Kirk, Surgeon T. Sinclair, 29, 79, 105, *106*, 135, 253, 281, 282, 283
  career, 106, 109
  retirement, 111
Knatchbull, Lt-Colonel W.M., 287
Knox, Dr Angela, *248*
Koch, Robert, 18, 32
Korean War, 117
Kyle, Dr Anne E., 186

La Mon bombing, 226–7
Laboratory Services, Directorate of, 167
Ladies' Committee, 72, 139, 173, 242–3
Lagan Valley Hospital, Lisburn, 190
Laird, Dr James D., 165, 271
Lamey, Professor Philip J., 204, 279
Lamki, Dr Harith M.N., 187, 268
Lamont, Mr Aeneas, 252
Lamont, Albert, 168
Langan, Dr Sinead, *248*
Langstaff, Colonel James W., 78, 285
Lannigan, Dr Robert, 266
Lanyon, Sir Charles, 12, 13
Larkin, René, *236*
Lassen, Dr, 214
Latimer, Dr G.D., *98*
Lattimore, Sister Elizabeth, 197
Laverty, Patt, 3
Lavery, Dr G. Gavin, *187*, 213, 215, 276
Lavery, Dr Hilary A., 273
Lavery, Mr, 86
Lavery, Mrs, *242*
Leggett, Dr Julian, *248*
Leman, Ralph, 95, 127, *137*, 165

Lemon, Reverend James A., 227
Lemon, Dr M.M. Vida, 211, 257
Lennon, Dr William, 152, 257
Lennoxvale, 144
Leonard, Mr Alan G., *201*, 202, 271
Leukaemia Research Fund, 169
Lewis, Dr Joseph T., 101, 102, 255, 281, 283
Lewis, Dr Michael A., 213, 265
Lewis, Pamela, 243
Linden, Mr G.J., 205–6
Lindsay, Professor James A., 59, 79, 97, 253, 281, 282
  career, 42
  construction committee, 69, 70
  retirement, 99
Linen Hall Library, Belfast, 5, 7
Linen Thread Company, 83
Lissue House, 138, 241
Lister, Joseph, 37, 38, 39
Little, Professor Robert, 251
Litvac, Marianne, 87
Livingston, Mr Reginald H., *180*, 181, 259, 284
Lizars, 126
Loan, Dr Paul B., 280
lock-wards, 15–16
Logan, Dr John S., 100, 151, 152, 258, 284
Logan, Dr T.S., *34*
Logan, Mr William C., 188, 269
Londonderry, 6th Marquess of, 77, 286
Londonderry, 7th Marquess of, 283
Losty, Wendy, 241
Loughridge, Mr James S., 140, 141, 182, 256, 281, 283, 285
  career, 116
Loughridge, Dr W.G. Gordon, 182, 268
Love, Professor Andrew H.G., 154, *181*, 206, 262, 281, 284
Love, Dr S. Harold S., 141, 197, 211–12, 259, 285
Lowry, Professor Brian, 119
Lowry, Professor Charles G., 55, 118, 119, 254, 283
Lowry, Ellen, 113
Lowry, Mr Henry C., 119, 255, 283
Lowry, Mr John H., 185, 264
Lowry, Dr Kenneth G., 213, 276
Lowry, Sister 'Lofty', 172, 177, 216
Lowry, Dr Patrick, *164*
Lowry, Professor William S.B., 269
Lurgan and Portadown Hospital, 174, 213
Lutton, Miss M.V., 90
Lying-In Hospital, 5
Lynch, Alice, *236*
Lynch, Dr Gerard, 166, 262
Lynch, Dr Patrick A., 252
Lynn, S.F., 30
Lyons, Dr Arnold R., 166, *166*, 261
Lyons, Mr James, 203
Lyons, Dr S. Morrell, 197, *198*, 199, 266, 281
Lyons, Mr W.B.T., 77, 286
Lyttle, Dr John A., 161, 266

Macafee, Professor Charles H.G., 118, 119, *119*, 186, 255, 283
McAlister, Sister Elizabeth, 217
McAllister, Mr Alex, *101*
McAllister, Dr Ian, *248*
McAteer, Dr Emer M., 213, 273
McBride, Dr Michael O., 160, 279
McBride, Dr Richard J., 213, 270

McBride, Dr William T., 199–200, 280
McCabe, Dr Thomas, 17, 251
MacCallum, Dr W.A. Gordon, 167, 266
McCance, Dr David R., 159, 279
McCann, Dr John P., 277
McCann, Dr J. Sydney, 104, 159–60, 257
McCarthy, Dr Gerard J., 279
McCaughey, Dr William T.E., 262
McCaw, Dr Ivan H., 103, 155, 255, 283
McCaw, Dr John, 103
McCaw Prize, 155–6
McCleery, Mr James B., 251
McClelland, Mr C. Joseph, 185, *187*, 273
McClelland, Dr Florence M., 212, 257
McClelland, Mr Richard, 6
McClements, Sister Judith, *183*
McCloud, Aileen, *236*
McCluney, Mr Robert, 6, 10, 250
McClure, Mr Harold Ian, 118, 119, 256, 281, 283
McCluskey, Dr David R., 155, 171, 274
McCombe, James, 83–4
McConnell, Mr Robert J., 111, 254, 283
MacCormac, Professor Henry, 18, 50, 251
MacCormac, Sir William, 18, 37, 38, 49–50, *50*, 252, 282
McCormack, Sister Joanna, 217
McCormick, Dr William O., 263
McCoy, Dr Eamon P., 214, 280
McCoy, Mr Gerald F.M., 185, 277
McCrea, Mr Robert S., 189–90, 260
McCreary, Alf, 219
McCrory, Reverend Joseph, 226
McCrory, Róisín, *234*
McCullagh, Dr W.M.H., *98*
McCullough, Sister Doreen, 172, 174, *176*
McCullough, Gwen, 165
McDade, W.J., 232
McDermott, Dr W., *98*
McDevitt, Professor Denis G., 267
McDonald, Dr Graeme H., 167, 277
McDonald, Meryl, *236*
McDonnell, Dr James, 4, 10, 44–5, 248, 250, 282
  Belfast Medical Society, 17
  career, 5–6
  first clinical lecture, 21
McDonnell, John, 21
MacElheran, William F., 30, 31, *31*, 286
McEvoy, Elma, *238*
McEvoy, Dr Joseph, 265
Macewen, Sir William, 39–40
McFarland, Miss Mary A., 141, 175, 176, 285
McFarland, Maureen, *183*
McGarry, Dr Philip J., 167, 278
McGeown, Professor Mary G., 262
McGimpsey, Mr John, 204
McGinnity, Mr Francis G., 188–9, 279
McGovern, Dr John Martin, 165, 279
McGowan, Mairead, 238
MacGowan, Mr Simon W., 198, 280
McGrath, Dr Kevin J., 213, 279
McGuigan, Mr James A., 195, 276
McGurk's Bar, 221
McIlhagger, George, 232, *232*, *233*
McIlrath, Dr Edwin M., *154*, 164, 263, 281, 284
McIlroy, Mr Jim, 197
MacIlwaine, Professor John E., 96–7, 99, 100, 254, 281, 282
McIntyre, James, 287

McKay, Dr Charles, 204
McKeag, Mr H.T.A., 122, 204
McKeagney, Nuala, *246*
McKee, Dr Raymond, *248*
McKee, William, 141, 245, *246*, 287
McKelvey, Frank, 27, 44, 52, 68, 99, 115, 118, 119, 129
McKelvey, Mr Samuel T.D., 183, 269
McKeown, Professor E. Florence, 167, 260
McKeown, Mrs, *242*
McKeown, Dr William, 120
McKibbin, Mr Robert, 251
Mackie, James, 97
Mackie, James, and Sons, 184
McKinley, Dr Andrew, *183*
McKinney, Sir Ian, *225*
McKinney, William, 287
McKinstry, Dr Charles Steven, 163, 276
McKisack, Dr Henry L., *48*, 79, 97, 107, 253, 281, 282, 283
  career, 48
  retirement, 99
MacLaughlin, Mr Francis A., 121, 189, 255, 281, 283
McLaughlin and Harvey, 73, 89, 93
McManus, Mr Kieran G., 195, 279
McMaster, Jacqueline, 241
McMath, Sister Thelma, *100*
McMechan, Mr Eric W., 112, 116, 256, 283
McMechan, Dr John, 251
McMillan, Geraldine, *236*
McMillan, Maureen, 165
McMordie, Beatrice, *236*
McMurray, Dr Terence J., 199, 276
McNally, Alan, *246*
McNeill, Dr Avril, 275
McNeill, J. Cuthbert, 206
McNeill, Dr Thomas A., 170–1, 266
McNern, Jennifer and Rosaleen, 221
McNicholl, Mr Brian P.G., 220, 280
McNulty, Dr John E., 276
McQuitty, Dr Mona, 186
McQuitty, Dr William B., 97, 97–8, 99, 253, 282
McQuitty Scholarship, 98
Macrory, Adam J., 53, 77, 287
McTier, Martha, 5, 54
McTier, Samuel, 5
McWatters, Mr, 129
MacWilliam, Dr E.U., *98*
McWilliams, Paul, 245
Magee, Miss, 135
Magee, Mr Reginald A.E., 141, 186–7, *187*, 264, 285
Mageean, Dr J.F., 205
Magill, Sir Ivan, 207, 209
Magnetic Resonance Imager (MRI), *162*, 163
Maguire, Mr Charles J.F., 188, 265
Mahony, Dr John D.H., 159, 266
Majury, Dr Clive, 206
Malcolm, Dr Andrew G., 6, 11, *20*, 22, 37, 51, 77, 251, 282
  History, 3, 19–20, *20*
Malcolm, Mr Henry Price, 111–12, 255, 281, 283
Malcolm Exhibition, 46
Malcolm Sinclair House, 239
Malone, J., 122
management *see* Board of Management *and* Committee of Management
Manley, Dr H.C., 135

maps
  1822, *xvi*
  1907, *64*
  1923, *88*
  1937, *91*
  1980, *143*
Markwell, Roy, 232, *233*
Marley, Dr John, 204
Marsh, John, 287
Marsh, Joseph C., 287
Marshall, Dr Andrew, 7, *7*, 250
Marshall, Miss Ann, 22, 285
Marshall, Dorothy, 101
Marshall, Professor James D., 21
Marshall, Dr Robert, *98*, 101, *101*, 113, 171, 255, 281, 283
  retirement, 156
Marshall, S., *98*
Marshall, Professor Thomas K., 160, 206, 262
Martin, John, 58–9
Martin, Mr John B., 279
Martin, Mr Norman S., 184, 257
Martin, Dr Peter, *248*
Martin, Mr Victor A.F., 151, 188, 262
Martin Children's Hospital, 135
Massereene Hospital, Antrim, 186
Mateer, Dr William, 251
Mater Infirmorum Hospital, 70, 141, 213, 220, 237, 245
Mattear, Dr John, 5
Maw, Dr Raymond D., 160, 271
Mawhinney, Dr Helen, 269
Mawhinney, Mr H.J. Dennis, 185, 276
Maxwell, Mr Robert J., 183, 276
Mayne, Dr Elizabeth E., 170, 268, 281
Meath Hospital, Dublin, 2
Medical Act (1858), 40
Medical Executive Committee, 141
Medical Executive Council, 213
Medical Institute, 44
Medical Records Department, 90, 147, 234
Medical Research Council, 153
medical staff
  after 1850, 46–51
  committee representation, 149–50
  doctors, 78
    Dispensary and Fever Hospital, 4–7, 16–20
    General Hospital, 26
    salaries, 5, 7, 10–11
  physicians, 151–5
  surgeons, 6, 78, 105–7, 180–3
    first woman House Surgeon, 107
  training, 6
  visiting physicians, 97–103
Medical Staff Committee, 74, 139, 184, 186
  almoners, 227
  anaesthetists, 211
  chairpersons, 153, 164, 169, 186, 281
  dentists on, 203
  enlargement, 149–50, 152
  Honorary Secretaries, 115, 128, 281
medical training
  beginnings, 20–2
  women students, 46, 54
Medical Women's Federation, 124
Megaw, Mr John, 206
Meharry, Joan, 237
memorial tablets, 75–7
Menarry, Eleanor, 243
metabolic medicine, 158–9
Methodist College, 44

Mewha, Miss Kate, 285
microbiology, 170–1
Microbiology Building, 145
Mid Ulster Hospital, 211
Mildred, Miss, 135
Millar, Dr J. Harold D., 151, 160, *160*, 258, 281, 284
Millar, Mr Robert, 201, 202, 270
Millen, Dr John L.E., 166, 259
Millfield, Belfast, *8*
Milligan, Dr Kevin R., 277
Mills, Dr J.O. Manton, 165, *187*, 268, 281
Mirakhur, Mr Meenakshi, 168, 277
Mirakhur, Professor Rajinder K., 211, 272
Mitchell, Mr Arthur B., *51*, 69, 79, 105, 107, 112, 118, 242, 253, 281, 282, 283
  AGM Address (1923), 109–10
  career, 51
Mitchell, Miss Christina, 205
Mitchell, Joyce, 239
Moffat, Dr William, 251, 287
Mollan, Professor Raymond A.B., 185, 271
Molloy, Jewel, 198
Molloy, Mr Patrick J., 197–8, *198*, 266
monasteries, 1
Montague, Anne, 172
Montgomery, Professor Desmond A.D., 151, *158*, 158–9, 258, 281, 284
Montgomery, Sir Frank P., 128, 139, 166, 255, 281, 283
Montgomery House, 128, 166
Moore, Anna L.C., 84
Moore, Austin, 184
Moore, Mr David, 10, 15, 17, 48, 77, 251
Moore, Eliza Jane, 84
Moore, George C., 84
Moore, James, 84
Moore, Dr James, 37, *48*, 48–9, 252, 282
Moore, Professor James, 264
Moore, Dr John, 45, 49, 252
Moorehead, Mrs, *242*
Morison, Dr E., *98*
Morison, Professor John E., 131, 257
Morrison, Dr Cyril C.M., 271
Morrison, Miss Elizabeth, 273
Morrison, Mr Ernest, 151, 180, 258, 281, 284
Morrison, Dr James D., 199, 267
Morrow, Mr Harry, 206
Morrow, Dr James I., 101, 161, 277
Morrow, Dr John S., 97, 98–9, *124*, 254, 282
Morrow, Sister Noel, *176*
Morrow, Dr W.F. Keith, 213, 215, *215*, 266
Morrow Memorial Lecture, 213
Morton, Dr William R.M., 261
mortuary, 90, *90*
Mulholland, A., and Sons, 28
Mulholland, Andrew, 14
Mulholland, Dr H. Connor, 157, 197, 270
Mulholland, St Clair Kelburn, 52, 81
Mulholland family, 52
Mulholland Wing, 52, *52*
Mullally, Mr Brian, 206
Murnaghan, Dr George A., 141, 187, 241, 269, 285
Murnaghan, Dr Mark, *248*
Murney, Dr Henry, 38, 49, 218, 252, 281
Murphy, Dr, 252
Murray, Mr James, 7, 231
Murray, R.W., 287
Murray Street, Belfast, 7
Musgrave, Henry, 69, 90, 93

Musgrave, Sir James, 90
Musgrave and Clark Clinic, *92*, 138, 158, *181*, 237
Musgrave Clinic, *90*, 93
Musgrave Park Hospital, 114, 152, 154, 221
  anaesthesia, 210, 212
  orthopaedics, 112, 183, 184, 185
  physiotherapy, 235
  radiology, 164
  surgery, 182
  TB, 194
Musgrave Wing, 90
Musson, Miss Anne E., 92, 133, *133*, 135, 172, 173, 285
Musson House, 92, *92*, 144, 149, 175

Napier, Seamus, 169
National Breast Screening Programme, 163
National Health Service (NHS), 66, 77, 85, 87, 119, 128, 131, 136
  chaplains, 226
  dentistry, 203
  established, 137–40
  nursing, 173
  reforms, 244
  reorganisation (1972), 140–1
  social workers, 230
National Insurance, 66
Naval Nursing Service, 113
Neil, Dr, 123
Neill, Dr Desmond, 101, *171*, 171–2
Neill, Harriette, 46
Nelson, Ida, 113
Nelson, Miss Jane, 285
Nelson, Dr Joseph, 56–7, *57*, 69, 120, 253, 282
Nelson, Professor M. Gerald, 128, 169, 170, 220, 256, 281, 283
  career, 131–2
  Medical Executive Committee, 140
Nelson, Dr Peter G., 192, 220, 269
neurology, 160–1
neuropathology, 168
neurosurgery, 115, 191–3
Nevin, Professor Norman C., 265
New Light, 6–7, 21
Newark, Professor F.H., 138
Newman, Lydia, 62
Newman, Margaret, 240
Ng, Dr Bing, *248*
Nichol, Andrew, 48
Nicholl, Dr Robert M., 212–13, 264
Nicholls, Dr D. Paul, 155, 274
Nightingale, Florence, 24, 39, 59
Nixon, Dr John W.G., 262
Norman C. Hughes Regional Burns Unit, 201
Norris, Dr William A., 166–7, 262
North and West Belfast District, 141–2, 175, 229, 245
North and West Belfast Unit of Management, 237
North Charitable Infirmary, Cork, 2
Northern Ireland Assembly, 187
Northern Ireland Blood Transfusion Service, 130, 194
Northern Ireland Council for Orthopaedic Development, 239
Northern Ireland Council for Postgraduate Medical Education, 159, 210
Northern Ireland Distinction Awards Committee, 159

Northern Ireland Fever Hospital and Radiotherapy Centre, 229
Northern Ireland General Health Services Board, 138
Northern Ireland Health Service, 231
Northern Ireland Hospitals Authority, 119, 149, 173, 186, 201, 216
  established, 128, 138, 139
  physiotherapy, 235
  plastic surgery, 200
  radiotherapy, 166
  and RVH, 140
  speech therapy, 239
Northern Ireland Housing Executive, 140
Northern Ireland Radiotherapy Centre, 128
Northern Ireland School of Physiotherapy, 235–6
Northern Ireland Tuberculosis Authority, 138, 152
Northern Whig Club, 5
nursing, 39, 78–9, 113, 132–5
  1948–66, 172–5
  accommodation, 68–9, 92, 133, 134, 144, 147
  care of, 174
  change of management system, 68–9
  Matrons, 78
  19th c., 59–63
  payment, 23
  pre-Nightingale, 22–4
  probationers, 134
  since 1966, 175–7
  State Registration, 135
  uniforms, 62–3, 134–5
Nursing Committee, 72
nutrition, 238
Nutt's Corner crash, 220

O'Brien, Professor Frank V., 168, 203–4
O'Brien, Miss, *242*
obstetrics and gynaecology, 53–5, 117–19, 185–7
occupational therapy, 224, 237–8
O'Connell Memorial, 38
Odling-Smee, Mr G. William, 183, *187*, 269
O'Doherty, Dr Ann J., 165, 277
O'Donnell, Dr Manus, 197
Official Unionist Party, 187
O'Hanlon, Sister Kate, 176, 220, *221*
O'Hara, Dr M. Denis, 167, 269
O'Hare, Dr John, *248*
O'Hare, Sean, 232
O'Kane, Mr Hugh O., 157, 198, 199, 268
Olpherts, Miss, 285
O'Neill, Dr Henry, 50–1, 58, 253
O'Neill, Dr J.S., 121, 203
O'Neill, Dr Tracy, *248*
operating theatres, 104–5, 145–6
Ophthalmic Hospital, 146
ophthalmology, 187–9
Orators, 21, 44–5, 282–4
Order of St John, 84
Orr, Dr Ian A., 199, 273
Orthopaedic Department, 112
orthopaedics and trauma, 183–5
Osterberg, Mr Paul H., 185, 263, 284
Otway, Miss, 61
Oulton, Plato, 287
Our Day, 84
outpatients *see* Austen Boyd Outpatient Building

Owens, Anne, 222
Owens, Dr P.D. Adrian, 202, 203

Page, Mr A. Brian, 188, 277
Pantridge, Professor James F., 113, 151, *156*, 156–7, 258, 284
Papanicolaou, George, 168
Park, Dr Richard, *248*
Parks, Professor T. George, 182–3, 267
Pathological and Bacteriological Laboratory Assistants' Association, 167
pathology, 57, 128–32, 167–70
patient controlled analgesia (PCA), 208
Patterson, Aileen, 240
Patterson, Dr George C., 157, *157*, 266
Patterson, Hugh, 232–3
Patterson, Muriel, 236
Patterson, Dr Victor H., 161, 274
Pedlow, Doreen, 113
Pedlow, Reverend Henry, 226
Pegram, A. Bertram, 80
Pemberton, Professor John, 260
Percy Thomas Partnership, 246
pernicious anaemia, 97
Pharmaceutical Society, 231, 232
pharmacology, 150–1
pharmacy, 231–4, *232*
Phillips, Dr Anne S., 199, 279
physiotherapy, 234–6
Piccioni, Felice, 48
Picken, Dr S.E., *98*
Pielou, Norma, 232
Pielou, Mr William D., 206
Pim, Joshua, 287
Pinkerton, Professor John H.M., 186, 187, 262
Pirrie, Dr John Miller, 46–7, 71, 252
Pirrie, Lady Margaret, 72, *72*, 80, 81, 110, 286
Pirrie, Lord *see* Pirrie, William James
Pirrie, Captain William, 46
Pirrie, William James, 47, 67, 68, *71*, 71–2, 74, 129
 memorial, 80–1
 Viscount, 87
Pirrie family, 71–2
plastic surgery, 200–2
Plenum System, 69–70, 73, 93
podiatry, 240–1
poliomyelitis, 214
Poliomyelitis Society, 145
Pollard, Mr, 3–4
Poole, Dr Desmond, 241
Poor House, 1, 2–3, 4, 9, 13, 54
 doctors, 4–7
Poor Law, 12, 229
Porter, Dr David C., 163, 257, 281, 283
Powell, Sir Philip, 246
Preliminary Training School (PTS), 175
Presbyterian Church, Non-Subscribing, 6–7, 21
prescriptions, 32–3
Press, Dr John R., 160, 275
Primrose, Mr William J., 191, 275
Princess Victoria, 221
Pritchard, Professor John Joseph, 260
Pro Tanto Quid, 131
Project 2000, 177
Prophet, Mr Arthur S., 203
psychiatry, 166–7
publications, 102–3
Pulendran, Dr Ramesh, *248*

Purce, Mr George R.B., 107, 113, *114*, 140, 196, 255, 283
 career, 114–15
 neurosurgery, 191
 thoracic surgery, 193
Purce, Dr Margaret, 107
Purce lecture, 193
Purdon, Dr Elias, 103
Purdon, Dr Henry S., 19, 47–8, 58, 103, 252
Purdon, Dr Thomas H., 18–19, *19*, 42–3, 251
Purdon Skin Ward, 103, 144
Purdysburn Hospital, 68, 70, 166, 214
Purdysburn House, 92

Quah, Dr Say P., *248*
Queen Alexandra's Military Nursing Service, 113
Queen's College, 17, 18, 19, *41*
 Faculty of Medicine, 22, 40–4, 46, 54
Queen's University Belfast, 22, 41, 66, 80, 167; *see also* Faculty of Medicine, QUB
 building committee, 141
 MPs, 111, 117–18
 nurse training, 177
Queen's Women Graduates' Association, 124
Quigley, Sir George, 245
Quin, Herbert, 115, 138, 144
Quin, Mr William, 251
Quin House, *137*, 143, *143*, 144, *146*, 148, 191, 204, 239
Quinn, Dr James T., 267

Radio Royal, 226
radiography, 94–5
radiology, 126–8, 133, 162–5
radiotherapy, 166
Radium Fund, 110–11
Rafferty, Dr Ciaran V., 213, 279
Ramsay-Baggs, Mr Peter, 204
Rankin, Mr David, 203
Rankin, Dr John C., 159, 254, 281, 282
 Electrical Department, 89, 126–7, 234
 VD clinic, 104, 127
Reade, Dr Thomas, 49
Red Cross Society, 84
Red Lion bombing, 221
Regional Child Mental Health Service, 241
Regional Intensive Care Unit, 214
Regional Joint Cleft Palate Clinic, 239
Reid, Dr Charles, 212, 257
Reid, Horace, 177
Reid, Dr James E., 210, 259
Reid, Professor James S., 43, *43*, 251
Reid, Leonard, 140
Reid, Dr Mark M., 270
Reid, Dr Robert, 135
Reina del Pacifico, 200, 220
relapsing fever, 9–10, 14
research fellowships, 139–40, 153
Resident House Officers, *248*
Respiratory Failure Unit (RFU), 214
Restrick, John, 232, *232*
Revive, 216
Richardson, Mr Andrew, 204
Richardson, Dr, 36
Richey, Dr Edmund E., 213, 266
Riddel, Eliza and Isabella, 82–3, 89
Riddel House, 144
Riddell, Dr James G., 271
Riordan, Mr Maurice G., 123
riots; *see also* Troubles

1798, 218
19th c., 38
1920s, 87
Ritchie, Dr James W.K., 270
road traffic accidents, 37, 110, 111, 216, 218, 219
Robb, Mr John D.A., 266
Robb, Miss M. Kathleen, 140, 141, 172, 175, 176, 285
Roberts, Dr Stanley D., 154, 264, 284
Robins, J. Wenlock, 74
Robinson, Dr Charles B., 166, 257
Robinson, Dr Holly, *248*
Robinson, Muriel, *164*
Robson, Sister Janet, *183*
Rocke, Mr Laurence G., 220, 278
Roddie, Professor Ian C., 263
Roddie, Mr Ken, *101*
Rodgers, Professor Harold W., 116, 180, *180*, 182, 256, 281, 283
Rodgers, J.S., 287
Rooney, Nichola, 241
Rosbotham, Susie, 234
Ross, Sister Gwen, *221*
Ross, Dr R.S., *98*
Ross, Dr Richard, 47, 252, 282
Ross, Dr T. Lawrence, 135
Roulston, Sister Rita, 174
Rowlands, Professor Brian J., 182, *183*, 275
Roy, Professor Arthur D., 182, 268
Royal Belfast Academical Institution, 16–17, 40, 52, 54; *see also* Belfast Academical Institution
Royal Belfast Hospital for Sick Children, 47, 50, 101, 115, 116, 138, *143*, 165, 175
 anaesthesia, 125, 211
 bereavement services, 241
 cardiac surgery, 197
 free funds, 140
 occupational therapy, 237–8
 opened, 92
 ophthalmology, 57
 plastic surgery, 201
 SNO, 176
 thoracic surgery, 195
Royal College of Nursing, 173, 175
Royal College of Obstetrics and Gynaecology, 117, 118, 186
Royal College of Physicians of Ireland, 154
Royal College of Surgeons in England, 50, 56, 180
 Faculty of Dentistry, 202
 Toynbee Lecture, 190
Royal College of Surgeons in Ireland, 5, 56, 108, 116, 163, 164, 187, 211
Royal Group of Hospitals, 138, 141, 175, 187, 249
 chaplains, 226
 reorganisation, 241–2
 social workers, 230
 structure, 245
Royal Hospitals Trust, 199, 236
 design competition, 246
Royal Institute of British Architects, 246
Royal Maternity Hospital, 68, *90*, 118, 138, 144, 186, 248
 anaesthesia, 212, 213
 clinical psychology, 241
 free funds, 140
 opened, 92
 SNO, 176

Royal Society, 19
Royal Society of Ulster Architects, 246
Royal Ulster Constabulary (RUC), 129
Royal University of Ireland, 41, 46, 55
Royal Victoria Hospital, 3, 57, *73*, 286, 287
  Administrative Officers, 287
  building programme, 148–9
    early 20th c., 87–93
    post-1945, 141–9
    1990s, *244*, 246–9, *247*
  charter, 70–1
  design and building of, *67*, 72–4
  finances, 30, 86
    Coronation Fund, 93
    donors, 79–84
    fundraising groups, 224–5
    under NHS, 139, 173
  medical practice, 150–1
    early 20th c., 96–7
  patient numbers, 87, 93, 95
  trust status, 244–6
  wards named, 79–84
  wards opened, 75–6
Royal Victoria Hospital Act (1947), 146
Royal Victoria Hospital Choir, 174, *174*
Royal Victoria Hospital League of Nurses, 172
Russell, Dr Beatrice, *101*
Russell, Mr Colin F.J., 182, 206, 273
Russell, Mr David, 205
Russell, Robert, 168
Rutherford, Dr E.D., 235
Rutherford, Mr William H., 220, *221*, 265
Ryan, Dr Thomas J., 155, 266

Sachs, Oliver, 161
St Paul, parish of, 226
St Thomas's Hospital, London, *39*
Salmon Report, 175
Samaritan Hospital, 119, 209, 212
Sanders, Dr James M., 16, 18, *18*, 251
Sansom, Canon Charles, 226
Sarsam, Mr Mazen A., 198, 279
Saunders, Mr Ian, 206
Saunsbury, Mr Philip, 205
Sawhney, Dr Bharat B., 161, 270
Sayers, John E., 146
Scher, Mr Eric, 205
School of Clinical Dentistry, 203
School of Clinical Medicine, 159
School of Dentistry, 143, 192, 202–3
School of Physiotherapy, 147
School of Radiography, 145, 165
Scott, Dr Eric, 212
Scott, Reverend Hugh, *225*, 226
Scott, Dr James H., 202
Scott, Mary, 172
Scott, Dr William E.B., 261
Seaver, Dean, 69
Shaftesbury, Anthony, 8th Earl of, 80
Shaftesbury, Harriet, Countess of, 80
Shaftesbury, 9th Earl of, 80
Shanks, Professor Robert G., 265
Share Music course, 161
Sharkey, Mr James A.M., 189, 279
Sharpe, Dr T.D. Emmett, 213, 277
Shaw, Reverend Gary R., 227
Shaw, George Bernard, 96
Shaw, Mrs Hetty Hamilton, 84
Shaw, William, 84
Shaw and Jamison, 84

Sheil, Dr, 251
Shepherd, Mr William F.I., 271
Shepherd, Dr William H.T., 163, 258, 283
Shepperd, Mr Harold W.H., 190, 264
Sheridan, Mr Sean, 205
Silvestri, Miss Giuliana, 279
Simmons, Rose, 238
Simpson, Professor David I.H., 170, *187*, 273
Simpson, James Young, 35
Simpson, John, *233*
Sims, Dr Marion, 50
Sinclair, Mr Samuel R., 259, 281
Sinclair, Professor Thomas, 29, 69, 79, 105, 111, 253, 281, 283
  career, 43
  MP, 118
  retirement, 108
Sinclair family, 28–9, 81
Sinclair Memorial Fund, 28
Sir George E. Clark Metabolic Unit, 144, 238
Sir Samuel Irwin Lecture Theatre, 148, *148*
Skelly, Dr Robert J., 263
Skin Department, 103
Slater, Mr Ronald M., 201, 268
Sloan, Dr James M., 167, 269, 281
Sloan, Mr Robert S.L., 203
Small, Mr James O., *201*, 278
smallpox, 32, 47, 55
Smiley, Dr Elizabeth, 195
Smiley, Dr James, 195
Smiley, Mr Thomas B., 113, 151, 196, 197, 258, 284
  career, 194–5
Smith, Professor J. Lorrain, 58, 128, 253, 282
Smith, Dr James W.T., 47, 252
Smith, Mr Ralph, 205
Smith, Dr Robert S., 47, 59, 253, 281
Smyth, Dr Edward T.M., 170, 274
Smyth, Mr Gordon D.L., 189, 190, *190*, 263
Smyth, Dr James C., 203
Smyth, Dr John A., 132, 156, 158, 172, 190, 255, 281, 283
Snow, John, 11
social workers, 229–31
Society of Apothecaries, London, 40
Society of Friends, 181
Society of Radiographers, 127
Society of Trained Masseuses, 234–5
South Belfast Group, 212
South Down Group, 213
South Tyrone Hospital, 212
speech and language therapy, 239–40
Spence, Robert T., 140, 141, *141*, 287
sports, 134
staff, 139, 145–6; *see also* medical staff *and* nursing
  house steward, 53
  Matrons, 285
  Medical Superintendents, 285
  RVH (1903), 77–9
  salaries, 31
Stafford, Dr Sarah, *248*
Stanfield, Mrs M., *242*
Stanford, Dr Charles F., 152, 155, 271
Stanley, Dr J. Clive, 213, 278
Stephenson, Dr Robert, 10, 17, 54, 250
Stephenson, Dr Samuel M., 6, *6*, 17, 250
stethoscope, 32
Steven, R. McDonald, 129, 167
Stevens, Dr Anthony B., 279
Stevenson, Professor Alan C., 257

Stevenson, Mr H. Morris, 151, 195, *195*, 196, 197, 210, 259, 281, 284
Stevenson, Mr Howard, 108, 111, 112–13, 118, 135, 195, 254, 281
Stewart, A.W., 160
Stewart, Mr David, 206
Stewart, Mr Ernie, 197, *198*
Stewart, Dr H. Hilton, 160, 214, 259
Stewart, Professor Horatio A., 37, 43, 252
Stewart, Jimmy, 222
Stormont Parliament, 118, 119
Stoy, Professor Philip J., 123, 202, *202*, 203
Strahan, Alex, 232, 233
Strain, Dr William, 206
Stranex, Dr Stephen, 280
strikes, 176
surgery, 104–5, 107–12, 178–9
  before anaesthesia, 14–16
  equipment, 108–9
  mortality rates, 109–10
  19th c., 37–40
  1940s, 116–17
Swallow, Dr Michael W., 161, 263
Swallow, Mr Neil, 205
Swan, Mr W. Marshall, 121, 203
Sweeney, Dr Louise E., 275
Swinson, Mr Terry, 204
Sykes, Donald, 241
Syme, Professor James, 48
Symington, Professor Johnston, 111, 126
Symmers, Professor William St C., 128–9, 130, 254, 282
Synod of Ulster, 21

Taggart, Dr Allister J., 274
Tait, Lawson, 39
Tate, John, 286
Taylor, Mr Alexander R., 192, 258
Taylor, Barbara, 238
Taylor, Dr D.R., 122
Taylor, Dr Ian C., 273
Taylor, Dr Maureen, 156
Taylor, Dr Robert H., 278
Templeton, Mr John, 185, 272
Territorial Army, 152
tetanus, 215–16
thermometer, 32
Thomas, Dr Paul S., 165, 266
Thompson, Dr Benjamin, 17, 251
Thompson, Elias H., 286
Thompson, Elizabeth, 236
Thompson, Judge H.M., 283
Thompson, James M., 287
Thompson, Dr Thomas, 251
Thomson, Captain H.B., 99
Thomson, Dr Samuel Smith, 7, *7*, 10, 250
Thomson, Professor William, 99, *99*, 113, 187, 254, 266, 281, 283
  retirement, 153
thoracic surgery, 193–5
Thornton, Dr Claire M., 278
Throne Hospital, 48, 78, 86, 112, 135–6, *136*, 144, 237
  bomb damage, 114
  established, 58–9
  Matrons, 132, 133, 135
  under NHS, 138
  plastic surgery, 200–1, 202, 204
  rheumatology, 152
  social workers, 229
Toner, Professor Peter G., 128, 167, 274

Training of Health Visitors Committee, 229
Training of Social Workers Committee, 229
Traub, Dr Anthony I., 187, 274
trench fever, 4, 14, 32
Trimble, Professor Elizabeth R., 172, 276
Trinity College Dublin, 7, 20
Troubles, 148, 160, 165, 175, 217–33
  head injuries, 192, 205
  nursing, 176
  surgery, 181
  trauma, 216
Truck Amendment Act (1887), 85
tuberculosis, 18, 23, 32, 59, 135–6, 152
  surgery, 194
Tuohy, Dr Owen, 203
Turkington, Dr John, *248*
Turkington, Dr Samuel I., *98*, 101–2, 255, 281, 283
Turner, Dr Graham, *248*
typhoid, 32
typhus fever, 4, 9, 14, 17, 32
Tyrone Crystal, 245

Ulster Academy of Arts, 133
Ulster Hospital, 104, 185
  anaesthesia, 211
  bomb damage, 114
  gynaecology, 119, 186
  pathology, 170
  plastic surgery, 200, 201, 202, 204
  radiology, 127, 163
Ulster Hospital for Women and Children, 97
Ulster Independent Clinic, 149
Ulster Medical Journal, 45, 119
Ulster Medical Society, 44, 47, 48, 102, 117, 153, 203
  Campbell Oration, 107
  established, 41
  first woman president, 124–5
  Purce lecture, 193
  Transactions, 49
Ulster Museum, 48
Ulster Polytechnic, 236, 237, 239; *see also* University of Ulster at Jordanstown
Union Fever Hospital, 12, 13, 21–2, 27, 70; *see also* Belfast City Hospital
Union Hospital, 12, 16, 51
Union Infirmary, 70
Unit of Management Executive Team, 245
United Irishmen, Society of, 4, 5, 7, 47, 52
University of Ulster at Jordanstown, 165, 167, 236, 238, 240; *see also* Ulster Polytechnic
Unni, Dr Varavoor K.N., *187*, 213, 270
UVF Hospital, 100

vaccines, 96
Valentine, Mr A.D., 206
Vallance-Owen, Professor John, 154, 264

Van Thal, Miss, 239
Vane, Tommy, 59
Varghese, Dr Grace, 271
Vaugh, Mrs, *242*
venereal disease, 15–16, 96, 104
venereology, 159–60
ventilation system, 69–70, 73, 93
Victoria, Queen, 28, 124
Victoria College, 54
Victoria Tower, 147
virology, 170
Virus Reference Laboratory, 170
von Richthofen, Baron, 43

Wade, Professor Owen L., 214, 260
Walby, Mr A. Peter, 191, 274
Wales, Mr John, 251
Wallace, Sister E.L.C., 177
Wallace, Mrs, 136
Walsh, Dr Maureen Y., 167, 275
Wang, Dr Jenn C., *248*
Waringstown Hospital, 114
Waters, Mrs, 78, 285
Watson, Dr Dorothy, 123
Watson, Dr Robert G.P., 155, 278
Watt, Dr Michael, 280
Watt, Dr Patrick C.H., 167, 277
Weathers, Mandy, *164*
Weaver, Dr John A., 139, 153, 156, 261, 281, 284
Webb, Dr Cecil H., 170, 277
Webb, Dr Samuel W., 157, 271
Webster, Mrs, 237
Weir, Dr Bob, *101*
Welbourn, Professor Richard B., 158, 181–2, 260
Welch, R.J., 75, 77, 78, 80, 81, 83, 105
Welfare Committees, 138
Wells, Charles, 181
Wells, Spencer, 39
West Wing, *65*, 69, 72–3, 77, 133
Wheeler, Mr James R., 51, 120, 150, 187, 189, 255, 281, 283
Wheeler, Mr Thomas K., 51, 253, 282
White, Dr, 5, 6
White Star Line, 82
Whiteabbey Hospital, 136, 173, 235
  anaesthesia, 210, 211, 213
  TB, 194
Whitfield, Dr Charles R., 186, 264
Whitla, Sir William, 42, *44*, 45, 47, 79, 97, 99, 150, 253, 281, 282
  career, 43–4
  Dictionary of Treatment, 33, 123–4
  Good Samaritan window, 44, 75–6, *76*
  MP, 118
  rebuilding, 66, 69, 70
  retirement, 98
Whitla Medical Building, 210

Whitlock, Mr Roy, 204, *204*
Wilkinson, Mr Alan J., 183, *187*, 275
Willis, Dr Jacob, 168, 264
Willix, Mr David, 129, 167
Wilson, Anne, 238
Wilson, Dr Carol M., 278
Wilson, Dr David B., *187*, 272
Wilson, Dr Herbert K., 270
Wilson, James, 217
Wilson, Dr Kaye, 181
Wilson, Marie, 176
Wilson, Professor Robert I., 112, 151, 184–5, 259, 284
Wilson, Mr Willoughby, *101*, 181, *181*, 260, 281, 284
Wilson, Dr W.M., 251
Winter Oration, 21, 44–5, 282–4
Withers, Mr Robert J.W., 112, *112*, 185, 256, 283
Womersley, Dr Richard A., 153–4, 259, 281
Wood, Mr Alfred E., 198, 273
Woodside, Mr Cecil J.A., 115, 255, 281, 283
Workhouse, 12, 13, 27, 37
Working Men's Committee, 69, 74, *85*, 85–7, 139, 225
  dental equipment, 121
  Million Shilling Fund, 93
  ward named, 84
Workman, Dr Charles, 253
World War One, 84, 87, 90, 113
  head wounds, 191
  massage, 234
  radiography, 126–7
  and RVH, 107–8
  shell-shock, 48
  VD, 96, 104
World War Two, 93, 101, 103, 104, 108, 111, 120, 124
  air raids, 113–14
  almoners, 228
  antibiotics, 96
  blood transfusion, 117, 130
  chest wounds, 193
  mortality rates, 191
  physiotherapy, 235
  and RVH, 112–14
Worrall, Catherine, *236*
Wright, Dr Almroth, 96, *96*, 129
Wright, Robert, 286
Wylie, Hazel, *236*

YMCA, 181
Young, George, 232
Young, Dr Hugh S.A., 270
Young, Professor John S., 130, 255
Young, Robert M., 90, 287
Young, Dr Shaun, 213
Young and McKenzie, 89, 90
Younger, Dr Jonathan, *248*